BIOTECHNOLOGY
AND
BIODEGRADATION

Current Titles in the
Advances in Applied Biotechnology Series

Also available:
Classics in Vision Research

ADVANCES IN APPLIED BIOTECHNOLOGY SERIES
Volume 4

BIOTECHNOLOGY AND BIODEGRADATION

EDITORS

Daphne Kamely   Ananda Chakrabarty
Gilbert S. Omenn

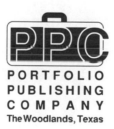

PORTFOLIO
PUBLISHING
COMPANY
The Woodlands, Texas

GULF PUBLISHING COMPANY
BOOK DIVISION
Houston ■ London ■ Paris ■ Zurich ■ Tokyo

ADVANCES IN APPLIED BIOTECHNOLOGY SERIES
VOLUME 4
Biotechnology and Biodegradation

Library of Congress Cataloging-in-Publication Data

Biotechnology and Biodegredation

Biotechnology and biodegradation
editors, Daphne Kamely, Ananda Chakrabarty, Gilbert Omenn.
p. 528 cm. – (Advances in applied biotechnology series; v. 4)
Papers presented at the International Workshop on Biotechnology and Biodegradation,
held in Lisbon, Portugal, June 1989.

1. Environmental biotechnology – Congresses. 2. Biodegradation – Congresses.
I. Kamely, Daphne. II. Chakrabarty, Ananda M., 1938- . III. Omenn, Gilbert S.
IV. International Workshop on Biotechnology and Biodegradation (1989: Lisbon, Portugal)
V. Series
TD192.5.B56   1989
628.4 – dc20
89-25490
CIP

Series ISBN 0-943255-08-2

ISBN 0-943255-06-6

On the Cover ———————————————————————

Kelp. a marine weed that produces a polysaccharide aliginate, which is widely used commercially in the food, chemical, and pharmaceutical industries. *Photograph provided by Dr. Ananda Chakrabarty.*

Table of Contents

Basic Science of Anaerobic Biodegredation

Molecular Genetics and Physiology of Aerobic Microorganisms with Biodegradative Potential

Methods and Applications in Biodegradation

Approaches to Closed and Open Systems

Experience with Field Applications:
Successes and Failures

Ecological Considerations and Risk Assessment

Foreword

Cleaning up the environment has become an increasingly important issue in industrialized countries. As pollution increases, authorities in various countries are seeking novel scientific and engineering solutions to the ever-increasing problems of industrial waste cleanup and water and air pollution. Environmental pollution is not limited to industrialized countries but is rapidly becoming a problem in lesser developed countries as well. Pollution and hazardous waste are now being debated as global issues both at national and international levels, by environmentalists and politicians, within and between governments. In fact, concern over the environment is an issue that has outgrown both geographical and political boundaries. At least one survey in the United States prior to the 1988 presidential election demonstrated that Americans cared more about a cleaner environment than any other issue, regardless of party affiliation.

The price tag of modern technology is high. Without efforts to clean the environment, the quality of life will deteriorate rapidly, resulting in an ultimate poisoning of the planet. Several physical, chemical, and thermal approaches to pollution control have been tried. They all leave something to be desired. Although some areas can be decontaminated by one procedure, the remedy may cause toxicity problems in other areas. For example, incineration transfers some pollution from solid waste into the air and into concentrated ash. Chemical decontamination sometimes breaks down compounds into more toxic components and can ruin equipment and other surfaces.

The costs of engineering cleanup plants and of treating large contaminated areas are staggering. Only governments can afford it, and even in desperation, certain areas were closed down as untreatable, namely Love Canal, New York, and Times Beach, Missouri. It will take years to try to clean up and restore Prince Williams Sound from the Alaskan oil spill. In fact, some scientists are arguing that the area will never be restored to its natural condition.

In this world of ever-increasing pollution, biological detoxification provides alternatives to conventional physical-chemical engineering techniques. Biodegradation is a process that has been going on in *nature* for years. Continuous biodegradation and regeneration is essential to life. Because biodegradation is a natural process, it poses less hazards to human health and the environment and is more acceptable to society than conventional treatment technology. Not only is biodegradation a natural process, but it is also selective, specific, and nontoxic. The reason biodegradation has received little attention in pollution control is that it is a slow process that occurs in *nature* over a long period of time. With the advent of biotechnology, it is now possible to accelerate this process and to look forward to applications of pollution treatment and large-scale decontamination. Researchers are now beginning to examine biodegradation at the molecular level, using the tools of biotechnology. Thus, they hope to unravel mechanisms that control the extent, rate, and other parameters of biodegradation. Ultimately, they wish to manipulate genes in order to achieve improved degradation of greater selectivity, efficiency, stability, and safety.

This international research workshop offers a spectrum of topics in biodegradation using the tools of biotechnology. The workshop covers the basic science aspects of biodegradation. Researchers in the field discuss not only the physiological characteristics of microorganisms but also the use of selective techniques that enhance the process of microbial evolution of biodegradative genes in *nature*. Similarly, the genetic characteristics of microorganisms allowing them to biodegrade both natural and synthetic toxic chemicals are emphasized, including the molecular techniques that allow selective assembly of genetic segments from a variety of bacterial strains to a single strain to enable the strain to degrade a number of recalcitrant chemicals. Methods needed to advance biodegradation research as well as the high-priority chemical problems important to the Department of Defense or to the chemical industry,have been discussed openly and candidly by various participants. Analytical techniques and practical applications of biodegradation are addressed by the participants from government, academia, and industry. Biotechnology provides a tremendous potential for the understanding of mechanisms that govern biodegradation. At the same time, new developments in biotechnology face a tangle of regulatory constraints. Scientists using the tools of biotechnology must comply with regulations and perform risk assessments. Thus, important contributions in the area of risk assessment and the present status of regulation governing environmental release of genetically engineered microorganisms have been included to provide the readers a wider perspective on the biotechnology of biodegradation.

Biotechnology was first used in the biomedical laboratory. Experiments were conducted in a contained laboratory. As biodegradation moves from the basic to the applied stage, experiments may need to be conducted in the open environment. The bacterial strains and their components need to be evaluated under varying environmental conditions for effects on stability, reproducibility, efficiency, effectiveness, and safety. As more results become available, it becomes possible to engineer improved biodegradable strains with the desirable traits, at the same time minimizing risks to human health and the environment. At these early stages of application, it is important to derive preliminary results from experience with early field applications, including successes and failures. Several researchers report promising results on biodegrading hazardous waste and toxic compounds both *in situ* and in contained bioreactors.

In this increasing world of regulatory burdens, this workshop will not be complete without a session on risk assessment. As more risk assessment information becomes available, it will become possible to engineer safer and more efficient microbial strains. Once released into the environment, these strains can carry out biodegradative functions and at the same time pose little or no hazards to human health and the environment.

—The Editors

The Editors

Daphne Kamely, Ph.D.
Scientific Advisor for Biotechnology
Department of The Army
United States Chemical Research,
Development, and Engineering Center
Aberdeen Proving Ground,
Maryland 21010-5423

Ananda Chakrabarty, Ph.D.
Professor
Department of Microbiology and Immunology
University of Illinois College of Medicine
Chicago, Illinois 60612

Gilbert S. Omenn, M.D., Ph.D.
Professor of Medicine and Environmental Health
Dean, School of Public Health and
Community Medicine
University of Washington
Seattle, Washington 98195

Acknowledgments

The workshop organizing committee wish to thank Drs. Isabel Sa Corriea and Julio Novais of the Instituto Superior Tecnico of Lisbon, Portugal, for their local organization and support. The organizers extend their appreciation to Dr. Joseph DeFrank and Mrs. Marcia Goforth for their technical and administrative assistance. The organizers also wish to thank the U.S. Army Chemical Research, Development and Engineering Center, the European Army Research Office, and the U.S. Air Force for their support.

Daphne Kamely
U.S. Army

Ananda Chakrabarty
University of Illinois Medical Center

Mirja Salkinoja-Salonen
University of Helsinki

Plenary Lecture

Protein Engineering and Biological Oxidation

Michael Smith

Biotechnology Laboratory
University of British Columbia
Room 237, Westbrook Building
6174 University Boulevard
Vancouver, British Columbia
Canada V6T 1W5

Introduction

It is clear that the best immediate hope for the use of microorganisms in biodegradation lies in organisms that already exist or in transgenic organisms that can be constructed by *in vivo* or *in vitro* gene manipulation. However, there is the possibility that protein engineering by the systematic *in vitro* mutagenesis of genes that encode specific enzymes will have a useful role. This could be to provide enzymes with more desirable general characteristics such as better stabilities under extremes of temperature or pH or resistance to metal ion toxicity; and it could also be to provide enzymes with established catalytic activities for new substrates or even to provide completely new catalytic activities.

Among possible targets for protein engineering studies, the heme proteins stand out as a particularly attractive group (Table 1). Apart from their basic roles in respiration, there are important functions in oxidative detoxification and drug metabolism, as manifested

Table 1
Some Roles of Heme Proteins in Biology

Electron Transfer	Oxygen Carrier
Eukaryote cytochromes *c*	Myoglobin
Prokaryote cytochromes *c*	Hemoglobin
Cytochrome *b* 5	Leghemoglobin
Cytochrome oxidase	
Cytochrome reductase	**Peroxidases**
	Catalases
Mono-Oxidases	Peroxidases
Cytochromes P-450	

by cytochromes P-450 and the role of peroxidases in the breakdown of lignins. Beyond the possibility of the use of protein engineering to define the basic functionality of the different classes of heme proteins lies the even more interesting objectives of creating enzymes with improved or new substrate specificity and of interconverting classes of heme proteins.

This presentation will describe protein engineering experiments on two examples of heme proteins: iso-1-cytochrome *c* and cytochrome *c* peroxidase, both mitochondrial proteins from the yeast *Saccharomyces cerevisiae*.

Studies on Phe-82 of Iso-1-Cytochrome *C*

Comparison of more than 90 eukaryote cytochromes *c* reveals that 23 amino acid residues are absolutely conserved out of the 103 residues in the protein.[1] These 23 residues can be divided into two groups, those with obvious function such as the two cysteine residues that are covalently linked to heme and the two ligands, His-18 and Met-80, and those residues with no obvious function. Among the latter is Phe-82, which has a putative but nonproven role in electron transfer.[2] A systematic analysis of the effect of replacement of this residue has been undertaken.[4-6] One surprising observation is that Phe-82 can be replaced by all 19 other residues, and the resultant mutant iso-1-cytochromes c will still support respiration *in vivo,* although its efficiency is substantially reduced in the case of the Cys-82 mutant (S. Inglis, A.G. Mauk, and M. Smith, unpublished results). Studies on the pure mutant cytochromes c have shown that an aromatic residue, Phe or Tyr, results in a higher redox potential, by approximately 50mV than does a residue such as Gly or Ser.[4] In addition, Phe or Tyr facilitate the transfer of an electron from ferrous cytochrome c to positively charged zinc cytochrome c peroxidase at a rate 10^4 greater than the Gly or Ser mutants.[5] Further, Ile or Leu at position 82 do not allow any faster electron transfer than do Gly or Ser.[6] Finally, an aromatic residue at position 82 is required for the high pK of the cytochrome c alkaline transition.[7] In summary, although Phe is not absolutely required at position 82 of cytochrome c, it is clear from these *in vitro* mutagenic studies that an aromatic residue at this position has a key role in establishing a number of characteristic properties of cytochrome c.

Cytochrome C Peroxidase

Because this enzyme can be crystallized readily, its three-dimensional structure is known at atomic resolution,[8] and this information has made the enzyme the primary tool for structure-function analysis of peroxidase activity. Two topics have been addressed to date, the site of the unusual free-radical species formed in the peroxide-oxidized enzyme[9] and the effect on enzyme function of replacing residues lying close to the enzyme-bound heme.[10-13] Replacement of Met-172 by Ser[10] and of Trp-51 and Trp-191 by Phe[11,12] coupled with selective deuteration of amino acid residues and ENDOR spectroscopy have shown that the radical lies on Trp-191.[13]

With regards to the enzymatic activity, replacement of Met-172 by Ser has no detectable effect on activity,[10] and replacement of Trp-191 by Phe greatly reduces activity.[12] However, replacement of Trp-51, a residue that lies close to the heme and to the distal His ligand, by Phe has the dramatic effect of shifting the pH optimum of the enzyme from pH 5.0 to pH 7.0 and also of increasing the specific activity four-to fivefold.[11] This provides an excellent example of the potential of *in vitro* mutagenesis for producing useful changes in enzyme function.

Conclusion

This presentation has provided a selective overview of the use and potential of *in vitro* mutagensis in the study and the modification of the properties of heme proteins. Extensive studies are being carried out elsewhere not only on cytochrome *c* and cytochrome *c* peroxidase but also on oxygen carrying proteins and on cytochrome P-450. Although practical applications of *in vitro* mutagenesis in the field of heme proteins has yet to be demonstrated, it is clear that these studies on this important class of proteins have a good chance of resulting in important functional insights and ultimately, in useful modified or new functions.

References

1. R.B. Cutler *et al.*, *Protein Eng.* **1**, 95 (1987).
2. T. Tanako and R.E. Dickerson, *J. Mol. Biol.* **153** (1980).
3. M.J. Zoller and M. Smith, *DNA* **3**, 458 (1984)
4. G.J. Pielak, A.G. Mauk, and M. Smith, *Nature* **313**, 152 (1985).
5. N. Liang *et al.*, *Proc. Natl. Acad. Sci. USA* **84**, 1249 (1987).
6. N. Liang *et al.*, *Science* **240**, 311 (1988).
7. L.L. Pearce *et al.*, *Biochemistry,* in press (1989).
8. B.C. Finzel, T.B. Poulos, and J. Krant, *J. Biol. Chem.*, 13027 (1984).
9. T. Yonetani, *J. Biol. Chem.* **240**, 4509 (1965)
10. D.B. Goodin, A.G. Mauk, and M. Smith, *Proc. Natl. Acad. Sci. USA* **83**, 1295 (1986).
11. D.B. Goodin, A.G. Mauk, and M. Smith, *J. Biol. Chem.* **262** (1987).
12. L.A. Fishel *et al.*, *J. Biochemistry* **26**, 351 (1987).
13. M. Sivaraja *et al.*, *Science* **241**, in press (1989).

Discussion

Newburgh: With respect to pH optimum of cytochrome *c* peroxidase, what is the charge effect on the surface of these mutant molecules?

Smith: I do not know. It is not a thing that we have done, either experimentally or theoretically. In some of our other studies on cytochrome *c* where we changed a surface residue, there have been calculations by Warshel, but we have not done anything on cytochrome *c* peroxidase.

Gunsalus: Have any of your mutants been looked at as crystals? Do the crystals hold up for cytochrome *c*?

Smith: For cytochrome *c*, yes. That is turning out to be a very amenable molecule for doing structure-function analysis and for looking at the crystal structure of the mutant. I think that Gary Brayer's laboratory is able to get crystals and do crystal structures almost quicker than you can do biochemical characterization. In fact, he has done about 20 different mutants not only at residue 82 but at other positions. There are some very interesting things coming out of this study. For instance, the glycine -82 mutant showed significant change in the skeleton. In terms of the crystal structure of the tyrosine mutant, it is interesting because there is not enough room in the molecule to put a phenol in to replace a benzene ring. Thus, there are two possibilities, one is the aromatic group moved out of the molecule or, alternatively, it displaces leucine -85. It turns out in fact that it does not displace leucine -85. The intriguing thing about that is some NMR studies of the mutant in the solution suggest that the opposite is happening. Thus, it may be one of these cases where in the solution the molecule has a different structure from that of the crystal. Another interesting case is a mutant that Fred Sherman's laboratory isolated by doing conventional mutagenesis on cytochrome *c*. It produced a mutant where leucine replaced a threonine that is in the region of the molecule close to a fixed water that sits very near the heme and that moves during oxidation and reduction. This leucine mutant turned out to be much more stable. I think it has the most dramatic increase on protein stability of any single amino acid replacement known, and so it was thought there would be a dramatic change in the shape of the molecule. The crystal structure has the same shape as the wild-type. So there is not an obvious answer as to why it is so much more stable. Thus, there are a number of interesting results. I believe that if you wish to obtain a quantitative interpretation of your data, you should know the crystal structure of the proteins you are working with, both mutant and wild-type. With respect to cytochrome *c* peroxidase, we have not done crystal structures. However, we would like to start working on them. The basic problem is that as you go into more detail, you need more equipment for getting the data out of the crystals. You need an area detector system and additional computer and graphics equipment to get the structure and interpret the data.

Newburgh: What about water? Are there any water molecules that are fixed in either of the monomers, or are they displaced in the pair when you get what appears to be the complex?

Smith: We do not have data on the cytochrome *c*, cytochrome *c* peroxidase complex. In the case of the mutant where the phenylalamine -82 is replaced by serine, we see an additional water molecule in the hole that is vacated by the benzene ring. We would like to see if we can put something like benzene sulfonic acid or something similar in that hole, to see if we can displace the water with a small ligand.

Clearly, the skeleton has not collapsed. There are many interesting things we would like to do.

Glaser: Would you care to comment on the thought that for the most part protein engineering is solely founded on thermodynamic considerations and as such gives a limited picture of what's really happening at the enzymatic level insofar that it does not adequately include the kinetic portion of the equation?

Smith: Well, again I think one has to accept that protein engineering is at a very nascent stage; I think there is going to be a lot of data collected that is uninterpretable. There is a debate among classical biochemists about whether one should do protein engineering with proteins for which one doesn't have a crystal structure. I would not take that position myself; I think there are a lot of valid questions one can ask that are based on just primary sequence. For instance, with respect to protein kinases, is it critical to have autophosphorylation of a tyrosine in the protein (which often occurs) for functionality? In terms of kinetic studies, I suspect we have to keep doing a lot more work on structures of the mutants. The thing I find most disturbing is researchers trying to make quantitative deductions from mutants where they have the structure of the wild-type protein, but they do not necessarily have the structure of the mutant protein. They assume the residues are going to sit in the same place. I think that is not always the case. With cytochrome c, in some of the mutant structures we find not only some movement in the vicinity of the amino acid residue that has changed but sometimes some movement in the molecule on the far side. I think that if you are taking an antagonistic position by saying that protein engineering is not telling us anything, I would say the proteins are very complex molecules. If you expect them to reveal all on the first attempt, then I think that is not fair. I think we will get there, but it is going to take time. I started out by saying that in the particular area of heme proteins, I think what already exists is going to give useful results. I also believe that ultimately, one should be able to design an enzyme or modify an existing one in a predetermined way to do something new. However, we are certainly not at that stage yet.

Glaser: Well, lest I be taken for an antagonist let me applaud your effort, but what I was concerned about was your studies in which you actually point out where the charge density is within the protein. I am not convinced, based on the data, that this is indeed the locus of the reactive radical.

Smith: Oh, in terms of the peroxidase? Let me start off by saying that I'm a genetic engineer, not a CCP expert. You are concerned about the horseradish peroxidase? Yes, I know that some people believe that maybe the radical ion is not on the heme. The slide was made a little while ago, and I realize that people are looking at this. With regards to the cytochrome c peroxidase, are you challenging the location on an amino acid residue?

Glaser: No, I know insufficient information about that system itself. I am just thinking of what we are looking at in terms of protein engineering. In many of the studies, we have very good pictures of the protein structure that we have elucidated from x-ray crystallography. This way we can correlate the information. I am just offering up the thought. We might be a little bit hesitant when we analyze our data as to what is truly happening. There is multiplicity of things that might actually occur under kinetic control.

Smith: Sure, but we'll always be in that position when we'll be looking at proteins. I feel that protein engineering may be going to help us to resolve some uncertainties or point out new problems that we did not know existed before.

Omenn: There might be at least two major reasons why your forecast that this work will take many years to be applied in the areas of biodegradation would be true. One is that the natural capacities are quite many and sufficient for most current tasks. The other would be that the techniques that you and others are developing need a good more time to become practical. There are some areas that you might predict would be useful sooner for the kinds of applications that researchers worry about, for example, insertions of the kind you illustrated to increase the thermal stability or the shelf life of a protein or the activity of an organism or to shift the pH optimum to work in particular environments. I wonder if you have any examples of these, or you would just like to make some general comments about these kinds of rather practical and probably quite feasible changes in the overall properties of the molecule?

Smith: Yes, obviously this point is very well taken. There are some very simple things where you can do something very useful. For example, we removed a cysteine group to make the cytochrome c molecule more stable. You might want to put a cysteine group in or some other group so that you can link protein to some insoluble support. That can be useful. Researchers are also using protein engineering to put cysteine in particular places so they can attach a heavy metal for doing isomorphous replacement studies. So there are those kind of practical things you can do. Regarding stability, that is a very interesting question. I think this is an area where there must be considerable data acquisition before we can predict what the benefit is. There has been a fairly serious assault on both lysozyme and subtilisin to generate commercially interesting proteins. There, research workers in genetic engineering companies are trying to place disulfide bonds in the protein on the presumption that the bonds would confer stability. They have been relatively unsuccessful in that quite often this has not increased stability or it has even decreased stability, although sterically the bond should fit. Although I am sure that it is going to be possible to engineer proteins to be more stable, it is not at all clear at the moment what the rules are for determining stability. We need much more quantitative and precise information for that sort of thing. Some researchers are working on changing pH optimum by changing the position of charge groups relative to active sites. I think these are certainly areas where one can carry out work, and I am sure that eventually we will get useful results.

Chakrabarty: I am not sure I heard you right. As you know, every time we find out a new gene, the first thing we do is the homology search to figure out any functionality. I was wondering if I heard you right when you said that you replaced all the amino acids of the homology region of all these cytochrome c, and you found out that even though you may replace all the amino acids, the functionality remains the same. Or would you care to speculate as to why these amino acids have been conserved in these cytochrome *c* molecules?

Smith: Yes, although we haven't replaced all the conserved residues, those that have been replaced are functional.

Chakrabarty: It did even though you replaced the amino acids that are homologous in all cytochrome *c*? Why do you think these amino acids have been conserved in all these cytochrome *c*?

Smith: I do not know. It is a big mystery to us. With cytochrome *c*, as I mentioned, there are 23 different conserved residues. Now, it is fairly obvious why some are conserved; for instance, there are the two ligands. There are the two cysteines that are covalently linked to the heme, and there are certain glycines and prolines that occur at bends between helices, but that still leaves approximately 14 or 15 that are conserved, and it is not obvious why. So far every one of those that we replaced by a variety of others has worked.

Chakrabarty: Do you feel that maybe you can replace an amino acid with cysteine or lysine or whatever? But maybe you did not necessarily replace that with another amino acid that would really distort the structure in such a way that you would see a difference?

Smith: We have not necessarily replaced a residue by 19 other ones. For the phenylalanine -82 we have, and for some of the other ones we have done a fairly substantial set because we are testing a hypothesis regarding hydrogen bonding or lipophilicity. But it is clear that at least the cytochrome *c*, under the conditions with that we are working, will tolerate quite a lot of substitutions in the naturally conserved positions. I do not know what this means. The trouble with our laboratory experiments is we are not really putting it in a selective environment in which it normally is where there is one gene copy in the chromosone. We are putting in a multicopy plasmid, and we are overproducing the protein. So it may be that under those conditions it will function reasonably well. I would not want to draw any physiological conclusions from saying we can get a functioning molecule by doing these replacements. It is just an observation that we get functioning molecules that may not pertain to whatever selective conditions existed during evolution. I end up by having protracted discussions with biologists on this question, and I feel that we are talking about two different things; what we are doing in the laboratory and what is happening with evolution.

Gunsalus: Well, I would agree that these are largely equilibrium experiments, thermodynamic experiments if you like. There are other ways of looking at the dynamics of the processes, and I think it is unfair to ask whether one can do structural analyses and get Kinetics from them.There are ways to do this, and one way is to change the temperature under which you do your x-ray analysis and that will see it, so you begin to find which groups move and how much. The other way, as you pointed out a while ago, is to pair molecules and see if you still get the binding and dynamics that you expect; so it is another step. It took a long time to convince

Perutz that he was not looking at the structure of the heme of the oxygen carrying protein but only at the majority of structures. There are a lot of other protein structures within the so-called crystal that Dr. Chakrabarty talked about.

Smith: I think that P-450 cam is one of the most exciting potential molecules for this kind of work. The potential for redesigning it so that it will oxidize different molecule from what it does normally, to me, is an exciting target for this particular area of work. There are researchers in Illinois who are interested in that kind of work.

Gunsalus: Of course the other thing is to make peroxidases out of them and not have to generate the first two electron reduction processes and to produce various kinds of hydroperoxides.

Kamely: Thank you for this wonderful session.

Basic Science of Anaerobic Biodegradation

1

The Anaerobic Microbiology and Biodegradation of Aromatic Compounds

L. Y. Young
*Department of Microbiology
and Department of
Environmental
Medicine
New York University
Medical Center
550 First Avenue
New York, NY 10016*

Max M. Häggblom
*Department of Microbiology
New York University
Medical Center
550 First Avenue
New York, NY 10016*

Biodegradation of substituted aromatic compounds takes place under a variety of anaerobic conditions. These reactions are mediated by photosynthetic bacteria, denitrifiers, sulfidogens, and methanogenic consortia; hence, it is a widespread phenomenon. Most of the information regarding ring modification and pathways of degradation has emerged from work on mixed cultures. These studies have demonstrated that side chains and ring substituents such as -OH and -Cl moieties are removed prior to further metabolism, which generally involves ring reduction, then ring fission. Pure culture work has begun to address the mechanisms of these ring transformations. These include activation of the benzoate to a CoA derivative, partial reduction of the phenolic ring structure, and anaerobic oxidation of the methyl ring substituent. From the environmental perspective, however, interactions among different species may be important for the biodegradation and removal of aromatic contaminants.

Introduction

Public concern about the health hazards associated with and the destruction of the environment by chemical contamination has led to a greater awareness of the problem and greater urgency in developing efficacious methods for the removal and treatment of these toxic contaminants. Microbiologically mediated processes are attractive because they hold the possibility of complete decontamination of toxic organic compounds to inocuous end products such as carbon dioxide and water. This is generally not the case with physical and chemical processes, which for the most part transfer the contaminant to a different compartment; thus, it remains to be further treated or disposed of.

Once the chemical contaminants have been released into the environment, if rapid loss and degradation does not occur, they may eventually find their way into anaerobic regions of the soil, sediment, or subsurface. A current concern is the contamination of groundwater by chemicals from leaking storage tanks and waste disposal sites. Deep aquifers are generally oxygen depleted, while many aquifers have regions of little or no oxygen.[1] Half the U.S. population (and three-quarters of the U.S. public water supply) is dependent on groundwater sources; thus, this country's chemical contamination is a serious public health problem. In this paper, the anaerobic degradation and transformation of substituted aromatic compounds is reviewed and discussed.

Background

The anaerobic fate of chemicals in the environment is better understood in the context of the anaerobic ecosystem. Carbon fixed into biomass is released back to the atmosphere as carbon dioxide via respiration and the reduction of oxygen to water. In the absence of oxygen, however, the fixed carbon can alternatively be mineralized to carbon dioxide with nitrate, sulfate, or carbonate serving as electron acceptors in oxidation-reduction reactions. Nitrogen or ammonia, hydrogen sulfide and methane, respectively, are the reduced products. The anaerobic contribution to the carbon cycle can be quite significant, as illustrated with several examples. In a salt marsh study, the sulfate mediated respiration of organic carbon was 12 times higher than that mediated by oxygen.[2] In a freshwater lake study, the methane released over a summer season accounted for up to one third of the annual carbon fixed.[3] Hence, the carbon cycle can be substantively impacted by the anaerobic component.

In the absence of oxygen, degradation of contaminants such as chlorinated and unchlorinated aromatic compounds cannot be mediated by the oxygenase mechanisms that have been thoroughly studied under aerobic conditions.[4] As a consequence, the anaerobic transformations of the aromatic ring structure would require very different mechanisms. Although other compounds, (for example, nitrates, sulfates, carbonates) can substitute for oxygen as an electron acceptor, they cannot substitute as the reactant in the oxygenase mediated reactions. The early literature reported that the aromatic structure of lignin,[5] benzoate, and other aromatic acids[6,7] are metabolized to gaseous end products in mixed cultures under methanogenic conditions. Benzoate, serving as a model compound, has since been shown to be susceptible to anaerobic ring fission mediated by pure cultures of denitrifying organisms[8,9] photosythetic bacteria,[10,11] and sulfidogens.[12,13]

Researchers involved in the first extended study to determine whether aromatic compounds other than benzoate and benzoate derivatives could be degraded looked at a series of lignin monomers (Table 1). The substantial and in some cases the complete conversion of the ring carbon to gaseous end products indicated that indeed the ring structure is cleaved. The stoichiometry of conversion and carbon balance data confirmed this observation.[14] Phenol and phenolic derivatives,[15-17] chlorophenols,[18] and phthalic acids[19,20] have also since been shown to undergo anaerobic decomposition. In all these cases, methanogenic mixed culture enrichments were used.

Mixed Cultures

That fission of the aromatic ring can take place is now a well-accepted phenomenon. Until relatively recently, the work has relied heavily, although not exclusively, on mixed cultures under methano-

Table 1

Degradation of Ligno-Aromatic and Related Aromatic Compounds in Methanogenic Enrichment Cultures[a]

Anaerobic Substrate	[c]n	Percent Conversion of Substrate Carbon to CO_2 and CH_4[b]
Vanillin	10	72 ± 1.4
Vanillic acid	8	86 ± 2.8
Ferulic acid	8	86 ± 2.8
Cinnamic acid	3	87 ± 8.1
Benzoic acid	5	91 ± 7.8
Catechol	10	67 ± 1.6
Protocatechuic acid	5	63 ± 1.8
Phenol	10	70 ± 3.2
p-Hydroxybenzoic acid	5	80 ± 2.7
Syringic acid	10	80 ± 1.6
Syringaldehyde	2	102 ± 13.3

[a]Adapted from Reference 14.
[b]Conversion results are reported as mean ± standard error.
[c]n=number of replicate measurements

genic conditions. Under physiological conditions, ring fission of benzoate is thermodynamically unfavorable:[21]

$$\Delta G^{0'}$$
$$C_7H_5O_2^- + 7H_2O \rightarrow 3CH_3COO^- + 3H^+ + 3H_2 + HCO_3^- \qquad +71 \text{ kJ/rk}$$

Methanogenesis, however, is energetically quite favorable,

$$3CH_3COO^- + 3H_2O \rightarrow 3HCO_3^- + 3CH_4 \qquad -93$$

and the role of the methanogens is thought to pull the reaction to the right, so that the net reaction of benzoate to methane and carbon dioxide is favorable.

$$C_7H_5O_2^- + 10H_2O \rightarrow 4HCO_3^- + 3CH_4 + 3H^+ + 3H_2 \qquad -22$$

Methanogens cannot metabolize the aromatic ring. Hence, the mineralization of the benzoate structure relies on an anaerobic food chain in which the benzoate is first metabolized and cleaved by one or more anaerobes, yielding aromatic acids. These in turn are further metabolized to methanogenic precursors such as acetate, carbon dioxide, or formate, which then are utilized by methanogens. A benzoate utilizer was successfully isolated only by growing it in coculture with a methanogen or sulfate reducer.[22]

Mixed methanogenic cultures have provided much information on the fate and the likelihood of degradation of a range of toxic aromatic compounds. In general, ring simplification takes place whereby removal of aliphatic side chains and of substituents such as -Cl, -OH, -OCH$_3$ takes place. Accumulated evidence suggests that in many but not all cases simplification to the phenol and benzoate structure occurs, which suggests that these structures may serve as key precursors to further ring reduction and ring fission reactions. Degradation of aromatic compounds under photosynthetic, denitrifying, and sulfidogenic conditions has not encompassed as many compounds. When information is available, some similarities emerge.

In *Rhodopseudomonas palustris*, the photosynthetic bacterium, aliphatic side chains of compounds such as ferulic, caffeic, 5-phenylvaleric, hydroxycinnamic, cinnamic, and phenylpropionic acids are cleaved, with a corresponding carboxyl group remaining and either a benzoic acid or 4-hydroxybenzoic acid serving as ring fission precursors.[11] This is similar to the reactions and the strategy mediated by a methanogenic consortia.[14]

p-Cresol (*p*Cr) degradation has been studied under methanogenic, denitrifying, and sulfidogenic conditions.[14,17,23,24] It is completely and stoichiometrically metabolized to CO$_2$ and CH$_4$ under methanogenic conditions[15] with 92 percent of the methyl group being oxidized to carbon dioxide.[17] Its degradative pathway under denitrifying conditions proceeds through *p*-hydroxybenzoic acid, which indicates that oxidation of the methyl group takes place.[25]

We undertook a systematic study of the degradation of *p*Cr under denitrifying, sulfidogenic, and methanogenic conditions using a single inoculum source in order to facilitate comparisons. Sediment from a freshwater pond in Athens, Georgia, was used as inoculum in triplicate anaerobic serum bottle cultures containing inorganic nitrate, sulfate, or methanogenic medium totaling 100ml. Initial pCr concentration was 1.0mM, and all incubations were at 30°C. Substrate loss was monitored by ultraviolet spectrophotometry; quantification of substrate and metabolites was measured by high-pressure liquid chromatography; N_2, CO_2, and CH_4 were analyzed by gas chromatography; nitrate and sulfate were determined by colorimetric procedures.[39]

Initial pCr utilization took 21 to 30 days of incubation, with unacclimated sediment for all three anaerobic conditions. After acclimation, pCr metabolism was complete with seven to 12 days. The amounts of electron acceptor used and/or gaseous end products formed are illustrated in Table 2. Under denitrifying conditions, stoichiometric conversion to gaseous end products was noted with 90 percent of the nitrate used converted to nitrogen gas and 5 percent to nitrous oxide (not shown). Similarly, significant amounts of sulfate were utilized coincident with pCr utilization in the sulfidogenic cultures; and 89 percent of the calculated amount of methane was produced in the methanogenic cultures.

Cultures well acclimated to pCr were then compared with parallel cultures that had not been acclimated to the aromatic substrate with regard to their ability to utilize putative intermediates of pCr degradation, p-hydroxybenzaldehyde (pOHbzald), p-hydroxybenzoate (pOHbzate). The initial rates of utilization of these compounds in acclimated and unacclimated cultures are shown in Table 3. Acclimated rates were significantly faster than unacclimated rates for pCr and pOHbzate with all three reducing conditions. The rate of pOHbzald utilization, however, is rapid in both acclimated and unacclimated cultures.

The transient appearance of pOHbzald and pOHbzate during the course of incubation in the cultures just described supports their role in intermediates in the degradative pathway. Figure 1 illustrates the metabolism of pCr, pOHbzald, and pOHbzate by pCr acclimated methanogenic cultures. A transient accumulation of pOHbzald and

Table 2
**Calculated and Measured Amounts of Electron Acceptor and/or Gaseous
End Products Formed With Complete Metabolism of 1.0mmol *p*-Cresol**

Condition	% of Expected
Denitrification	
Nitrate used	90
N$_2$ produced	84
Sulfidogenic	
Sulfate used	78
Methanogenic	
Total gas	68
CH$_4$	89

Adapted from Reference 39.

Table 3
**Initial Rates of Substrate Utilization With Cultures Acclimated or
Unacclimated to *p*-Cresol Metabolism**

Substrate Added (0.5mM)	Denitrification accl.	unaccl.	Methanogenesis accl	unaccl	Sulfidogenesis accl	unaccl
p-cresol	105.00*	26.25	51.25	0	43.75	0
p-OHbenzoate	56.25	12.50	52.50	5.00	8.75	0
p-OHbenzaldehyde	99.75	75.00	100.50	84.75	115.75	126.25

Adapted from Reference 39.

*p*OHbzate was observed in the *p*Cr fed cultures. In the *p*OHbzald fed cultures, *p*OHbzate and benzoate were both produced and then utilized. The initial time of onset suggests that benzoate is formed from *p*OHbzate. In the denitrifying and sulfidogenic cultures, the transient appearance of *p*OHbzald and *p*OHbzate was also observed. Benzoate, however, was not detected. These results suggest that the initial reactions for *p*Cr metabolism under denitrifying, sulfidogenic, and methanogenic conditions are similar, in which an oxidation of the

Figure 1. The metabolism over time of *p*-cresol and suspected *p*-cresol intermediates, *p*-hydroxybenzaldehyde and *p*-hydroxybenzoate, by *p*-cresol acclimated methanogenic cultures. Adapted from Reference 39.

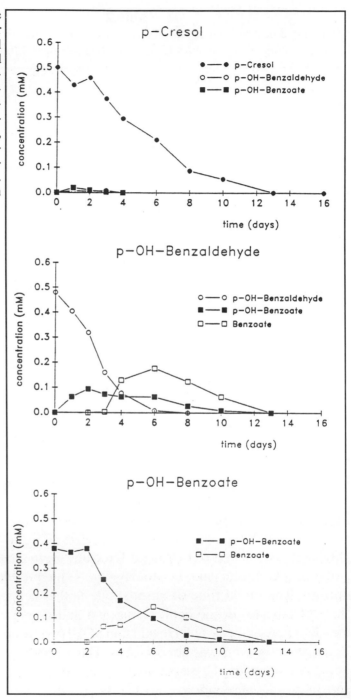

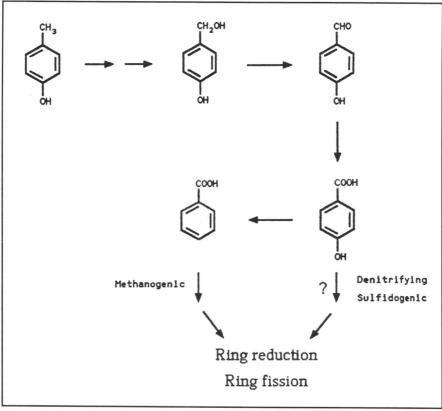

Figure 2. Tentative scheme of *p*-cresol metabolism under methanogenic, denitrifying, and sulfidogenic conditions. Adapted from Reference 39.

methyl group of *p*Cr to the carboxylic acid moiety takes place prior to ring fission. An additional dehydroxylation step was apparent under methanogenic conditions that was not observed with the other cultures. The tentative pathway is summarized in Figure 2, which is a similar scheme that was suggested for a sulfidogenic mixed culture [24] and suggests that a common strategy for degradation of this methyl phenol may exist in anaerobes of widely different physiology.

Of much interest recently is the anaerobic or reductive dechlorination of the aromatic ring that has been reported for chlorobenzoates, chlorophenols, and chlorobenzene compounds.[4,18,26] The studies were all carried out under methanogenic, mixed culture conditions. For the chlorobenzoate isomers, dechlorination proceeds to benzoate, which

then undergoes ring fission and mineralization.[4] For pentachlorophenol, -Cl, the *ortho* position is first removed, then the para followed by
the meta.[18] Complete metabolism to methane and carbon dioxide
takes place, presumably through a phenol intermediate, although this
was not confirmed. The dechlorination of the pentachlorophenol
required mixing together cultures that had been separately acclimated
to 2-, 3- or 4-chlorophenol. Methanogenic cultures also dechlorinated
hexachlorobenzene. In this case, however, chlorine is removed from
four positions on the ring, leaving the three dichlorophenol isomers
that are not metabolized any further.[26] Although reductive dechlorination is readily demonstrated in methanogenic enrichment cultures, it
should be noted that aerobic organisms also have been shown to
mediate the reaction (see Figure 3).

Pure Cultures

As more pure cultures of anaerobes capable of aromatic degradation are isolated and studied, a better understanding of the mechanism of ring degradation is emerging. For benzoic acid degradation as
mediated by the photosynthetic bacterium *R. palustris*, its uptake and
initial activation has been shown to be linked to the formation of a
benzoyl-CoA thioester.[11,27] Cell-free extract assays determined that
its formation from benzoic acid is very rapid and complete. Radiolabeled benzoic acid was virtually completely converted to the CoA
thioester within 15 seconds.[11] The apparent K_m was estimated to be
less than 1μM, thereby providing the organism with a highly efficient
uptake mechanism. Growth, then, can be maintained on even small
amounts of the aromatic compound in the natural environment. The
initial activation of benzoate to the CoA thioester apparently is also
observed in some denitrifying strains.[28]

The initial reactions involved in the degradation of trihydroxyl-
ated aromatic acids appear to follow a somewhat different strategy
than that for benzoic acid. Using an isolated pure culture *Pelobacter
acidigallici*, the compounds gallic, 2,3,4,-trihydroxybenzoic and 2,4,6-
trihydroxybenzoic acids were first decarboxylated to the correspond-

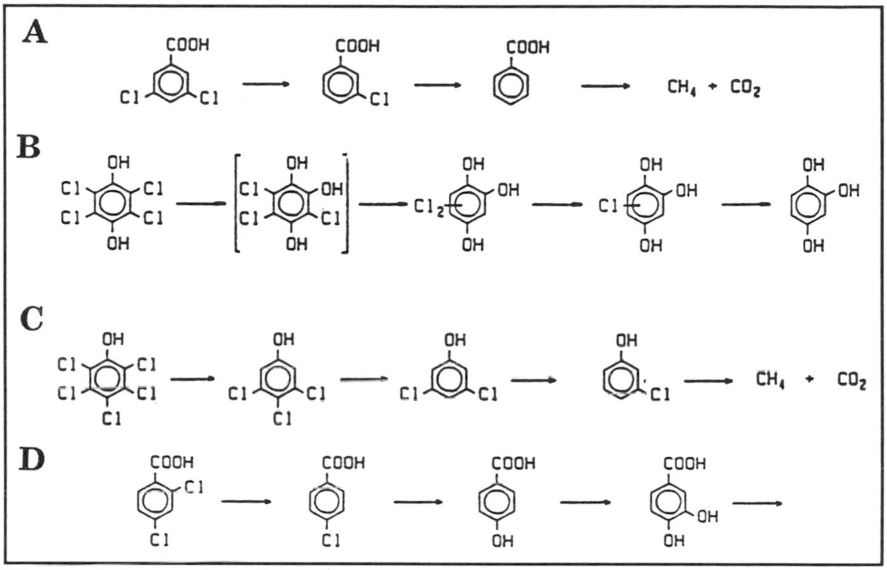

Figure 3. Examples of reductive dechlorination under anaerobic and aerobic conditions: **Anaerobic: A.** Degradation of 3,5-dichlorobenzoate by anaerobic microbial consortia. Adapted from Reference 36. **B.** Pathway of PCP degradation by a mixture of anaerobic sludges. Adapted from Reference 18. **Aerobic: C.** Suggested sequence for dechlorination of TeCH by *Rhodococcus* sp. CP-2. Adapted from Reference 37. **D.** Degradation of 2,4-dichlorobenzoate by *Alcaligenes denitrificans* NTB-1. Adapted from Reference 38.

ing trihydroxybenzene. The resulting pyrogallol (2,3,4-trihydroxybenzene then underwent an isomerization to phloroglucinol (2,4,6-trihydroxybenzene). By using cell-free extracts, it was determined that phloroglucinol is reduced to dihydrophoroglucinol in the presence of nicotinamide-adenine dinucleotide phosphate.[29] Whether the dihydrophoroglucinol is the direct precursor to ring fission is not known. However, analysis of products formed indicates that ring fission of the aromatic structure yielded stoichiometric conversion to acetate, with three moles of acetate produced for each mole of phloroglucinol converted.[30] That such a phloroglucinol reductase is not unique is suggested by the fact that the same reaction has been observed in separate studies with a *Coprococcus*[31] (Figure 4) and a *Eubacterium*.[32]

For more reduced aromatic compounds such a *p*-cresol, as suggested by the mixed culture studies described earlier, initial

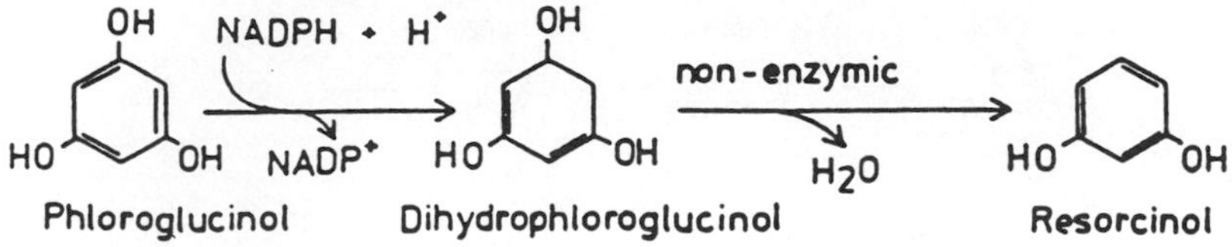

Figure 4. Reduction of phloroglucinol by the anaerobe *Coprococcus*. Adapted from Reference 31.

reactions appear to oxidize the methyl substituent to the carboxylic acid. This is an oxidative set of reactions occurring under anaerobic conditions. We have reported on a denitrifying pure culture recently biotyped as an *Achromobacter* sp., which stoichiometrically oxidizes *p*-cresol to *p*-OHbzate.[23,25,33] The oxidation is obligately coupled to nitrate reduction, and such activity is only observed in cells grown under denitrifying conditions. The pathway for the methyl group oxidation sequentially forms the *p*-OH- benzyl alcohol, then the *p*-OH-benzlaldehyde followed by the corresponding *p*-OH-benzoic acid. This is evidenced by the observation of the downstream interme-diates when an upstream intermediate is added in cell suspension studies. It is further underscored by the stoichiometry of nitrate reduction. For every mole of *p*-cresol oxidized, one mole of nitrate is reduced. When induced cell suspensions are given the more oxidized benzylalcohol intermediate, one third less reducing capacity is avail-able and, quantitatively, one third less nitrate is reduced. Similarly, when the benzaldehyde is the added intermediate, two thirds less nitrate is reduced.

A partially purified *p*-cresol methylhydroxylase enzyme was shown to mediate the oxidation of *p*-cresol to the benzylalcohol and then to the benzylaldehyde. Oxidation of the *p*-OH-benzaldehyde to *p*-OH-benzoic acid was mediated by an NAD⁺–dependent dehydro-genase. The methylhydroxylase required an alkyl substituted phenol ring with a hydroxyl group in the *para* position.[33] The pathway is summarized in Figure 5. Because sulfidogenic and methanogenic mixed cultures mediate a similar sequence of reactions, it would be of interest to know if a related *p*-cresol methylhydroxylase is respon-

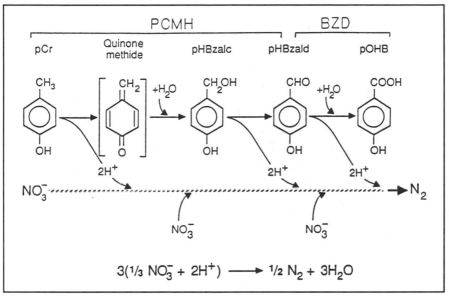

Figure 5. Summary of the anaerobic oxidation of p-cresol by a denitrifying isolate as mediated by p-cresol methylhydroxylase (PCMH) and benzaldehyde dehydrogenase (BZD). Adapted from References 23 and 33.

sible. This mechanism has also been described in a pseudomonad under aerobic conditions.[34]

Conclusions

It is important to recognize the need for more pure culture studies in that much needs to be understood with regard to the anaerobic mechanisms and enzymes that mediate ring alteration and ring fission. The diversity of physiologically different anaerobes is in contrast to the similarity of some of the known pathways for aromatic catabolism. Whether the shared strategy has a common ancestry is not known. It is also important to recognize that it was from the mixed culture work that the phenomenon became established. In addition, certain pathways have been shown thus far only to operate in mixed cultures. This is most clearly demonstrated by the mineralization of 3-chlorobenzoate to methane and carbon dioxide.[35] Dechlorination yields benzoate, which is metabolized to acetate, and then further transformed to methane. Each of these steps is mediated by a separate species that, for the most part, cannot catalyze any other step. The complete degradation of 3-chlorobenzoate, therefore, requires the interaction of different species in this anaerobic microbial food chain. Ideally, what we learn from any of these studies should be ultimately translated into application for treatment. In that respect, we then come full circle back to mixed cultures; that is, there is a need to understand and optimize the wanted activity of the desirable organism against a background of a mixture of many different species, whether in an environment or in a treatment process.

Acknowledgments

This work was supported inpart by NSF CES-8605143, EPA CR-814611 and NIH ES-04895.

References

1. G. Bitton and C.P. Gerba, in *Groundwater Pollution Microbiology*, G.Bitton and C.P. Gerba, Eds. (John Wiley & Sons, New York, 1984), pp. 1-7.
2. R.W. Howarth and J.M. Teal, *Limnol. Oceanogr.* **24**, 999 (1979).
3. R.F. Strayer and J.M. Tiedje, *Limnol. Oceanogr.* **23**, 1201 (1978).
4. S. Gibson and J.M. Suflita, *Appl. Environ. Microbiol.* **52**, 681 (1986).
5. C.S. Boruff and A.M. Buswell, *J. Am. Chem. Soc.* **56**, 886 (1934).
6. D. Tarvin and A.M. Buswell, *J. Am. Chem. Soc.* **56**, 1751 (1934).
7. F.M. Clark and L.R. Fina, *Arch. Biochem.* **36**, 26 (1952).
8. R.J. Williams and W.C. Evans, *Biochem. J.* **148**, 1 (1975).
9. B.F. Taylor, W.L. Campbell, and I. Chinoy, *J. Bacteriol.* **102**, 430 (1970).
10. P.L. Dutton and W.C. Evans, *Biochem. J.* **113**, 525 (1969).
11. C.S. Harwood and J. Gibson, *J. Bacteriol.* **165**, 504 (1986).
12. F. Widdel, Ph.D. thesis, Universitat Gottingen, 1980.
13. F. Widdel and N. Pfennig, in *Bergey's Manual of Systematic Bacteriology, Vol. 1, 9th Ed.*, N.R. Kreig and J.H. Holt, Eds. (Williams and Wilkins, Baltimore, 1984), pp. 663-679.
14. J.B. Healy and L.Y. Young, *Appl. Environ. Microbiol.* **38**, 84 (1979).
15. L.Y. Young and M.D. Rivera, *Water Res.* **19**, 1325 (1985).
16. S.A. Boyd *et al.*, *Appl. Environ. Microbiol.* **46**, 50 (1983).

17. D.J. Roberts and P.M. Fedorak, *Can. J. Microbiol.* **33**, 335 (1987).
18. M.D. Mikesell and S.A. Boyd, *Appl. Environ. Microbiol.* **52**, 861 (1986).
19. D.R. Shelton, S.A. Boyd, and J.M. Tiedje, *Environ. Sci. Technol.* **18**, 93 (1984).
20. O.A. O'Connor and L.Y. Young, *Environ. Toxicol. Chem.*, **8**, 569 (1989).
21. J.G. Ferry and R.S. Wolfe, *Arch. Microbiol.* **107**, 33 (1976).
22. D.O. Mountfort and M.P. Bryant, *Arch. Microbiol.* **37**, 441 (1983).
23. I.D. Bossert, M.D. Rivera, and L.Y. Young, *FEMS Microbiol. Ecol.* **38**, 313 (1986).
24. W.J. Smolenski and J.M. Suflita, *Appl. Environ. Microbiol.* **53**, 710 (1987).
25. I.D. Bossert, M.D. Rivera, and L.Y. Young, *FEMS Microbiol. Ecol.* **38**, 313 (1986).
26. B.Z. Fathepure, J.M. Tiedje, and S.A. Boyd, *Appl. Environ. Microbiol.* **54**, 327 (1988).
27. P.J. Whittle, D.O. Lunt, and W.C. Evans, *Biochem. Soc. Trans.* 4, 490 (1976).
28. U. Schennen, K. Braun, and H.J. Knackmuss, *J. Bacteriol.* **161**, 321 (1985).
29. E. Samain, G. Albagnac, and H.C. Dubourguier, *Arch. Microbiol.* 144, 242 (1986).
30. B. Schink and N. Pfennig, *Arch. Microbiol.* **133**, 195 (1982).
31. T.R. Patel, K.G. Jure, and G.A. Jones, *Appl. Environ. Microbiol.* **42**, 1010 (1981).
32. L.R. Krumholz *et al., J. Bacteriol.* **169**, 1886 (1987).
33. I.D. Bossert *et al., J. Bacteriol.*, **171**, 2956 (1989).
34. D.J. Hopper and D.G. Taylor, *J. Bacteriol.* **122**, 1 (1975).
35. J. Dolfing and J.M. Tiedje, *Arch. Microbiol.* **149**, 102 (1987).
36. A. Horowitz *et al., Dev. Ind. Microbiol.* **23**, 435 (1982); J. Suflita *et al., Science* **218**, 1115 (1982).
37. M.M. Häggblom, D. Janke, and M.S. Salkinoja-Salonen, *Appl. Environ. Microbiol.* **55**, 516 (1989).
38. W.J.J. van den Tweel *et al., Appl. Microbiol. Biotechnol.* **25**, 289 (1986).
39. M.M. Häggblom *et al., Microbial Ecology,* in press.

Discussion

Schink: In one of your schemes I saw again this reductive transformation of phenol to cyclohexanol that has been repeated through the literature hundreds of times. Is there any experimental evidence of that? I know it came up with Evans about 12 or 13 years ago and was repeated by Bakker in the Netherlands; I do not see any way how such a reaction should occur. I think it is just a side reaction of something else that we do not understand, because whatever we know so far about that reductive transformation of an aromatic nucleus is always occurring with benzoid derivatives after binding to CoA. Without that, I do not see how to run such a reaction. So is there any more reliable evidence after these original ideas about it that supports that reaction? What do you think?

Young: You are right, the evidence that is available comes from mixed cultures for the most part and comes from detection of metabolites and not quantitative detection of metabolites; if they are there, then it is put into the pathway. How much was there was not important at that point. In terms of more specific evidence and clear-cut mechanisms, that remains to be definitively shown. That is where I think we have to proceed to pure culture work to get the uneqivocal evidence of the mechanism and the pathway. The mixed culture work has been very useful, but there is always the question of who is doing what, what kind of reactions are the major reactions, and which are the minor reactions. So it is a good question; I do not know of any hard evidence beyond what you have indicated.

Gunsalus: Does this answer your question?

Schink: Yes.

Gunsalus: Who has the next question?

Glaser: I have several questions. One having to do with Patel's conversion of the phloroglucinol. The last step was indicated as being nonenzymatic. What is the basis for that? Did he actually check into that with any kind of detail?

Young: They did see that product. Their conclusion was that this occurred nonenzymatically, and it was not pursued much further. So I cannot enlighten you on that particular step very well. Sorry.

Glaser: The conversion of the phenol to a carboxylic acid intermediate seems to be contrathermodynamic. Any comments on that?

Young: Somebody in the audience may be able to help me on that. This question did come up with Barbara Genthner's work at the Environmental Protection Agency laboratories, Gulf Breeze has shown this mechanism in a very lucid study.

Glaser: It is the phenolic acid?

Young: Yes, the phenol is carboxylated. It has been shown in her system; it has been shown by Joseph Winters in anaerobic digester enrichments; and it has been shown by Juergen Wiegel in sediments systems. So it was not an isolated report. There seems to be a growning set of information, which suggests that this may be of the ways phenol proceeds to degradation.

Glaser: Sure.

Schink: If I could just comment on that point. The reaction is endergonic and needs about 20 kilojoules per mole. It has been shown in pure culture by Andreas Tschech, so it is pretty well studied in the meantime.

Young: So, therefore, further degradation downstream would have to be energetically highly favorable in order to keep the process going.

Glaser: The final question then would be in your studies. I have noticed you have confined most of your thoughts to conversion of starting materials to products. Any word on inhibition or inhibitors that you have encountered?

Young: Inhibition of the degradation?

Glaser: Yes. The reason why I asked the question is that coming more from the engineering side and treatment development side, one of the problems we find with anaerobic organisms and their use in treatment schemes is their inhibition in more complex situations.

Young: By other elements in the wastestream?

Glaser: Yes.

Young: Well, we have not pursued that. I know that people at Drexel

University, for instance, Dick Speece, have looked extensively at the inhibition of degradation.

Glaser: Are you worried about intermediates or compounds that happen to be present?

Young: You are talking about metal or other things that may come in the wastestream, right?

Glaser: Yes, it is unfortunately a global problem for which little is understood because one does not have the opportunity to understand and study the wastestream in the detail that one does for studies such as yours.

Gunsalus: Do you have a problem with nitrite inhibition of your systems?

Young: Not so far.

2

Selecting and Developing New Microbes: Anaerobes

Bernhard Schink

Universität Tübingen,
Mikrobiologie I
Auf der Morgenstelle 28
D-7400 Tübingen
West Germany

The degradative capacity of anaerobic bacteria isolated from or active in natural or "semi-natural" environments has expanded considerably in the recent past. In many cases, new varieties to known pathways of attack on recalcitrant compounds were found; in other instances, entirely new pathways were established that differ basically from the well-described aerobic or oxygenase-dependent modes of substrate activation. In some cases, for example with nonionic surfactants or phenolic compounds, anaerobic degradation proved to be even more efficient than aerobic mineralization. The biochemical versatility of anaerobic bacteria is by far greater than what was expected only some few years ago, and several new reaction types have been discovered, mostly in newly isolated natural inhabitants of usual anoxic environments.

Introduction

A comparison of energy yields of aerobic and anaerobic biomass degradation (here exemplified by glucose) demonstrates convincingly why anaerobic microbes are primarily applied thus far in degradative rather than synthetic processes:

$$C_6H_{12}O_6 + 6\,O_2 \rightarrow 6\,CO_2 + 6\,H_2O$$
$$\Delta G_0' = -\,2870 \text{ kJ/mol}$$

$$C_6H_{12}O_6 \rightarrow 3\,CO_2 + 3\,CH_4$$
$$\Delta G_0' = -\,390 \text{ kJ/mol}$$

The small amount of energy available to anaerobic microorganisms (approximately 15 percent of that obtained by aerobes, according to the equation just presented) gives rise to only small amounts of biomass formed. This helps to keep sludge production low, a problem that becomes more and more difficult to solve in densely populated areas. Moreover, products such as methane or ethanol, acids, and so forth can be formed that might be of interest for either energy generation or solvent production purposes.[1]

However, the low energy yield of anaerobes compared with aerobes also implies some drawbacks. Low growth rates and yields make an anaerobic microbial population less flexible in adapting to changing environmental conditions, changes in substrate availability, or recovery after shock loads of, for example, toxic compounds. For these reasons, the application of anaerobic microorganisms such as to waste treatment was for a long time considered to be less efficient than aerobic processes. These shortcomings of anaerobes compared with aerobes have recently been overcome by the development of reactor systems that maintain high amounts of biomass, independent of the retention time for the treated waste material.

Also, the degradative capacity of anaerobic bacteria was thought to be considerably smaller than that of aerobes. All compounds that are aerobically attacked by oxygenase reactions should be recalcitrant in the absence of oxygen because there is in the anaerobic world no equivalent to oxygen, with its very specific properties.[2] Work done during the last 15 years in microbial ecology and physiology has changed this view drastically: many compounds thought so far to be nondegradable in the absence of oxygen proved to be well degradable; some of them are even better degradable without oxygen than when they are in the presence of oxygen.[1]

All these "new" degradative capacities of anaerobic bacterial communities were discovered by enrichment or isolation from natural sediments or from sewage digestors and other technical systems; no case has become known so far in which, for example, genetic manipulation has conferred new important degradative capacities to a known anaerobic bacterium. This was also the approach taken in my own laboratory during the recent six years. Consequently, my contribution does not deal with the "development" of "new" microbes; this is being done by several laboratories in the world today. Rather, I would like to stress the fact that numerous unknown degradative or other metabolic capacities exist in "old" nature. These activities are "new" to us and only need to be detected and studied under defined conditions after isolating the responsible bacteria by suitable methods. The following examples are taken from our group's recent work to support this hypothesis.

Ether Linkage Cleavage

The degradation of polyethylene glycol by fermenting bacteria enriched and isolated from polluted marine sediment was first reported by our group.[3] Acetaldehyde was the first degradation intermediate detected;[4] this suggests that cleavage of the ether linkage is accomplished by an enzyme analogous to diol dehydratase, which shifts the terminal hydroxy function to the C-atom vicinal and then to the linkage oxygen, thus transforming the ether linkage into a comparably unstable halfacetal structure. We succeeded recently in demonstrating the polymer-degrading enzyme at low activity in cell-free extracts. All the polyethylene glycol-fermenting anaerobes isolated so far exhibit high diol dehydratase activities in cell-free systems. Obviously, the polymer-degrading enzyme has been derived from an additional copy of the diol dehydratase enzyme and has undergone considerable modification which, on the one hand, allows polymer degradation but, on the other hand, also confers high instability to the enzyme, which has so far precluded its successful measurement in cell extracts. We consider this the most probable way in which degrada-

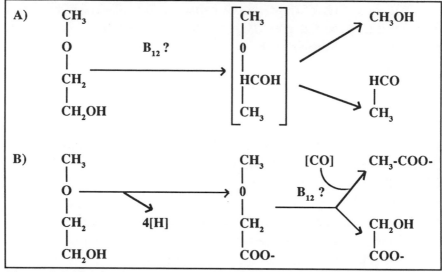

Figure 1. Different pathways of methoxyethanol degradation used by different combinations of fermenting bacteria. (A) *Pelobacter venetianus/Acetobacterium malicum* combination; (B) syntrophic oxidation and subsequent ether cleavage by *Acetobacterium* sp.

tion of polyethylene glycol could evolve in the considerably short time of approximately 30 years that this substrate has been in the environment.[5]

The suggested pathway implies that anaerobic degradation of polyethylene glycol-containing nonionic surfactants can proceed only from the free hydroxyl end and is limited to a great extent by membrane permeability of the substrate and its intermediate products.[6]

Also, another synthetic dialkylether, methoxyacetate, was recently found to be degraded in the absence of oxygen. Similar to polyethylene glycol degradation, a B_{12} coenzyme is likely to be involved in this ether linkage cleavage reaction as well.[7] Hints for such a pathway have been obtained recently with homoacetogenic bacteria growing on natural methylphenyl ether compounds.[8]

The discovery of anaerobic methoxyacetate cleavage opens another pathway for anaerobic degradation of methoxyethanol, an important solvent in the chemical industry (Figure 1): diol dehydra-

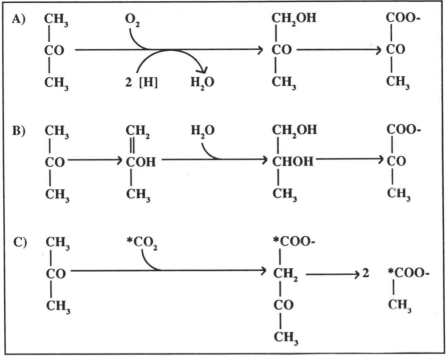

Figure 2. Different pathways of acetone degradation. Explanation is given in the text.

tase-catalyzed ether linkage cleavage was proved recently with a *Pelobacter venetianus* strain,[9] whereas primary oxidation to methoxy-acetate and subsequent demethylation was suggested earlier;[10] however, it could be proved experimentally only recently.[7]

Ketone Degradation

The literature on degradation of ketones, especially acetone, is small but not free of contradictions. Acetone is degraded aerobically by bacteria [11] and mammalian liver cells[12] via oxygenase-dependent hydroxylation to acetol and subsequent oxidation (Figure 2, A). An oxygen-independent primary attack by reversion of a diol dehydratase reaction (Figure 2, B)[13] has never been established unequivocally. We isolated several new strains of bacteria that degrade acetone in the absence of oxygen with either nitrate[14] or sulfate as electron acceptor. Moreover, a syntrophic methanogenic culture was also described that converts acetone to $2\ CH_4$ and $1\ CO_2$ via intermediate formation of two acetate residues.[15] In all cases, the substrate molecule was activated by a carboxylation reaction that could be demonstrated by experiments with labeled $^{14}CO_2$ (Figure 2, C). Numerous efforts in our laboratory to isolate aerobic bacteria that use the originally described oxygenase-dependent pathway have failed so far; all aerobic isolates, even if enriched in the (nearly) complete absence of CO_2 depended on CO_2 addition for degradation of this substrate but did not need CO_2 when growing with acetate. It appears from these results that the originally reported oxygenase-dependent pathway is the exception rather than the rule, even in well-aerated environments, and that oxygen-independent attacks on the ketone molecule can well compete with the oxygenase-dependent pathways, at least under the selection conditions applied in our enrichment cultures.

Degradation of Aromatic Compounds

At least four different pathways for degradation of mononuclear aromatic compounds are known today which, depending on the last aromatic structure detectable before ring cleavage, are known as the benzoate pathway, the phenol pathway, the resorcinol pathway, and the phloroglucinol pathway.[16] With this, the anaerobic pathways differ basically from the aerobic ones that all merge, independent of the original substrate, into only two common intermediates, catechol or protocatechuate. The various carboxy-, hydroxy-, and amino derivatives of bezene are channeled into the four intermediate pathways by interesting modification reactions, for example, decarboxylations, transcarboxylations, reductive dehydroxylations, or reductive (and hydrolytic ?) deaminations. These ring modifications are of interest for several reasons. First, they represent chemically new and exciting reaction types that are worth being studied in more detail. However, they might also be of interest for possible applications in preparative organic and bioorganic chemistry: suitable enzymes for site-specific ring modifications might be applied in this field, especially if these enzymes can be cloned and produced cheaply in large quantities.

Although the rates of substrate conversion and growth by these anaerobic degraders of aromatic compounds are low, anaerobic degradation of phenols, nitroaromatics, and aniline derivatives may prove to be better applicable in treatment of specific industrial waste waters than the common aerobic treatment because the formation of polymeric side products from phenol radicals by reactions with excess oxygen can be avoided.

How to Select for Unknown Microbes or Who Wins the Game?

The classic enrichment technique in batch culture with comparably high substrate concentrations always selects for those bacteria that can grow the fastest under the respective conditions. This statement appears trivial at first sight; however, it needs to be considered very seriously. Neither energy efficiency nor substrate affinity or the most simple degradation pathway have anything to do with the outcome of such an enrichment experiment. Only growth velocity counts; for example, the incubation temperature that influences growth rates quite differently with different bacteria has a much more striking effect than may be expected. A basically different strategy is the enrichment in continuous culture, for example, a chemostat, which selects at low dilution rates for slow-growing bacteria with high substrate affinity, thus far better mimicking the conditions in a natural ecosystem than the batch culture enrichment does. A direct dilution of the inoculum material in a tube series over several steps allows detection of those representatives for a certain degradative activity that are the most numerous ones in the respective environmental sample.

We enriched for fermentative glycerol degraders by all three approaches with freshwater sediment as inoculum. In batch culture, fast-growing facultative anaerobes always developed that formed acetate and 1,3-propanediol. The same happened in a continuous culture enrichment before the medium flow was started. However, after several volume changes at a mean residence time of one day, propionate was found as the predominant fermentation product. The bacterium isolated from this culture represents a new species that is specialized on only glycerol as substrate and ferments glycerol to only propionate and traces of molecular hydrogen.[17] Direct stepwise dilution of the same sediment sample used for the enrichments previously described showed that the propionate former was the numerically predominant bacterium that was outcompeted in the lower dilution tubes by the fast-growing facultative anaerobes.

The two metabolic types of isolated anaerobes differ considerably in the total free energy change of the reaction catalyzed as well as in the adenosine 5'=triphosphate (ATP) yield:

3 Glycerol →
$$\text{Acetate}^- + \text{Formate}^- + 2\ \text{H}^+ + 2\ \ \textbf{1,3-Propanediol} + \text{H}_2\text{O}$$
$$\Delta G_o{'} = -216 \ \text{kJ per mol reaction}$$
$$= -72 \ \text{kJ per mol glycerol}$$
$$\rightarrow 2/3 \ \text{ATP per glycerol}$$

Glycerol → Propionate⁻ + H⁺ + H₂O
$$\Delta G_o{'} = -150 \ \text{kJ per mol}$$
$$\rightarrow 5/3 \ \text{ATP per glycerol}$$

This example shows that different enrichment strategies may yield metabolically quite different bacteria with the same medium, the same substrate, and the same inoculum material and that even the inoculum size can have a dramatic effect on the outcome of the enrichment experiment.

In the case presented here, we ended up with two types of bacteria that both ferment glycerol to fermentation products of industrial interest, namely, 1,3-propanediol and propionate.

Similar effects have to be expected with other substrates that might give rise to more interesting biochemical sidepaths. Our simple enrichment experiment can also help to explain why degradation pathways studied with enriched or pure cultures often come to results quite different from those obtained by tracer experiments in sediment or sludge samples.

Conclusions

In recent years, research on anaerobic degradability of organic compounds has led to the discovery of many unusual or novel reaction types in anaerobic biochemistry. This research has also shown that in many cases more than one pathway exists to solve a certain degradation problem. I am convinced that there are many more "unusual" reactions possible in the anaerobic world that are only waiting to be discovered. To me, the search for unknown processes in nature looks more promising than constructing new pathways from existing genetic elements. Nature has invested a lot of phantasy into creating many more processes in general biochemistry than our biochemical textbooks can list; constructions of our own, however, will never go beyond those processes we know.

For nearly 50 years, the classic citric acid cycle was the only way to oxidize acetate; anaerobes have developed two variants of it as well as a completely different, noncyclic pathway, all of which were discovered only recently.[18] The same is true for autotrophic CO_2 fixation: Two new pathways entirely different from the Calvin cycle have been elucidated in the last ten years.[19] How long did researchers try unsuccessfully to transfer nitrogen fixation into cellulolytic bacteria before a bacterium with both abilities was isolated from the gland of Deshayes in shipworms?[20] I think we still can learn a lot from nature before we start to "improve" it.

References

1. B. Schink, in *Biology of Anaerobic Microorganisms*, A.J.B. Zehnder, Ed. (John Wiley and Sons, New York , 1988), pp. 771.

2. B.G. Malmstom, *Annu. Rev. Biochem.* **51**, 21 (1982).
3. B. Schink and M. Stieb, *Appl. Environ. Microbiol.* **45**, 1905 (1983).
4. A. Strag and B. Schink, *Appl. Microbiol. Biotechnol.* **25**, 37 (1986).
5. D.P. Cox, *Adv. Appl. Microbiol.* **23**, 173 (1978).
6. St. Wagener and B. Schink, *Appl. Environ. Microbiol.* **54**, 561 (1988).
7. B. Schuppert and B. Schink, *Arch. Microbiol,* submitted.
8. K. De Weerd *et al., Appl. Environ. Microbiol.* **54**, 1237 (1988).
9. K. Tanaka and N. Pfennig, *Arch. Microbiol.* **149**, 181 (1988).
10. K. Tanaka, E. Mikami, and T. Suzuki, *J. Ferment. Technol.* **64**, 305 (1986).
11. D.G. Taylor *et al., J. Gen. Microbiol.* **118**, 159 (1980).
12. B.R. Landau and H. Brunengraber, *Trends Biochem. Sci.* **12**, 113 (1987).
13. H. Rudney, *J. Biol. Chem.* **210**, 361 (1954).
14. H. Platen and B. Schink, *J. Gen. Microbiol.* **135**, 883 (1989).
15. H. Platen and B. Schink, *Arch. Microbiol.* **149**, 136 (1987).
16. B. Schink and A. Tschech, in *Microbial Metabolism and the Carbon Cycle*, S. Hagedorn, Ed. (Harwood Academic Publishers, Chur, Switzerland, 1988), pp. 213.
17. R. Schauder and B. Schink, *Arch. Microbiol.*, in press.
18. R. Thauer, *Eur. J. Biochem.* **176**, 497 (1988).
19. H. G. Wood, S.W. Ragsdale, and E. Pezacka, *FEMS Microbiol. Rev.* **39**, 345 (1986).
20. J.B. Waterbury, C.B. Calloway, and R.D. Turner, *Science* **221**, 1401 (1983).

Discussion

Omenn: I think that you have made a very noteworthy point that there are extensive metabolic capabilities in nature yet to be discovered and characterized. The problem of trying to interpret the potential usefulness of these systems is to have some kind of a clue or even a strategy for accessing what the quantitative capacity of some of these pathways might be and whether these bacteria under realistic growth conditions will really have turnover rates that would be significant in microcosms or other controlled environments or even in other applications. In other words, to go from the metabolic biochemistry to at least thinking about whether the bacteria might be useful in various kinds of applications. Could you give us guidance on that?

Schink: There is no doubt that the establishment of such a system will take a longer time than that for an aerobic one because the cell yield per transformation reaction is small; it takes a long time to establish a sufficient amount of biomass to run the business. But once you have that, then just due to the fact that they get only a small amount of energy from it, they actually have to transform a lot of substrate to maintain, for instance, the energy demand of the running metabolism in the cell. So if you look at the metabolic activity in terms of transformation rates in micromoles turned over per time and milligrams of protein, you end up in the same range as with aerobic bacteria. With our enzyme assays, we find about .5 to $1\mu M$ substrate transformed per milligram protein per minute, which is pretty well what you expect with an aerobic bacterium as well. The problem is if there is also a mutual dependence on other bacteria, then the establishment of two or even three or four bacteria cooperating in such a system takes even longer. That is for sure a problem that has been overcome to some extent by the establishment of suitable reactor systems that bind the biomass in the system; that makes the substrate transformation rate more or less independent of the bacteria's growth rate.

Young: Your talk nicely underscored the importance of these multiple species interactions in anaerobic environments and the fact that we must again diverge from the single-substrate, single-organism concept. My question is very different, however. I would like to ask you whether you care to speculate as to why it has been so difficult to isolate the anaerobic reductive dechlorinating enzyme. To date Tiedje's laboratory at Michigan State has the only isolate that can anaerobically dechlorinate. I know that many people are trying but have not been successful thus far.

Schink: The approach is still a problem. I just pointed it out with this dechlorinaton concept. If you compare that system with an aerobic system you would probably call it a type of cometabolic activity because the bacteria may get some energy from the system, but they cannot grow with it. Especially with this bacterium, researchers do not know what it is growing on. Once they find a good electron source on the one side and a good source for running the anabolic metabolism at the same time, I think then it should not be a problem at all. At the moment, we do not know what these bugs grow on. I think that it is fine that Tiedje and co-workers have grown the bacteria with pyruate and yeast extract and whatever else, but it is not the reaction the bugs are running in nature. They could not yet show definitely that this reductive dechlorination actually gives the bacteria sufficient energy to live on. I think that is our problem in general with all these systems. We do not really know how to select for bacteria that take advantage of exactly that type of reaction. Once we know that, it should be a lot easier.

3

Anaerobic Degradation of Aromatic Hydrocarbons

J. Zeyer
P. Eicher
J. Dolfing
R.P. Schwarzenbach
Swiss Federal Institute for
Water Resources and Water
Pollution Control
EAWAG/ETH
CH-6047 Kastanienbaum
Switzerland

Toluene and *m*-xylene were rapidly mineralized in a denitrifying laboratory aquifer column operated under continuous flow conditions in the complete absence of molecular oxygen. A bacterium, tentatively identified as a *Pseudomonas* sp., was isolated from this column. This organism mineralized toluene and *m*-xylene under pure culture conditions with nitrate or nitrous oxide as the sole electron acceptors. Carbon balance studies using 0.3mM [ring-UL-^{14}C]toluene revealed that more than 50 percent of the radioactivity was evolved as $^{14}CO_2$.

Introduction

Aquifers near infiltration zones of polluted rivers or in the proximity of leachate plumes from landfills often change from aerobic to denitrifying, sulfate-reducing, and eventually methanogenic conditions.[1-3] It is well established that some aromatic compounds such as phenol and benzoate are metabolized under both aerobic and anaerobic conditions.[4-6] It is assumed that the presence of a functional group (that is, hydroxy- or carboxy-substituent) facilitates the anaerobic breakdown of the aromatic ring. However, aromatic hydrocarbons such as benzene, toluene, and xylene have no functional groups. The existence of anaerobic catabolic pathways for aromatic hydrocarbons has been controversial for many years.[5-7] Data from field studies in polluted aquifers have suggested that a slow anaerobic degradation of aromatic hydrocarbons may take place,[1,2] but clear evidence for a microbial metabolism of benzene, toluene, and xylene in the absence of molecular oxygen has been presented only recently. Wilson and co-workers[8] found a slow mineralization of [^{14}C]toluene to $^{14}CO_2$ in anaerobic aquifer material incubated in the laboratory. Grbic-Galic and Vogel[9,10] reported degradation of [^{14}C]benzene and [^{14}C]toluene to $^{14}CO_2$ in a methanogenic microbial culture originally enriched on ferulic acid. Lovley[11] demonstrated that the mineralization of toluene in anaerobic aquatic sediments was coupled to iron reduction.

Experiments with a denitrifying aquifer column in our laboratory revealed that toluene and *m*-xylene are rapidly mineralized under continuous flow conditions in the absence of molecular oxygen. Carbon balance studies using up to 0.3mM ^{14}C-labeled substrates showed that more than 80 percent of the added radioactivity was evolved as $^{14}CO_2$ within eight days.[12-14] The courses of the $^{14}CO_2$ evolution from the column after applying [methyl-^{14}C]toluene and [ring-UL-^{14}C]toluene, respectively, were identical and therefore did not allow any conclusions on the pathway. Toluene and *m*-xylene metabolism in this laboratory aquifer column was coupled to the reduction of nitrate to nitrite. Metabolism was not affected upon the replacement of nitrate by nitrous oxide. However, nitrite was a poor electron acceptor for anaerobic toluene and *m*-xylene mineralization.[12-14]

Experiments were performed to identify intermediates of the anaerobic toluene mineralization in the laboratory aquifer column. The effluent of the toluene degrading column was frequently analyzed by high pressure liquid chromatography and by gas chromatography, but no major metabolites were detectable.[12-14] To force the accumulation of intermediates in the toluene degrading column, an isotope-dilution technique was applied. [A continuous flow of 0.25mM toluene into the column was supplemented with an aliquot of [ring-UL-^{14}C]toluene and an excess (2.6mM) of a suspected intermediate acting as a carrier. The effluent of the column was collected, and the carrier was extracted and tested for the incorporation of ^{14}C from the degradation of [ring-UL-^{14}C]toluene.] This technique led to an accumulation of [ring-UL-^{14}C]benzoate originating from [ring-UL-^{14}C]toluene;[14] however, it remains unclear whether benzoate is an intermediate of the anaerobic toluene metabolism or just a product of a side reaction.

A bacterium was isolated from the toluene and *m*-xylene degrading laboratory aquifer column. It was tentatively identified as a *Pseudomonas* sp. and designated strain T.[15] Cells of strain T were yellow-pigmented, gram-negative, motile rods. Strain T was able to grow on acetate, pyruvate, fructose, and glucose with nitrate or nitrous oxide as the sole electron acceptor. The generation time on pyruvate was in the range of five to seven hours. This microorganism was able to mineralize toluene and *m*-xylene in the complete absence of molecular oxygen when nitrate or nitrous oxide was used as an electron acceptor (see Table 1 legend).[15] A carbon mass balance established after incubating strain T anaerobically with 0.3mM [ringUL-^{14}C]toluene is presented in Table 1. After two weeks, about 50 percent of the radioactivity initially added to the oxygen-free cultures was recovered as $^{14}CO_2$. A large part of the toluene was sorbed to the butyl rubber stoppers and could only be recovered by extraction. The nonvolatile residues in the toluene degrading microbial cultures (referred to as [^{14}C]metabolites in Table 1) were partially extractable with ethyl acetate at pH 2, but an analysis by high pressure liquid chromatography or gas chromatography revealed no major metabolite. The overall recovery of ^{14}C in all cultures was greater than 80 percent.

To study the degradation of toluene in the absence of molecular oxygen, media were routinely made oxygen-free by heating and subsequent cooling under a nitrogen atmosphere. In addition, some experiments were performed in media that were not only oxygen-free but also chemically reduced with FeS (see Table 1 legend).[15] Strain T was able to mineralize toluene under these conditions (see Table 1), which suggests that not even traces of molecular oxygen were involved in the anaerobic degradation of toluene. This conclusion was confirmed by experiments with cell suspensions. Cells of strain T were anaerobically (under a N_2O atmosphere) precultured in the pres-

Table 1.
Degradation of [Ring-UL-^{14}C]Toluene by strain T*

^{14}C Balance After an Incubation Time of Two Weeks (%)

Medium and electron acceptor	[^{14}C]toluene recovered in culture	^{14}CO$_2$ evolved	[^{14}C]metabolites recovered in culture	[^{14}C]toluene sorbed to stopper
Oxygen-free (nitrate)	<1	51	17	22
Oxygen-free (nitrous oxide)	<1	57	23	14
Reduced with FeS (nitrate)	<1	47	24	9

*Experimental procedures are summarized as follows: Cultures (30ml) were incubated in 50ml serum flasks sealed with butyl rubber stoppers. The oxygen-free medium consisted of basal medium (pH 7.5)[13] supplemented with 0.3mM [ring-UL-^{14}C]toluene as the sole source of carbon and energy. The sole electron acceptor provided was either 10mM nitrate (with N$_2$ in the headspace) or 26mM nitrous oxide (corresponding to a saturated aqueous solution). Some media were supplemented with FeS (22mg/l) to bind traces of oxygen residues. Resazurin (which was added as a redox indicator) was decolorized within hours in these media. The cultures were acidified to pH 2 at the end of the incubation and purged with air. [^{14}C]Toluene and ^{14}CO$_2$ were trapped in isobutanol and 0.1 N NaOH respectively. After purging, the nonvolatile [^{14}C]metabolites in the culture were quantified. In addition, the butyl rubber stoppers were extracted with ethyl acetate to recover the sorbed [^{14}C]toluene. The amount of radioactivity in all samples was determined in a liquid scintillation counter. Experimental procedures are also described in detail elsewhere.[17] All numbers represent mean values of at least 2 independent determinations.

ence of toluene, harvested, suspended in phosphate buffer, and incubated with toluene either aerobically or anaerobically (under a N$_2$O atmosphere). Toluene was not degraded in the aerobic cell suspension but rapidly mineralized in the anaerobic suspension.

A number of hypothetical intermediates of the anaerobic toluene degradation have been postulated by various authors; a scheme of some of the proposed pathways is presented in Figure 1. A degradation through *p*-cresol was suggested by Vogel and Grbic-Galic[10] because they detected traces of [hydroxy-^{18}O]*p*-cresol in a methano-

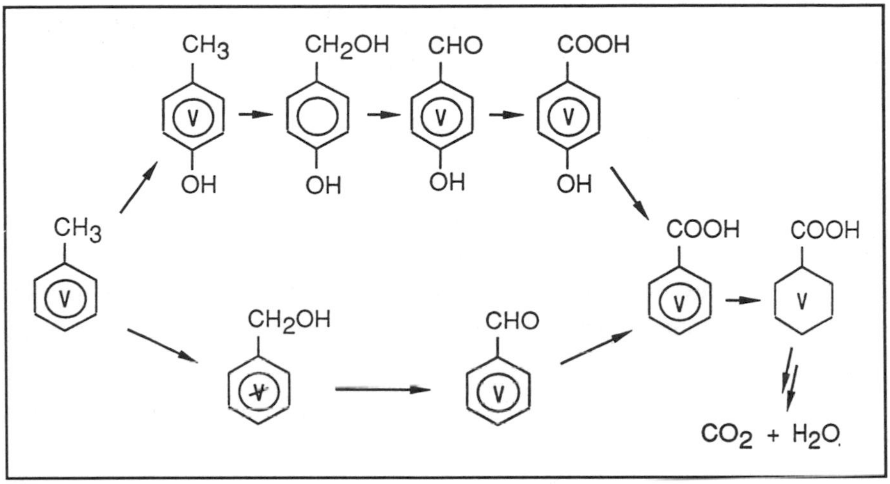

Figure 1. Proposed pathways of the anaerobic degradation of toluene. (V), intermediate degradable by strain T. (Ⅴ̷), intermediate not degradable by strain T. Degradability of p-hydroxybenzylalcohol was not tested.

genic culture incubated with toluene and ^{18}O-labeled water. Furthermore, the anaerobic conversion of p-cresol to p-hydroxybenzoate, the turnover of p-hydroxybenzoate to benzoate, and the anaerobic mineralization of benzoate through cyclohexanecarboxylic acid (see Figure 1) is well documented in the literature.[5,6,16] The alternative pathway of toluene degradation through benzyl alcohol, benzaldehyde, and benzoate (see Figure 1) is very common under aerobic conditions;[7] however, speculations on the occurrence of such a catabolic sequence under anaerobic conditions have never been confirmed experimentally.[9,14] The anaerobic degradation of benzoate and phenol is often initiated by a direct reduction of the aromatic ring,[5,6] but a microbial transformation of toluene to methylcyclohexane was never observed. Moreover, methylcyclohexane was not degraded in the laboratory aquifer column, whereas benzoate was rapidly mineralized.[14]

We investigated the ability of strain T to use some of the postulated intermediates (see Figure 1) as carbon sources in the presence of nitrate as the only electron acceptor (the degradation studies were performed in oxygen-free basal medium supplemented with 1.0mM carbon source [only 0.5mM for benzaldehyde due to the severe growth inhibitory effect on strain T] and with 10mM nitrate as the sole electron acceptor).[15] Rapid growth was detectable with p-cresol, p-hydroxybenzaldehyde, p-hydroxybenzoate, benzoate, cyclohexanecarboxylic acid, and benzaldehyde, whereas benzylalcohol did not serve as a growth substrate. These data, however, have to be interpreted with great care because growth studies may be impeded both by uptake and induction effects. Furthermore, substrates may be degradable even though they are not intermediates of the catabolic sequence of interest. Based on these results, a particular route for the anaerobic toluene degradation by strain T cannot yet be suggested. In particular, the mechanism of the initial catabolic step through which the molecule is activated remains obscure. Presently, we are focusing our efforts on the elucidation of this pathway.

Acknowledgments

This research was supported by grants from the European Communities (Project COST 641) and Ciba-Geigy AG.

References

1. R.P. Schwarzenbach *et. al.*, *Environ. Sci. Technol.* **17**, 472 (1983).
2. M. Reinhard, N.L. Goodman, and J.F. Barker, *Environ. Sci. Technol.* **18**, 953 (1984).
3. G.G. Ehrlich *et al.*, *Dev. Ind. Microbiol.* **24**, 235 (1983).
4. M. Tiedje, S.A. Boyd, and B.Z. Fathepure, *Dev. Ind. Microbiol.* **27**, 117 (1987).
5. W.C. Evans and G. Fuchs, *Ann. Rev. Microbiol.* **42**, 289 (1988).
6. L.Y. Young, in *Microbial Degradation of Organic Compounds*, D.T. Gibson, Ed. (Marcel Dekker, New York, 1984), pp. 487-523.
7. D.T. Gibson and V. Subramanian, in *Microbial Degradation of Organic Compounds*, D.T. Gibson, Ed. (Marcel Dekker, New York, 1984), pp. 181-252.
8. B.H. Wilson, G.B. Smith, and J.F. Rees, *Environ. Sci. Technol.* **20**, 997 (1986).
9. D. Grbic-Galic and T.M. Vogel, *Appl. Environ. Microbiol.* **53**, 254 (1987).
10. T.M. Vogel and D. Grbic-Galic, *Appl. Environ. Microbiol.* **52**, 200 (1986).
11. D.R. Lovley *et al.*, *Nature* (London) **339**, 297 (1989).
12. E.P. Kuhn *et al.*, *Environ. Sci. Technol.* **19**, 961 (1985).
13. J. Zeyer, E.P. Kuhn, and R.P. Schwarzenbach, *Appl. Environ. Microbiol.* **52**, 944 (1986).
14. E.P. Kuhn *et al.*, *Appl. Environ. Microbiol.* **54**, 490 (1988).

15. J. Dolfing *et al.*, manuscript in final preparation.
16. I.D. Bossert and L.Y. Young, *Appl. Environ. Microbiol.* **52**, 1117 (1986).

Discussion

Buswell: Do you know whether the cell is permeable to benzyl alcohol, or is impermeability the reason why strain T does not grow on this compound?

Zeyer: Yes, you are right, it might be an uptake problem, and we did not check uptake. That is why these degradation studies do not give us solid evidence on the pathway. What we checked is toxicity because some of the metabolites are rather toxic to strain T. We grew strain T on pyruvate and, at a given moment, we added one of the suspected intermediates; we determined the inhibition of growth in the presence of this intermediate.

Chakrabarty: Does this strain have any aerobic pathway genes for toluene degradation?

Zeyer: I do not know anything about the genes involved in the aerobic pathway, but the strain is able to degrade toluene under aerobic conditions. If you grow the strain in the presence of nitrous oxide, you have some 60 percent $^{14}CO_2$ evolution from ^{14}C-labeled toluene. If you grow the strain in the presence of molecular oxygen, you have some 35 percent $^{14}CO_2$ evolution. There is obviously an aerobic and an anaerobic pathway, but the enzymatic system induced under anaerobic conditions is not able to handle toluene in the presence of oxygen, and vice versa.

Chakrabarty: I was wondering whether there is any hybridization of the DNA from this strain with any of the known toluene genes? What I am aiming at is if you have some of these genes from the aerobic pathway when you grow the cells in the presence of toluene under aerobic conditions. Isolate the RNA and hybridize them with the toluene gene probes, then you could figure out if the aerobic toluene degradation genes are in fact expressed during toluene degradation under anaerobic conditions.

Zeyer: Yes, I agree, but we have not yet done such experiments.

Kukor: Do you know which of the aerobic toluene pathways your strain uses when it grows on toluene in the presence of oxygen?

Zeyer: No, we do not know, but it is kind of suspicious that the culture turns yellowish under those conditions. I would not exclude the possibility that we have one of the pathways going through aldehyde. We have not yet done any enzymatic studies and we do not have any solid evidence for a certain pathway.

Ribbons: Could you tell me the yields of labeled carbon dioxide that you would get with respect to the methyl-labeled toluene and ring-labeled toluene?

Zeyer: Yes, in presence of nitrous oxide, we got some 65 percent $^{14}CO_2$ from methyl-labeled toluene and approximately 60 percent $^{14}CO_2$ from ring-labeled toluene.

Ribbons: Could you then tell me if the ring-labeled toluene is uniformly labeled or specifically labeled?

Zeyer: It is uniformly labeled. We are not surprised that we have more CO_2 evolution from methyl-labeled toluene because the methyl group could be oxidized to a carboxy group and then be decarboxylated at an early step.

Molecular Genetics and Physiology of Aerobic Microorganisms with Biodegradative Potential

4

Recruitment of *tft* and *clc* Biodegradative Pathway Genes: Modes of Evolution

correspondence
Wayne M. Coco
Uday M.X. Sangodkar
Randi K. Rothmel
Ananda M. Chakrabarty
Department of Microbiology and Immunology
The University of Illinois
College of Medicine
Chicago, IL 60680

Pseudomonas putida can utilize a simple chlorinated compound 3-chloro-catechol (3-*clc*) through elaboration of a plasmid pAC27 encoded pathway. The *clc* genes are clustered as an operon termed *clcABD*. The positive regulatory gene *clcR* maps close to but is transcribed divergently from the *clcABD* operon. A similar genetic organization for catechol (Cat) degradation has been shown, where the *catB* gene of the *catBC* operon and its divergently transcribed *catR* regulatory gene show appreciable homology to *clcB* and *clcR*. This suggests that *clc* genes evolved by diverging from an extant, regulated catechol pathway.

In contrast, a strain of *P. cepacia* (AC1100) was isolated from a chemostat under strong selection in the presence of 2, 4, 5-trichlorophenoxyacetic acid (2, 4, 5-T). This strain is characterized by: (1) marked genetic instability specific to the *tft* genes of the 2, 4, 5-T pathway, (2) several copies of the insertion sequence, RS1100, and (3) lack of detectable hybridization of either RS1100 or of the *chq* locus in the *tft* pathway with DNA from several species of pseudomonads. Apparently, bacteria under such conditions may require a mode of evolution distinct from that observed in the evolution of the *clc* pathway.

Introduction

Synthetic chemicals play an ever-increasing role in the highly industrialized world in which we live. Their post–World War II production has been estimated to have doubled every 10 years in the United States alone, and there is growing concern about their environmental and health impact.[1]

Because chlorinated aromatic chemicals are often the most environmentally and biologically stable of such compounds and are among the most toxic substances known, there is great interest in elucidating the pathways for their biodegradation and the mechanisms of evolution of such pathways. In the past several decades, a variety of hypotheses have been put forth to explain aspects of the molecular evolution of metabolic pathways. Early reviews on the subject included those by Hegeman and Rosenberg[2] and Clarke and Slater.[3] Notable elements of several of such hypotheses include Horowitz's retroevolution hypothesis;[4] gene duplication and divergence; and the intergenetic, plasmid-assisted recruitment of genes.[5,6] More recently, constraints have been described that explain the events leading to the rapid evolution of duplicate genes in a given bacterium, and specific molecular events have been proposed to begin explaining the repertoire of mechanisms available for divergence above and beyond the selection of random point mutations.[7,8] However, the effect of the availability of parent genes in the rhizosphere or how the strength of selective pressure might effect the likelihood of the evolution of a given biodegradative pathway by differing modes of evolution has been difficult to evaluate. For the purposes of this paper, a mode of evolution is defined as a characteristic sequence of genetic events coupled with selective pressure resulting, of course, in the establishment of a viable metabolic pathway in a population. Preliminary evidence for the evolution of the 2, 4, 5-T (*tft*) degradative pathway of *Pseudomonas cepacia* AC1100 and the 3-chlorocatechol (*clc*) pathway of *P. putida* by two distinct modes of evolution is presented in this chapter.

The Evolution of the *CLC* Pathway From the *CAT* Pathway

Benzoate degradation and the cat *genes.* Benzoate is produced in large quantities in nature by several mechanisms including as an intermediate and/or breakdown product of some plant terpenes (for example, benzoin gum). It is thus thought to have been available in the environment on the evolutionary time scale corresponding to the emergence of such benzoate-producing systems. Not surprisingly, biochemical pathways for the degradation of benzoate have evolved and are widespread among free-living soil bacteria.[9] The most widely observed pathway for the degradation of benzoate is through catechol to ß-ketoadipate, which is directly convertible into the two Krebs cycle substrates succinate and acetyl-coenzyme A.[9] Indeed, the enzymes involved in this catabolic pathway have been studied for more than 40 years.[10] Benzoate is first converted through chromosomally encoded dioxygenase and then dehydrogenase activities to catechol. Catechol, in turn, is subject to four further enzymatic conversions to yield ß-ketoadipate (Figure 1). The four enzymes have been identified and named dioxygenase I, muconate lactonizing enzyme I, muconolactone isomerase, and hydrolase I. The structural genes responsible for these enzymes have been cloned from the chromosomes of various bacterial genera[11,12] and have been assigned the designations *catA*, *catB*, *catC*, and *catD*, respectively (see Figure 1). In *P. putida*, *catB* and *catC* occur as a *catBC* operon, which is inducible in the presence of benzoate and is under the positive control of a regulatory gene, *catR* (Figure 2).[13]

Biodegradation of a chlorinated benzoate in Pseudomonas putida. The ß-ketoadipate pathway is used extensively by microorganisms for the degradation of a variety of aromatic compounds.[14] In a series of steps quite analogous to those in the benzoate pathway, the substituted benzoate, 3-chlorobenzoate (3Cba), is degraded by reactions that result in the readily utilizable ß-ketoadipate (Figure 1).[15] In order to degrade this compound, the same dioxygenase and dehydrogenase that act on benzoate are thought to convert 3Cba to 3-chlorocatechol (Clc).[16] The conversions of Clc to maleylacetate is deter-

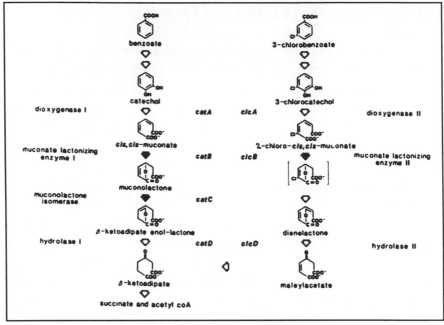

Figure 1. The catechol and 3-chlorocatechol degradative pathways.

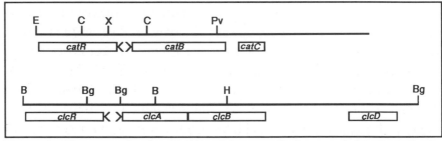

Figure 2. The operonic organization of the *cat* and *clc* structural and regulatory genes.

mined by the genes *clcA*, *clcB*, and *clcD*, which encode the enzymes dioxygenase II, muconate lactonizing enzyme II, and hydrolase II, respectively. Finally, maleylacetate is readily converted to ß-ketoadipate by a putatively chromosomally encoded function. Note that when muconolactone is 2-chloronated, its dehydrogenation to dienelactone and the concomitant loss of the chlorine from the lactone ring (Figure 1) are spontaneous and rapid under physiological conditions.[15] As might be expected, no enzyme as been found to catalyze this step. In *P. putida,* the three *clc* genes exist as a plasmid-borne *clcABD* operon under the positive control of the regulatory gene *clcR* (see Figure 2).[17,18]

The apparent functional homologies between *catA, catB,* and *catD* and the corresponding *clcA, clcB,* and *clcD* gene products are obvious (Figure 1). Indeed, significant stretches of amino acid residue sequence identity do exist between CatA and ClcA as well as between CatB and ClcB, but only sparingly between CatD and ClcD.[19-21] The lack of similarity between CatD and ClcD is not surprising because their respective substrates, an enol-lactone and a diene-lactone, are quite different. Further support for the evolution of the *clc* genes from *cat* gene ancestors is found in the relative catalytic efficiencies and substrate ranges of the respective proteins. For example, if the enzymatic activity of CatB to its canonical substrate, *cis, cis*-muconate, is assigned a value of 100 percent, its activity toward the ClcB substrate, 2-chloro-*cis, cis*-muconate, is only seven percent. On the other hand, the activity of ClcB toward CatB's substrate is 50 percent relative to its activity toward its own substrate.[21] Similar arguments have been made for the evolution of *clcA* from *catA* as well as for both *clcA* and *clcB* based on subunit size and, as mentioned previously, sequence homologies.[19,21] In addition, the levels of Cat and Clc proteins in fully induced cell is three percent and 30 percent of total cellular protein, respectively. This has been suggested as further support for the evolution of the *clc* pathway from the *cat* patyway because the loss of catalytic efficiency accompanying a recent increase in substrate range of the respective enzymes would be expected to have been compensated for by an increase in protein production.[19] Based on such considerations, a strong case can be made for the relatively recent divergent evolution of *clcA* and *clcB* from their respective catechol-degrading ancestor genes in the *cat* pathway.[19]

The LysR family of transcriptional activator proteins and the apparent relationship between catR-catBC and clcR-clcABD. In 1987, Plamann and Stauffer[22] published the nucleotide sequence of *metR,* a 276 amino acid long regulatory protein that is divergently transcribed from and is closely linked to *metE*, a structural gene in the methionine biosynthetic pathway. Shortly thereafter, Henikoff used the computer-translated MetR sequence as a query in a search of several DNA data banks. The approximately 50 million nucleotides in these data banks were computer-translated in all six frames on both strands. The 16 polypeptides deemed homologous by their search parameters were then themselves used as queries, and an additional two sequences were fished out for a total of 18.[23] Four of these 18 proteins were clearly spurious and another five were NodD activator proteins from various rhizobia and were considered as one member for the purpose of analysis. The characteristics of the remaining set, when taken as a whole, yielded clear patterns of a related protein family. Of the ten different members, six, AmpR, LysR, IlvY, CysB, NodD, and MetR, are known bacterial transcriptional activators whereas the other four, LeuO (one each from *Salmonella* and *Escherichia coli*), TfdO, and AntO, are closely linked to the structural genes from which they earn their name designations but have as yet undetermined functions. Four of these six confirmed regulators are known to be autoregulated.[23] All of the members contain a confirmed or highly suspected helix-turn--helix DNA-binding motif starting an average of 20 amino acids in from the N-terminus. Except for the 251 residue CatM,[24] each of the members, for which there is a completely determined sequence, is close to 300 amino acids in length. The highest homologies within the family are concentrated toward the N-terminal end of each protein, with scattered but conserved homologies throughout the rest of the primary sequences. This conservation of small stretches of homology was taken to be an indication of similar protein folding within the family.[23] The decrease in C-terminal homology was postulated to be due to the need for recognition of widely varying inducers in the disparate pathways represented. Inducers range from small molecules such as diaminopimelic acid and O-acetylserine for LysR and CysB to large compounds like ß-lactamase and vitamin B_{12} for AmpR and MetR, respectively.[23] One quite provocative observation is that all but one of these are divergently transcribed from the gene or operon they control (CysB being the exception). However, the spacing between transcriptional starts varies from 25-base pair (bp) in the case of *metR-metE* to the 266-bp reported for *nodD-nodA*,[25] and there are no obvious recurring DNA motifs that might indicate a consensus for a LysR-family DNA binding site.[23] Since the publication of this search in September 1988, at least 13 additional known or suspected LysR family regulatory proteins have been determined by further computer searches using new search parameters and/or more recent sequence data banks. Many of the genes found also function in biodegradative pathways and/or are transcribed divergently from and are closely linked to at least one gene they regulate (S. Henikoff, personal communication, 1989; I.P. Crawford, personal communication, 1989).

In 1987, the complete nucleotide sequence of the *clcABD* operon was determined and published along with approximately 400-bp of the upstream region.[17] A computer search of this upstream region revealed the N-terminus of a truncated open reading frame with consensus homology to the LysR regulator family (S. Henikoff, personal communication). Further, we have shown[18,26] that *clcR* maps immediately upstream of the *clcABD* operon. Interestingly, the recently sequenced *catR* also encodes a LysR family member that is divergently transcribed from and is closely linked to the *catBC* operon.[18] Ongoing research in our laboratory continues to indicate that *clcR* is the LysR-type activator, which is transcribed divergently from the *clcABD* operon. The above characteristics of *clcR-clcABD* and *catR-catBC* suggest that the former pathway for a chlorinated substrate and its regulatory gene appear to have evolved directly from the latter.

The Molecular Genetics of AC1100

The involvement of foreign genes in the 2,4,5-T pathway. P. *cepacia* is widely cited as among the most catabolically diverse of known bacteria.[27-29] In 1982, a pure culture of *P. cepacia* designated AC1100 was isolated from a chemostat after selection with 2, 4, 5-T as the major growth substrate. Strain AC1100 is unique in its ability to utilize 2, 4, 5-T as its sole source of carbon and energy.[30] In an effort to characterize this newly evolved *tft* pathway, Tn5 mutagenesis was performed, and a 2, 4, 5-T⁻ mutant, PT88, was isolated.[31,32] PT88 was shown to be defective in the further catabolism of the intermediate, 5-chloro-2-hydroxyhydroquinone (CHQ).[32] This mutant was complemented by the pCP13-cosmid library clone of AC1100 genomic DNA, pUS1, which contains a 25-kb insert. The genes necessary to complement PT88 were subcloned from pUSI to a 4.3-kb fragment and required a 290-bp fragment located 1.3-kb upstream for efficient expression. This locus was shown to encode the enzymatic activity needed for the conversion of CHQ and was designated the *chq* locus.[33] Our current understanding of the AC1100 2, 4, 5-T pathway thus involves the conversion of 2, 4, 5-T to 2, 4, 5-trichlorophenol and its further oxidative dechlorination to CHQ, which is ultimately metabolized to CO_2. This oxidative dechlorination is analogous to the mechanism of degradation of pentachlorophenol observed in *Rhodococcus chlorophenolicus*[34] as well as in a *Flavobacterium* sp.[35] It should be noted, however, that the cloned *chq* locus does not hybridize with the DNA from either strain. In fact, when the *chq* locus is used as a probe, no hybridization is found when many scores of known bacteria, nor microbes isolated from soil on *Pseudomonas* Isolation Agar or Luria agar are screened (J. Johnson, personal communication, 1989). Thus, it appears that the ancestor gene(s) of the *chq* locus may have diverged widely or may have been recruited from one or more taxonomically distant sources. A published example[33] of the lack of hybridization of *chq* to nine different strains of pseudomonads, including three strains of *P. cepacia* is shown in Figure 3.

AC1100 contains a foreign repeated sequence. On analysis of the DNA flanking the Tn5 insertion in PT88, the mutant just described, a genetic element was located and shown to be present at high copy number in the AC1100 genome. The nucleotide sequence of this element, designated RS1100, was found to share characteristics of insertion sequence elements (IS elements). RS1100 is 1477-bp long, with 38-39-bp inverted repeats flanked by 8-bp direct repeats and contains a single large open reading frame that has structural similarity to the Mu and other transposases.[36] IS elements have long been

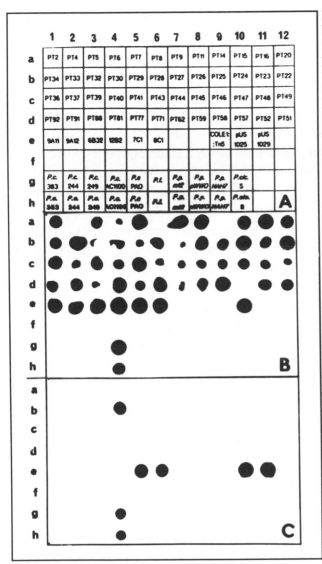

Figure 3: Colony hybridization analysis using ^{32}P-labeled DNA probes of RS1100 and the *chq* locus (as described in reference 33). Panel A: cultures used for hybridization. Rows a to d contain Tn5 mutants of AC1100. Strains 1 to 6 in row e contain spontaneous 2, 4, 5-T⁻ mutants of AC1100. Colony "COLE1::Tn5" (row e, number 9) is a vector containing no AC1100 DNA. Plasmids pUS1025 and pUS1029 (row e, numbers 10 and 11) are *E. coli* AC80 grown vectors containing RS1100 and *chq* regions, respectively. Rows g and h are, respectively, *LB* and glucose minimal media grown colonies of various *pseudomonas* species and, where known, the contained plasmids. *P.A.; P.aeruginosa; P.C., P. cepacia; P. cic., P. cichorii (ATCC43388); P. f., P. fluorescens; P. p., P. putida.* Panel B: Hybridizations of the strains in panel A with RS1100 as the probe. Panel C: hybridizations of the strains in panel A with the *chq* locus as the probe.

implicated in mediating evolutionary processes (for an early review, see reference 8). They are known sites for homologous and illegitimate recombinations; they mediate genetic rearrangements, plasmid-

plasmid and plasmid-chromosome fusions, gene mutations, deletions, transfers, and can possess promoter elements that can activate surrounding genes.[36-40]

RS1100 has been recently shown to transpose from the AC1100 genome onto the plasmid, pKT240 and is able to activate the promoter-less *aphC* gene of the vector, thereby conferring streptomycin resistance in both *P. cepacia* and *E. coli*. In addition, RS1100 has also been shown to mediate the transfer of a fragment of AC1100 chromosomal DNA onto pKT240.[41] Gaffney and Lessie[37] described a *P. cepacia* strain 249 in which 12 IS elements were found, at least some of which were characterized as transposing at high frequency. These transpositions caused a number of chromosomal and plasmid rearrangements and several auxotrophic mutants. High frequencies of transposition are by no means limited to *P. cepacia* and are reported, for example, at frequencies of 10^{-1} to 10^2 for IS*R1* in *Rhizobium lupini*.[42] It is perhaps, then, not unexpected to find that the 2, 4, 5-T$^+$ phenotype is lost from 50 percent of a population of AC1100 in less than 20 generations on nonselective media.[30] Nor is it unexpected to observe varying patterns of RS1100 locations on loss of the 2, 4, 5-T degradative function or even on independent culturing of the AC1100 wild-type strain.[41]

There are, however, some quite provocative differences between what is thought to be the normal incidence and organization of IS elements in bacteria and that found in AC1100. AC1100 chromosomal DNA can be cleaved with restriction endonucleases that recognize few sites on the AC1100 genome (for example, *Dra*I, *Sep*I, and *Xba*I). When the digested genome is analyzed by pulsed-field electrophoresis, the resulting bands are summed to determine a size for the AC1100 chromosome of 4×10^6-bp, which is comparable to that of *E. coli*. When these bands are probed with RS1100, bands summing to only 1.3×10^6-bp show hybridization to this IS element.[43] Although it has not been determined whether the RS1100-free segments are contiguous, it appears two thirds of the AC1100 chromosome is devoid of RS1100 elements. Comparing the number of bands hybridizing (10 of 24 for *Sep*I digests and 9 of 27 for *Xba*I) with the estimated number of RS1100 elements (30 to 100s) makes this by no means a statistically expected configuration. Reasons for this apparent localization of RS1100 might include a target-site specificity requirement that the majority of the *P. cepacia* chromosome does not fulfill. Further supporting the idea of RS1100 localization is the extremely low rate (less than 10^{-6}) of spontaneous auxotrophic mutations in AC1100, even when large, presumably RS1100 mediated chromosomal deletions are observed (unpublished results). A similar localization of repeated sequences has been reported in *Rhizobium japonicum* or *Bradyrhizobium* in which RSRjα and RSRjß (1) are clustered mainly around the *nif* and *nod* genes and/or not among essential genes, (2) possess characteristics of IS elements, and (3) are not observed to result in the production of auxotrophic mutants. A notable difference, however, is that transposition has yet to be observed for RSRjα and RSRjß, and the documented deletion of the *nif* and *nod* genes is thought to occur by a single cross-over mechanism and only on heat treatment.[40]

In order to determine the ancestral origin of RS1100, the DNA from several known strains of pseudomonads was screened for hybridization using RS1100 as a probe (see, for example, Figure 3). These efforts were expanded to include several degradative plasmids[36] and well over 5000 soil isolates (reference 30 and J. Johnson, personal communication, 1989). In each case, the hybridizations yielded negative results.

Modes of Evolution

The evidence just presented and elsewhere[18,19,21] indicates that *clcA*, *clcB*, and, perhaps, *clcR* evolved from *catA*, *catB*, and *catR*, respectively. Although the evidence for *clcD* arising from *catD* is less conclusive, their similarity of subunit size and reaction mechanisms, coupled with their active site sequence identities, allows at least the plausibility of this contingency. Regardless, the relative youth of the *clc* pathway (see previous discussion) together with both the observation of the regulation of the *clcABD* operon, and the similarity of G + C content among *clc* genes, suggests that *clcD* was readily available in the genetic milieu in which it evolved. Thus, the development of the *clc* pathway from an extant *cat* pathway can easily be envisaged to have occurred by mechanisms such as gene duplication concomitant with, or followed by relocation onto a plasmid by legitimate or illegitimate recombination or IS element–mediated events and the fine tuning mechanisms of divergence cited earlier. Many of the genes in the analogous protocatechuate (Pca) biodegradative pathway have been shown to have similar relatedness with the *cat* pathway genes[12] and appear also to have evolved from an extant ancestor of the *cat* pathway. Another example of this mode involves the similarly analogous 2,4-dichlorophenoxyacetic acid biodegradative pathway (*tfd*) genes. The *tfdC* gene, as well as the LysR family regulatory protein-encoding *tfdO*, show higher identity to their respective *clc* gene counterparts than to the respective *cat* genes.[23,43,45] Evidence for the interpathway borrowing of enzymes includes early work by Wu, and coworkers.[46] Their observations in *Aerobacter aerogenes* 1033 demonstrated that growth on xylitol was made possible by the constitutive expression of the gene encoding the host ribitol dehydrogenase. Further mutation of this gene increased the activity of the dehydrogenase specifically toward xylitol. An additional mutation resulting in constitutive expression of a putative D-arabitol transport system allowed still further reduction of doubling time on xylitol. Central to the concept of this mode of evolution, however, is that the ancestor genes necessary were readily available and that the *cat* pathway, perhaps including its regulation, required only divergence to meet the needs of a new substrate. Finally, although the borrowing of a readily available gene for a catabolic function may define a mechanism of recruitment, the acquisition of a majority of the enzymes for a novel pathway by divergence from readily available sources defines one mode of evolution. One of the expected hallmarks of such an evolutionary mode is the traceability of ancestor genes to, for example, few or closely related donors, if not to within the same species.

In contrast to that just described, the biodegradative pathway in AC1100 appears to have evolved after the IS element–assisted recruitment of otherwise unavailable genes from a foreign host. Support for this idea includes (1) the lack of hybridization of the *chq* locus with many pseudomonads, degradative plasmids, likely gene donors, and soil isolates, (2) the ability of RS1100 to carry intervening chromosomal DNA during transposition,[41] (3) the fact that both the *chq* locus and RS1100 remain untraceable despite exhaustive efforts to find a hybridizing laboratory strain or soil isolate, (4) the localization of RS1100 to a limited area of the chromosome indicating, perhaps, the site specificity for RS1100 for a quite foreign genome, (5) the mapping of the *chq* locus to such a RS1100-populated region, and (6) the occurrence of RS1100 on plasmids of AC1100 but not on the plasmids of other tested pseudomonads, further suggesting the newness of this IS element to this genus. These genes may have been recruited from distantly related soil communities such as from anaerobes or even fungi (see, for example, reference 8) and/or from a variety of different genera. Proof of these assertions must, of course, await positive identification of the original donor genes and their host(s).

The similarities of the respective substrates and reaction mechanisms in Tfd, Pca, and Clc biodegradation to those used in the degradation of catechol suggest the rationality of the recruitment of the *cat* genes in the evolution of the former functions. The same rationale would offer the 2, 4-dichlorophenoxyacetic acid biodegradation pathway (*tfd*) genes as reasonable progenitors for the *tft* pathway genes. Further, these ubiquitous genes are known to be available as plasmids in soil microorganisms[47] and were therefore present in the chemostat in which AC1100 evolved. It is thus noteworthy that no hybridization is found between the *chq* locus and the *tfd* genes. It can be inferred that the probability of the events necessary to evolve *tft* genes by this route was so low as to render this contingency untenable. This lack of ready availability of the suitable *tft* ancestral genes is key to the concept of a distinct mode of evolution. That is, when the probability of events necessary to assemble or evolve the needed genes are sufficiently rare, the previously described "extension" or "relaxed" mode of evolution with plasmid transfer and conventional recombinational events is inefficient. As described, IS elements provide several additional types of interactions, often at high frequency, through which the chance of recruitment and/or expression of foreign genes is enhanced. The indicated scarcity of progenitor genes for the development of this pathway in *P. cepacia* appears to have necessitated such an IS element–assisted recruitment mechanism.

Central to the evolution of any pathway is selective pressure. The rarer the events necessary to recruit, express, and fine-tune the genes for a given pathway, the longer or more intense such pressure might have to be. Consistent with the terminology discussed here, the acquisition of a foreign gene mediated by an IS element cannot be considered a mode of evolution. However, the evolution of a pathway, which necessitates the IS element–assisted assemblage of DNA from distant or diverse sources, or the IS element-assisted recruitment of genes separated by large distances on a foreign chromosome, accompanied by the strong selection needed to favor and establish in a population such rare events does represent a distinct mode of evolution. We believe the preliminary evidence just described for the events involved in the evolution of the *tft* pathway implicate a mode of evolution distinct from that implicated for the *clc* pathway.

Acknowledgments

This work was supported by Public Health Service Grant ES 04050 from the National Institute of Environmental Health Sciences, Grant (DMB) 87-21743) from the National Science Foundation, and in part by the cooperative agreement CR-812911-02 from the U. S. Environmental Protection Agency.

References

1. A.M. Chakrabarty, in *Biodegradation and Detoxification of Environmental Pollutants*, A.M. Chakrabarty, Ed. (CRC. Press, Boca Raton, Florida, 1982), pp. 127-139.
2. G. D. Hegman and S.L. Rosenberg, *Ann. Rev. Microbiol.* **24**, 429 (1970).
3. P.H. Clarke and J.H. Slater, in *The Bacteria Volume X: The Biology of Pseudomonas*, J.R. Sokatch and L.N. Ornston, Eds. (Academic Press, Inc., Orlando, Florida, 1986), pp. 71-144.

4. N.H. Horowitz, *Proc. Natl. Acad. Sci. USA* **31**, 153 (1945).
5. S.T. Kellogg, D.K. Chatterjee, and A.M. Chakrabarty, *Science* **214**, 1133 (1981).
6. J.S. Karns et al., in *Genetic Control of Environmental Pollutants*, G.S. Omenn and A. Hollaender, Eds. (Plenum Press, New York, 1984), pp. 3-22.
7. L.N. Ornston and W.K. Yeh, *Proc. Natl. Acad. Sci. USA* **76**, 3996 (1979).
8. S.N. Cohen, *Nature* **263**, 731 (1976).
9. L.N. Ornston, *J. Biol. Chem.* **241**, 3795 (1966).
10. R.Y. Stanier et al., *J. Bacteriol.* **59**, 129 (1950).
11. M.S. Shanley et al., *J. Bacteriol.* **165**, 557 (1986).
12. L.N. Ornston and W.K. Yen, in *Biodegradation and Detoxification of Environmental Pollutants*, A.M. Chakrabarty, Ed. (CRC. Press, Boca Raton, Florida, 1982), pp. 105-126.
13. M.L. Wheelis and L.N. Ornston, *J. Bacteriol.* **109**, 790 (1972).
14. R.Y. Stanier and L.N. Ornston, *Adv. Microbiol. Physiol.* **9**, 88 (1973).
15. W. Hartmann, W. Reineke, and H.-J. Knackmuss, *Appl. Environ. Microbiol.* **37**, 421 (1979).
16. E. Dorn and H.-J. Knackmuss, *Biochem. J.* **174**, 73 (1978).
17. B. Frantz and A.M. Chakrabarty, *Proc. Natl. Acad. Sci. USA* **84**, 4460 (1987).
18. R.K. Rothmel et al., in *Annual Meeting of the American Society for Microbiology*. (New Orleans, 1989), Abstract K-60, p. 91.
19. E.L. Neidle et al., *J. Bacteriol.* **170**, 4874 (1988).
20. B. Frantz et al., *J. Bacteriol.* **169**, 704 (1987).
21. B. Franz, T. Aldrich, and A.M. Chakrabarty, *Biotech. Adv.* **5**, 85 (1987).
22. L.S. Plamann and G.V. Stauffer, *J. Bacteriol.* **169**, 3932 (1987).
23. S. Henikoff et al., *Proc. Natl. Acad. Sci. USA* **85**, 6602 (1988).
24. E. Neidle, C. Hartnett, and L.N. Ornston, in *89th Annual Meeting of the American Society for Microbiology*. New Orleans, 1989), Abstract H-102.
25. T.T. Egelhoff et al., *DNA* **4**, 241 (1985).
26. D. Ghosal et al., *Proc. Natl. Acad. Sci. USA* **82**, 1638 (1985).
27. R.W. Ballard et al., *J. Gen. Microbiol.* **60**, 199 (1970).
28. T.G. Lessie and T. Gaffney, in *The Bacteria, The Biology of Pseudomonas ,Vol. 10*, J.R. Sokatch and L.N. Ornston, Eds. (Academic Press, Orlando, Florida, 1986), pp. 439-481.
29. R.Y. Stanier, N.J. Palleroni, and M. Doudoroff, *J. Gen. Microbiol.* **43**, 159 (1966).
30. J.J. Kilbane et al., *Appl. Environ. Microbiol.* **44**, 72 (1982).
31. P. Tomasek et al., in *Biotechnology for Solving Agricultural Problems*, P.C. Augustina, H.D. Danforth, and M.R. Bekst, Eds. (Martinus Nijhoff , Dordrecht, Netherlands, 1986), pp. 355-368.
32. P.J. Chapman, U.M.X. Sangodkar, and A.M. Chakrabarty, in *Annual Meeting of the Society of Environmental Toxicology and Chemistry*. (Pensacola, Florida, 1987), pp. 127.
33. U.M.X. Sangodkar, P.J. Chapman, and A.M. Chakrabarty, *Gene* **71**, 267 (1988).
34. J.H.A. Apajalahti and M.S. Salkinoja-Salonen, *J. Bacteriol.* **169**, 5125 (1987).
35. J.G. Steiert and R.L. Crawford, *Biochem. Biophys. Res. Commun.* **141**, 825 (1986).
36. P.H. Tomasek et al., *Gene* **76**, 227 (1989).
37. T.D. Gaffney and T.G. Lessie, *J. Bacteriol.* **169**, 224 (1987).
38. T. Barsomian and T.G. Lessie, *Mol. Gen. Genet.* **204**, 273 (1986).
39. D.E. Berg and M.M. Howe, Eds., *Mobile DNA* (ASM Press, Washington, D.C., 1989).

40. K. Kaluza, M. Hahn, and H. Hennecke, *J. Bacteriol.* **162**, 535 (1985).
41. R. Haugland, U.M.X. Sangodkar, and A.M. Chakrabarty, *Mol. Gen. Genet.*, in press.
42. U.B. Priefer *et al., Cold Spring Harbor Symp. Quant. Biol.* **45**, 87 (1981).
43. W.M. Coco *et al.*, in *Pseudomonas 1989 Meeting* (Chicago, 1989), Abstract 112K.
44. K.-L. Ngai *et al., J. Bacteriol.* **169**, 699 (1987).
45. D. Ghosal and I.-S. You, in *Abstracts of the Annual Meeting of the American Society for Microbiology,* (New Orleans, 1989).
46. T.T. Wu, E.C.C. Lin, and S. Tanaka, *J. Bacteriol.* **96**, 447 (1968).
47. R.H. Don and J.M. Pemberton, *J. Bacteriol.* **145**, 681 (1981).

Discussion

Gunsalus: Do any of you or Nick Ornston have any structure data on folding of any of these enzymes in the *ortho* pathways?

Chakrabarty: Well, Nick has been collaborating with a number of biophysicists to look at the x-ray crystallographic data of a number of ortho pathway enzymes such as the MLEI, DLH, and so forth. Because many of these enzymes have now been purified and crystallized, structural data are becoming available.

Buswell: What sort of activity do the cholorocatechol cleavage enzymes and the chloromuconate lactonizing enzymes exhibit towards the various chlorinated and nonchlorinated substrates?

Chakrabarty: Actually, Nick Ornston published a paper last year, and before him, Hans Knackmuss published a paper showing that although the *ortho* pathway enzymes for catechol or *cis, cis*-muconate had little activity (about seven percent or so) toward the chlorinated catechol and muconate, the plasmid-specified enzymes for chlorocatechol or chloromuconate degradation had about 50 percent activity toward the nonchlorinated substrates.

Salkinoja-Salonen: Because the pathway of the AC1100 is so similar to pentachlorophenol degradation as has been described by our group or Ron Crawford, did you check for genetic homology with these organisms?

Chakrabarty: You know that you sent us some DNA from the *Chlorophenolicus* organism, and we got the *Flavobacterium* strain from Ron Crawford. All these bacteria appear to have a similar pathway for chlorophenol catabolism; we hybridized these DNA with both RS1100 and the 2,4,5-T degrading gene called *chq*, but in no case did we see any hybridization.

Salkinoja-Salonen: No homology with any of these bacteria?

Chakrabarty: That is right, no obvious hybridization between our cloned 2,4,5-T genes and the genomic digests of the pentachlorophenol degrading strains that you and Ron Crawford have worked with.

Ribbons: I wonder if you would give me some feel for the numbers game in selecting mutants, for example, which can grow with, let's say, 3-chlorobenzoic acid the way the parents could not. You indicated that the chromosomal enzymes for the benzoate oxygenase will normally tolerate 3-chlorobenzoic acid and hydroxylate it to catechol in two steps, which involves probably at least three or four genes. Then there are three critical reactions for the utilization of the 3-chlorocatechol, that involves, presumably, the evolution of three different genes, three different specificities, and on top of that, the regulation of those genes, if it is in the same kind of situation as for the regular catechol pathway that involves two regulatory situations. So we are talking about five genetic events, at least.

Chakrabarty: In most cases, Doug, bacteria recruit and evolve genes that are only absolutely necessary, and where it may already have chromosomal genes that can be useful, then they use those genes. This sometimes causes problems when the genes are transferred to a different host. For example, if you introduce pJP4 into *Pseudomonas aeruginosa*, even though all the 2,4-D genes are expressed, it does not utilize 2,4-D because it has a reductase missing. *Alcaligenes eutrophus* has this reductase, so it presumably did not need to recruit this gene in pJP4, assuming that pJP4 evolved in a host like *A. eutrophus*. Thus, the pAC27 plasmid has only 3-chlorocatechol degradative genes but no benzoate dioxygenase or maleyl acetate reductase genes, as they appear to be chromosomal in *P. putida*. As I mentioned to you, the chlorocatechol (*clc*) genes are strikingly similar to the chromosomal catechol genes in terms of their organization and homology between *catR* and *clcR*, *catA* and *clcA*, *catB* and *clcB*, and so forth. We refer to this sort of evolution as relaxed evolution in contrast to the gene recruitment for the 2,4,5-T pathway, where the 2,4,5-T genes show no homology with other analogous genes. Thus, we think that evolution under strong selection pressure, which we call directed evolution, may bypass the requirement for genetic relatedness, leading to acquisition of genes from any sources.

Janssen: Could you comment or speculate on the mechanism that causes selective insertion of RS 1100 in the AC1100 chromosome, and is there a clustering of catabolic genes in this region?

Chakrabarty: At this point in time, the only thing we know is that there are a large number of copies of RS1100 on the plasmids and chromosome of AC1100, but even all the chromosomal copies, estimated to be at least 50, presumably more, are present only on one segment (about 1300kb, or one third) of the chromosome. We have shown that during transposition of RS1100, large segments of chromosomal DNA are carried with RS1100. Whether this type of event allows the recruitment of 2,4,5-T genes from nonpseudomonal ancestors is an open question, but we are interested in knowing the ancestry as well as the mode of transposition of RS1100, both in AC1100 as well as in other microorganisms. We have also demonstrated by pulsed field gel electrophoresis studies that at least two 2,4,5-T genes map near the RS1100 copies, but whether all the catabolic genes are clustered in this region or not is presently unknown.

5

Design of New Pathways for the Catabolism of Environmental Pollutants

correspondence
K. N. Timmis
Division of Microbiology,
GBF–National Research Centre
for Biotechnology
Braunschweig
Federal Republic of Germany

F. Rojo
Centro de Biologia Molecular
CSIC y UAM
Madrid, Spain

J.L. Ramos
Estación Experimental
del Zaidin
CSIC, Apto 419
18080 Granada, Spain

Experimental evolution of new catabolic activities in microbes constitutes a powerful approach toward obtaining organisms that are capable of degrading toxic chemicals.

Detailed in this review are two current strategies for the evolution of novel or improved biodegradative routes for aromatic compounds. One strategy outlined involves stepwise restructuring of exisiting pathways, thereby gaining new substrate specificities, whereas the other method mentioned involves the construction of a new pathway brought about by the combination of enzymes derived from different pathways in different microorganisms.

Introduction

Over the past few decades enormous quantities of industrial chemicals have been released into the environment. A large number of them, particularly those structurally related to natural compounds, are readily degraded by soil and water microorganisms. However, a significant proportion, mainly those having novel structural elements or substituents found rarely in nature (xenobiotics), are only catabolized slowly and thus tend to persist and accumulate in the environment. Certain compounds, particularly those that exhibit some degree of toxicity, contribute substantially to environmental pollution. Recent environmental catastrophes have underscored the acute danger that industrial chemicals can constitute for our biosphere. However, the existence of many waste dump sites containing highly toxic substances and large-scale chronic pollution certainly represent a more important long-term hazard. Clearly, in addition to terminating current production of the more toxic and persistent industrial chemicals, it is essential to exploit more effectively the biodegradative capacities of soil microorganisms in order to diminish the consequences of existing and continuing environmental pollution.

Fortunately, soil and water microorganisms collectively exhibit remarkable capacities to degrade a wide range of noxious organic chemicals[1] and to evolve degradative activities toward new compounds.[2] On the other hand, the evolutionary process can be extremely slow, particularly where the acquisition of multiple catalytic activities is necessary. In such cases, the evolution of new metabolic activities in the laboratory may be helpful,[3-6] because the frequency and type of genetic events needed (for example, mutation, alteration of gene expression, and gene transfer) can be carefully controlled and selective conditions can be optimized.[8]

There are basically three experimental approaches to the laboratory evolution of metabolic pathways, namely:

(1) Long-term chemostat selection, which often involves progressive replacement of a mineralizable substrate by a recalcitrant analogue.[8]

(2) *In vivo* genetic transfers, in which genes of critical enzymes of one organism are recruited into a pathway of another organism through experiments involving natural genetic transfer processes, such as transduction, transformation, and especially conjugation.[9] This approach is sometimes facilitated by

the fact that the genetic information for recently evolved pathways is frequently located on transmissible plasmids or transposons[10,11] genetically promiscuous elements that readily move from one replication unit to another within the same cell. Thus, once a critical enzyme has evolved in one organism, its gene can be easily transferred to others and become recruited into related or unrelated existing or evolving pathways. Moreover, once a new pathway has emerged in one organism, it can be readily transferred to others.

(3) *In vitro* evolution, in which cloned and well-characterized genes are selectively combined in a new host in order to evolve a new or improved pathway.[12-14]

Although all three approaches constitute powerful experimental tools to effect desired phenotypic changes in microbes, *in vitro* evolution has the added advantage of being highly controlled as well as producing predictable changes and enabling multiple genetic changes to be effected in a single step, often without the need to directly select the final phenotype desired.[7] However, *in vitro* evolution does require detailed information on the genetics and biochemistry of the key elements of the pathways and the enzymatic steps to be manipulated. In contrast, chemostat selection and *in vivo* evolution can often be carried out without prior extensive characterization. In this brief review, we will discuss genetic manipulation strategies for the rational evolution of new catabolic phenotypes in soil bacteria.

Strategies for *In Vitro* Evolution of Catabolic Pathways

In general, evolution of new metabolic potential involves the acquisition of new or modified enzymatic activities.[3,13-15] However, because the synthesis of many enzymes is carefully regulated and occurs only in response to the appearance of specific induction signals (for example, the appearance in the medium of the cognate substrate of the enzyme or pathway), the acquisition of new specificities of regulators of gene expression can also be important.[3,13,14] *De novo* evolution of a protein with a radically new activity often involves a number of genetic events (mutations, recombinations, fusions, and so forth), most of which cannot be predicted *a priori*. Thus, evolution of new phenotypes will generally involve the acquisition of new enzymatic or regulator specificities (for substrates and effectors, respectively) through mutational alteration of existing proteins or through recruitment of new proteins from different organisms. The ability of enzymes and regulators to undergo a relaxation of their specificities without loss of function[3,13] and the existence of enzymes exhibiting catalytic activities toward a broad range of structurally distinct substrate molecules[12,16] are of critical importance to evolution.

Two general strategies have been developed for the laboratory evolution of catabolic pathways for recalcitrant compounds by means of genetic manipulation.[7] If the chemical exhibits substantial structural analogy to compounds that are readily degraded, the initial strategy of choice is to identify the steps of the known pathway that are nonpermissive for the chemical in question, and then to modify these such that they become permissive. This approach generally leads to an expansion of the substrate profile of the pathway. The expansion can be horizontal in that more analogues of a single class of compounds are metabolized (see following section, as a result of the recruitment of isofunctional enzymes from other pathways[12] or as a result of the mutational alteration of the substrate specificities of existing key enzymes.[13,14] Pathway expansion can also be vertical in that the existing pathway is used as a base onto which are grafted additional enzymes that extend the pathway upward.[12,17] Alternatively, if an existing pathway for related compounds is not known, new pathways can be conceived and appropriate component enzymes can be sought in bacteria found in natural habitats. Once the feasibility of a new route is established, the corresponding enzymes can be recruited into a single bacterium (or a consortium) by the cloning of their structural and regulatory genes and by the combination of such genes in appropriate host organisms.[18]

Rational Restructuring of Catabolic Pathways by Sequential Modification

Pseudomonas putida bacteria carrying TOL plasmid pWW0 are able to degrade and utilize as sole source of carbon and energy several alkylbenzenes including toluene, *m*- and *p*-xylenes, 3-ethyltoluene and 1,3,4-trimethyl-benzene.[19] Metabolism of these compounds is initiated by progressive oxidation of the methyl side chain substituent of carbon-1 (upper pathway), followed by oxidation of the aromatic carboxylic acid thereby formed to short chain carboxylic acids, pyruvate, and aldehydes (*meta*-cleavage pathway; see Figure 1). Such bacteria can also grow on the corresponding alkylbenzoates but not, however, on either 4-ethyltoluene or 4-ethylbenzoate. Other bacteria able to metabolize benzenes and benzoates are readily isolated from soil but these also cannot generally degrade the 4-ethyl-substituted analogues. In order to identify the metabolic impediments to degradation of 4-ethyltoluene and to determine whether these may be overcome by appropriate genetic modification, we have carried out a substrate/effector study of the enzymes and regulators of the TOL catabolic pathway. In order to be able to exploit more than once growth of modified bacteria on 4-ethyl-substituted compounds as part of the strategy to select desired genetic changes, we initially focused on the *meta* cleavage pathway before turning to the upper pathway.

Expression of the TOL plasmid genes is regulated at the transcriptional level.[20] The upper pathway operon is induced by toluene/xylenes and their alcohol derivatives and this induction is mediated by the *xylR* gene product positive regulator (Figure 1).[20] Expression of the *meta*-cleavage operon is induced by benzoate/toluates, and this induction is mediated by the *xylS* gene product positive regulator. The promoters of the two operons and their accompanying regulatory determinants have been localized and sequenced, and the operon transcriptional start sites have been identified.

In order to examine the inducer specificity of the positive regulator of expression of the *meta* cleavage operon, the promoter of this operon *Pm* was fused in a cloning vector to *lacZ*, which encodes

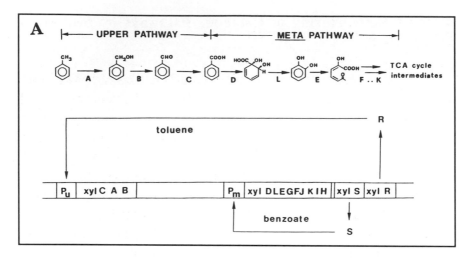

ß-galactosidase, a readily assayed test enzyme used extensively in gene expression studies.[13]*Escherichia coli* K-12, carrying this hybrid plasmid, plus another containing *xylS*, the gene of the positive regulator of transcription from *Pm*, synthesizes ß-galactosidase when benzoate is present in the growth medium but not when a noninducer such as salicylate is present. Using this system, a large number of

Figure 1. (Facing Page) The TOL plasmid–encoded pathway for the degradation of alkylbenzenes and the experimental broadening of its substrate range. **A.** The TOL catabolic pathway is shown for the substrate toluene, but 3- and 4-methyltoluene (*m*- and *p*-cresol, respectively); 1,3,4-trimethylbenzene; and 3-ethyltoluene are degraded in a similar fashion. The organization into two operons of the genes encoding the catabolic enzymes is shown, as are the regulatory circuits controlling transcription of these operons. The XylS positive regulator stimulates transcription of the *meta* operon when activated by benzoate or alkylbenzoates (that is, the substrates of the *meta* operon), whereas the XylR positive regulator stimulates transcription of the upper operon when activated by toluene or another upper operon substrate. **B.** 4-Methylbenzoate is both an effector molecule that activates the XylS protein as well as a substrate for the *meta* pathway. 4-Ethylbenzoate does not serve as an effector for the XylS protein regulator of the catabolic operon promoter *Pm* (see Table 1) and thus fails to induce synthesis of the catabolic enzymes. Isolation of a mutant that produces a XylS protein analogue that is activated by 4-ethylbenzoate results in the synthesis of all catabolic enzymes in response to the presence of 4-ethylbenzoate in the bacterial culture medium. However, this compound is only metabolized as far as 4-ethylcatechol, because the latter inactivates the ring cleavage enzyme C23O. The isolation of a mutant that produces a C23O analogue resistant to inactivation by 4-ethylcatechol eliminates the final metabolic block and permits complete degradation of 4-ethylbenzoate through the *meta* pathway.

benzoate analogues were tested for their ability to provoke synthesis of ß-galactosidase through activation of the XylS protein regulator. The structural features of benzoate analogues critical for their interaction with the regulator were thereby analyzed (Table 1). From this study, it became clear that whereas a number of benzoate analogues activate the XylS protein and induce synthesis of the *meta* pathway enzymes, 4-ethylbenzoate does not.[13]

In order to select *xylS* mutants that produce regulators having broader inducer specificities, a hybrid plasmid was constructed in which the *Pm* promoter was fused to a gene specifying resistance to tetracycline (Figure 2). This gene is expressed, and thus host bacteria are resistant to tetracycline *only* when the XylS protein is activated by benzoate or one of its analogues. Bacteria spread on a nutrient agar plate containing tetracycline and 4-ethylbenzoate (or some other ordinarily noninducing benzoate analogue) are killed because the XylS protein is not activated. The plating of a large number of such bacteria and the inclusion of a strong mutagen such as ethylmethane

Table 1
Activation of XylS and XylS Mutant Proteins by Benzoate Analogues

Benzoate Analogue	Induction Ratio (relative increase in ß-galactosidase)	
	XylS	XylS4
None	1	1
2MB	18	37
3MB	17	14
4MB	4	10
2,3MB	10	12
3,4MB	5	8
2,4MB	1	5
2,5MB	1	1
3,5MB	1	1
4EB	1	8

Note: *Escherichia coli* K-12 bacteria containing two plasmids, one carrying a *Pm::lacZ* fusion and the other carrying either *xylS* or the mutant *xylS* allele *xylS4* were cultured in L-broth containing or lacking the benzoate analogue indicated in the left-hand column. ß-galactosidase levels were subsquently measured, and the ratio plus analogue/minus analogue (induction ratio) was determined. A value of 1 indicates that the analogue did not induce synthesis of ß-galactosidase and thus does not serve as an effector of the XylS or mutant XylS proteins, whereas values greater than 1 indicate that the analogue served as an inducer. Abbreviations: B, benzoate; M, methyl; E, ethyl.

sulfonate in the plate result in the isolation of a few tetracycline-resistant colonies (Figure 2). Some of these colonies produce mutant XylS proteins that are activated by new effector molecules such as 4-ethylbenzoate.[13,14]

One such *mutant xylS* gene, *xylS4* , was transferred to *P. putida* bacteria carrying the TOL plasmid (Figure 2). This derivative also failed to grow on 4-ethylbenzoate but did degrade the compound to 4-ethylcatechol (Figure 1). Thus, the catabolic enzymes are synthesized in this derivative, and 4-ethylbenzoate is transformed to 4-ethylcatechol, but the *meta*-cleavage enzyme does not permit further metabolism.[14] Characterization of the *meta*-cleavage enzyme, catechol 2,3-dioxygenase (C23O), revealed that 4-ethylcatechol is in fact a suicide substrate that causes irreversible inactivation of the enzyme.

It was reasoned that if a single amino acid change in C23O could render it resistant to inactivation by 4-ethylcatechol and that if this was the only further change needed to permit the complete degradation of 4-ethylbenzoate via the TOL plasmid–encoded pathway, then the appropriate C23O mutants might be obtained by selecting directly for growth of bacteria on 4-ethylbenzoate. A large number of *P. putida* bacteria carrying the TOL plasmid and the *xylS4* gene were plated on a minimal medium containing ethylmethane sulfonate and 4-ethylbenzoate as the sole source of carbon and energy (Figure 2). Several colonies grew under these conditions, and all were subsequently shown to be able to use 4-ethylbenzoate as a source of carbon and energy and to produce altered C23O enzymes that exhibited increased resistance to inactivation by 4-ethylcatechol.[14]

Although *P. putida* bacteria carrying a derivative TOL plasmid containing the *xylS4* mutation and the *xylE* mutation conferring 4-ethylcatechol resistance on C23O are able to grow on 4-ethylbenzoate as sole carbon source, they are not able to grow on 4-ethyltoluene. An analogous approach was therefore taken to analyze the effector and substrate specificities of the XylR protein regulator and catabolic enzymes, respectively, of the upper pathway.

A fusion between *lacZ* and the upper pathway operon promoter *Pu* permitted analysis of the effector specificity of the XylR protein. This study revealed that the effector specificity of this protein is extremely relaxed and that XylR is activated by a wide range of alkyl- and chlorotoluenes, including 4-ethyltoluene, and by methyl- and chlorobenzylalcohols. Thus, failure to metabolize 4-ethyltoluene is not due to a lack of synthesis of the catabolic enzymes (M.A. Abril, C. Michan, K.N. Timmis, and J.L. Ramos, *J. Bacteriol.*, in press).

Analysis of the substrate specificities of the three upper pathway enzymes, toluene oxidase, benzylalcohol dehydrogenase, and benzaldehyde dehydrogenase, revealed that although the latter two had rather relaxed substrate specificities and transformed the correspond-

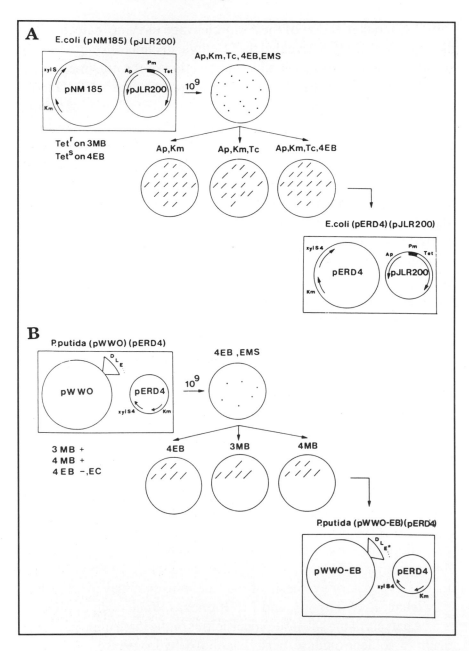

ing 4-ethyl-substituted intermediates, toluene oxidase had little to no activity on chlorotoluenes or 4-ethyltoluene. It seemed therefore that

Figure 2. (Facing Page) Sequential mutational elimination of metabolic barriers to the degradation of 4-ethylbenzoate through the TOL plasmid–specified *meta* pathway. **A.** Selection of mutant XylS proteins activated by new effector molecules such as 4-ethylbenzoate. *Escherichia coli* K-12 (pNM185; pJLR200) bacteria were spread on nutrient agar plates containing ampicillin, kanamycin, tetracycline, 4-ethylbenzoate, and the mutagen ethylmethane sulfonate (EMS). After incubation of the plates, two classes of clones appeared: one class that grew on tetracycline plates lacking 4-ethylbenzoate (most of these contained a mutation in the *Pm* promoter, so that the *tet* gene was expressed constitutively), and another class that grew only on tetracycline plates containing 4-ethylbenzoate. Mutants of the latter type contained plasmids such as pERD4 that carry mutant *xylS* genes (for example, *xylS4*) whose products are activated by 4-ethylbenzoate (see Table 1). **B.** Isolation of mutants producing C23O analogues resistant to inactivation by 4-ethylcatechol. *Pseudomonas putida* (pWW0; pERD4) bacteria were spread on minimal medium containing 4-ethylbenzoate as sole source of carbon and energy and the mutagen EMS. After incubation of the plates, six clones appeared, five of which grew on 4-ethylbenzoate and 3- and 4-methylbenzoate, whereas the other grew only on 4-ethyl- and 4-methylbenzoate. All clones contained mutant *xylE* genes (*xylE**) that encode C23O enzyme analogues exhibiting resistance to inactivation by 4-ethylcatechol.

the barrier to 4-ethyltoluene degradation in such bacteria resided in the narrow substrate specificity of a single enzyme, the first in the pathway. Again reasoning that a single mutation might eliminate this barrier and enable bacteria to metabolize 4-ethyltoluene, we plated out a large number of bacteria on a minimal medium containing the mutagen ethyl methane sulfonate (EMS) and having 4-ethyltoluene as sole source of carbon and energy. Mutants growing on this medium arose at a frequency of approximately 10^{-8}. Such mutants co-transferred with the TOL plasmid their new phenotype to other bacteria and produced an altered toluene oxidase that attacks 4-ethyltoluene (M.A. Abril , C. Michan, K.N. Timmis, and J.L. Ramos, *J. Bacteriol.*, in press).

The TOL plasmid–encoded pathway for the degradation of alkylbenzenes had thereby been rationally restructured to enable it to process 4-ethyltoluene by sequential mutational modification of three elements, resulting in relaxation of the effector specificity of the XylS protein, an increase in the resistance of catechol 2,3-dioxygenase to inactivation by 4-ethylcatechol, and a broadened substrate specificity of the initial enzyme of the pathway, toluene oxidase.

Figure 3. (Facing Page) Unproductive misrouting of substituted catechols by *ortho*- and *meta*-cleavage enzymes. **A.** Degradation of chloro- and methyl-substituted aromatics often involves as a first step their conversion to corresponding catechol derivatives. Chlorocatechols are degraded through *ortho*-cleavage pathways but may be misrouted into a *meta*-cleavage pathway in bacteria containing a *meta*-cleavage enzyme. As a result, they are channeled to dead-end metabolites that in some cases (such as that from 3-chlorocatechol) are highly reactive and inactivate the *meta*-cleavage enzyme. On the other hand, methylcatechols are normally degraded through *meta*-cleavage routes, although they can be transformed by *ortho*-cleavage pathways, eventually forming methyllactone derivatives as dead-end metabolites. **B.** Effect of misrouting substituted catechols. Bacteria were grown in minimal medium containing 4-methylbenzoate (5mM) as sole source of carbon and energy. When the cultures reached an absorbance of $A_{660} = 0.5$, they were diluted 10-fold with fresh medium containing both 4-methylbenzoate and either 3-chlorobenzoate (left) or 4-chlorobenzoate (right) at the indicated concentrations, and incubation was continued for a further 20 hours. The final A_{660} was measured and plotted against the concentration of 3- and 4-chlorobenzoate initially present in the fresh medium. The strains used were: *Pseudomonas putida* KT2440 (TOL) (o; possesses a *meta* pathway for degradation of methylbenzoates); *Pseudomonas* sp. B13(TOL) (Δ; possesses TOL plasmid *meta* pathway and an *ortho* pathway for 3-chlorobenzoate; B13 derivative FR1 (pFRC20P) (Δ; lacks a *meta* pathway but possesses *ortho* pathways for degradation of both chloro- and methylbenzoates).

Designing New Catabolic Pathways: Patchwork Assembly of Enzymes and Regulatory Systems

The redesigning of an existing pathway is a relatively straightforward experimental approach to evolve a pathway for the degradation of a recalcitrant compound. However, this approach will not always be sufficient, in which case it may be necessary to construct a new pathway by rationally combining in patchwork fashion a series of catalytic activities derived from different organisms.

Individual substituted phenols and benzoates have a significant level of toxicity but nevertheless can be degraded via catechol by microorganisms in soil and in wastewater treatment plants. Industrial wastes, however, frequently contain mixtures of chloro- and methyl- substituted phenols and benzoates. Such mixtures are not only difficult to degrade but also tend to destabilize phenol- and benzoate-degrading microbial communities. The problem lies in the existence of both *ortho*- and *meta*-cleavage routes for de-

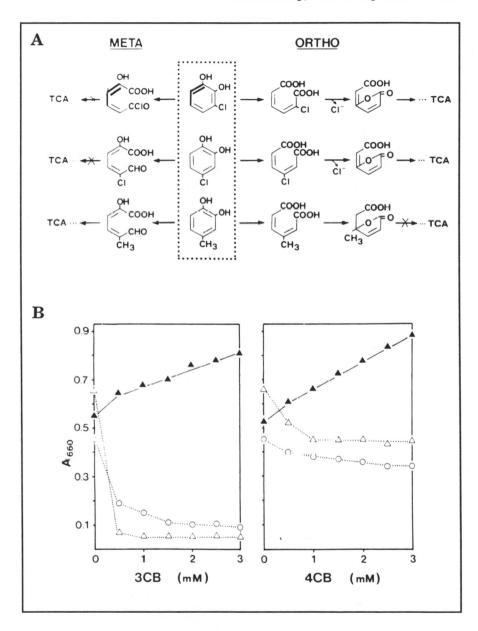

gradation of catechols. Catechol and chlorocatechols are generally subjected to *ortho* fission, whereas methylcatechols suffer *meta* fission (Figure 3). Although both pathways may exist in individual microorganisms, only one is usually functional at any given moment according to the substrate that is available. However, when both chloro- and methylcatechols are formed from mixtures of chloro- and methylaromatics, both pathway types are functional, often in the same organism, and the catechols will be subjected to both types of cleavage. Whereas *ortho* cleavage of chlorocatechols leads to their productive metabolism, *ortho* cleavage of methylcatechols leads to the formation of dead-end products. Similarly, whereas the *meta* cleavage of methylcatechols leads to their productive metabolism, the *meta* cleavage of chlorocatechols leads to the formation of either dead-end products or reactive products that inactivate C23O, the ring cleavage enzyme.[21-23] The nonproductive misrouting of catechol cleavage products during simultaneous metabolism of chloro- and methyl-substituted aromatics constitutes a sort of biochemical anarchy and eventually perturbs the productive metabolism of aromatics by the cell or the community to such an extent that cell death or disruption of the community may occur (Figure 3).[18,22]

One potential solution to this problem is the construction of catabolic routes for chloro- and methylaromatics that employ only one type of catechol ring fission mode. *Pseudomonas* sp. B13 possesses only *ortho*-cleavage routes for catechols; it can grow on 3-chlorobenzoate and acquires the ability to grow on 4-chlorobenzoate when it recruits the TOL plasmid–encoded relaxed substrate specificity toluate dioxygenase through transfer of the *xylDLS* genes of the TOL plasmid.[9,12] In order to create a stable B13 derivative that is able to degrade 4-chlorobenzoate, the cloned TOL genes were inserted into transposon Tn5, and the hybrid element was subsequently transposed into the B13 chromosome.[18] The derivative thereby obtained, FR1 (Figure 4), grew on 3- and 4-chlorobenzoate but not on 3- or 4-methylbenzoate. The latter two compounds were, however, cometabolized via *ortho* cleavage to the dead-end products 2- and 4-methyl-2-enelactone, respectively (Figure 4).[18,24] In order to effect mineralization of the dead-end products of *ortho* cleavage of 3- and 4-methylbenzoate, it was necessary to identify and recruit additional enzymes. The

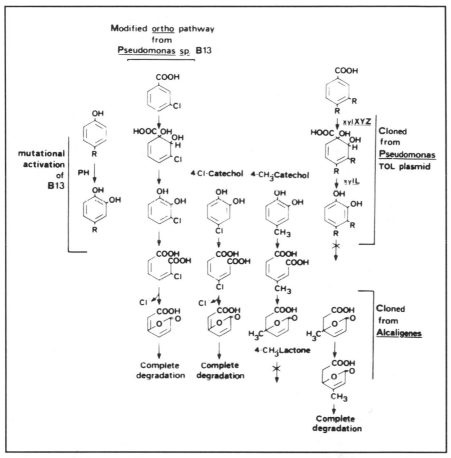

Figure 4. Constructed pathway for the simultaneous degradation of chloro- and methylaromatics. The route is based on the modified *ortho* pathway for 3-chlorobenzoate of *Pseudomonas* sp. B13. Introduction into B13 of the TOL plasmid genes coding for toluate 1,2-dioxygenase (*xylD*) and dihydroxy-cyclohexadiene carboxylate dehydrogenase (*xylL*), together with that of the positive regulator of the *xylDL* operon (*xylS*), expands the degradation range to include 4-chlorobenzoate and permits transformation of methyl-benzoates to methyl-2-enelactones, which are accumulated as dead-end meta-bolites. Recruitment of a 4-methyl-2-enelactone isomerase from *Alcaligenes eutrophus* allows transformation of 4-methyl-2-enelactone (the intermediate of 4-methylbenzoate catabolism) to 3-methyl-2-enelactone (bottom right), which is completely degraded by other enzymes of B13. Mutational modification of expres-sion of the phenol hydroxylase of B13 further extends the degradation capacities to chlorophenols and methylphenols. The final route is thereby composed of five different pathway segments derived from three different organisms.

methyl-2-enelactones that accumulated during metabolism of methylbenzoates were therefore isolated and used to select organisms able to use such compounds for growth. This resulted in the isolation of an *Alcaligenes* sp. capable of growing on 2- and 4-methyl-2-enelactone.[24] Growth on 4-methyl-2-enelactone involves isomerization of 4-methyl-2-enelactone to 3-methyl-2-enelactone. Because *Pseudomonas* sp. B13 is able to grow on 3-methyl-2-enelactone, it was reasoned that recruitment of the isomerase function of the *Alcaligenes* sp. into FR1 would allow it to grow on 4-methylbenzoate. An *Alcaligenes* gene bank was therefore prepared in a wide host range, mobilizable cosmid vector and mass-transferred into FR1 by conjugation. Transconjugants that were able to grow on 4-methylbenzoate were readily isolated; the hybrid cosmid present in one of these was designated pFRC20P[18] (Figure 4). Cell-free extracts of these transconjugants exhibited enzymatic activities that converted purified 4-methyl-2-enelactone to 3-methyl-2-enelactone. High levels of activity were measured both in 4-methylbenzoate-grown cells and in acetate-grown cells, although highest levels were obtained in 4-methylbenzoate grown cells. This indicates that expression of the isomerase is regulated in these constructions but that the basal level of synthesis is high.

Pseudomonas sp. B13 is able to grow on phenol and, after adaptation, on 4-chlorophenol as its sole source of carbon and energy; catabolism is via an *ortho*-cleavage route, with catechol or 4-chlorocatechol as intermediates.[25] The phenol hydroxylase involved also transforms 3- and 4-methylphenols in cell-free extracts and produces from these substrates the corresponding methylcatechols.[25] In principle, therefore, an appropriate derivative of B13 such as FR1(pFRC20P) that can mineralize 4-methylcatechol possesses all of the enzymes necessary to grow on 4-methylphenol as sole source of carbon and energy. However, although phenol is a growth substrate for this derivative, 4-methylphenol is not.[18] Spontaneous mutants could nevertheless be selected that grow on 4-methylphenol (see Figure 4; frequency 10^{-7} to 10^{-8}). Measurement of phenol hydroxylase levels in such mutant bacteria grown in succinate, phenol, or 4-methylphenol revealed little or no enzyme in succinate-grown cells and high activities in bacteria grown on phenol or 4-methylphenol. Synthesis of this enzyme is therefore specifically regulated.

Figure 3   shows that addition of a chloroaromatic such as 3-chlorobenzoate to bacteria [for example, *P. putida* KT2440 (TOL) or *Pseudomonas* sp. B13(TOL)] that are actively degrading a methylbenzoate through a *meta* ring-fission pathway resulted in inhibition of cell growth as a result of misrouting of 3-chloro-catechol into the *meta* pathway and irreversible inactivation of the key enzyme of the pathway, C23O,[21] by the ring-fission product of 3-chlorocatechol, which is a highly reactive acylhalide. Addition of 4-chlorobenzoate to such cells had a less severe impact on growth because the dead-end product that forms as a result of misrouting of 4-chlorocatechol into the *meta* pathway is less reactive (Figure 3). Addition of 3- or 4-chlorobenzoate to FR1(pFRC20P) bacteria growing on 4-methylbenzoate had no inhibitory effect and in fact promoted further growth of the cultures (Figure 3). Moreover, the B13 derivative degraded simultaneously the chloro- and methylben-zoates in the given mixtures.

Thus, a novel *ortho* cleavage strain for the degradation of mixtures of 3- and 4-chloro- and 4-methylbenzoates has been constructed by the patchwork assembly of four pathway segments (Figure 4), namely, (1) the TOL plasmid toluate dioxygenase and following *cis*-diol dehydrogenase, which transform methylbenzo-ates to methylcatechols; (2) the B13 chlorocatechol-1,2-dioxygenase and choromuconate cycloisomerase, which convert methylcatechols to methyl-2-enelactones; (3) the *Alcaligenes eutrophus* 4-methyl-2-enelactone isomerase, which converts 4-methyl-2-enelactone to 3-methyl-2-enelactone; and (4) the B13 3-methyl-2-enelactone path-way, which completes the catabolic route. This pathway was further expanded through activation of the synthesis of a relaxed substrate specificity phenol hydroxylase. The newly evolved strain meta-bolizes chloro- and methyl-substituted phenols and benzoates exclu-sively via *ortho*-cleavage routes, tolerates shock loads of one type of substituted benzoate or phenol while utilizing the other as a carbon source, and degrades both types simultaneously when present together.[18]

Concluding Remarks

Current levels of environmental pollution urgently necessitate, among other measures, much greater exploitation of microbial degradative activities. Unfortunately, some chemicals possess structural elements or substitutents that confer on the molecule a high degree of resistance to enzymatic attack or are present in mixtures that are incompatible for the effective degradation of the toxic component. Soil microorganisms have the capacity to evolve enzymes capable of attacking most classes of organic chemicals, but the evolution of new catabolic pathways proceeds very slowly where multiple genetic changes are required and where the selection pressures may only be effective in selecting the last genetic change to occur.

A major advantage of experimental evolution of pathways is that laboratory selection conditions [for example, antibiotic treatment), when selecting acquisition of a hybrid plasmid containing the gene of an enzyme to be recruited or a mutant regulatory protein (see above), may be totally unrelated to the ultimate phenotypic change desired (for example, catabolism of an aromatic compound). Effective selection procedures can thus be *custom designed* for each of the individual genetic changes required.[18] Successive changes can either be effected in the organisms to be evolved or be effected in different organisms and subsequently combined sequentially or simultaneously in the organism selected to carry out the biodegradative activity. In this way, the evolutionary process can be substantially accelerated. The cloning of genes of proteins having useful characteristics such as relaxed substrate specificities, both for the purpose of genetic and functional analysis and for their transfer into organisms to be evolved, generates "evolutionary modules" for further experiments. Growth in the number of different modules available will increasingly facilitate the design and experimental evolution of new and more complex pathways.

In the experiments we have described, existing pathways were restructured by mutational alteration of protein specificities so that the modified proteins recognized new substrates/inducers, and novel metabolic routes were created by the patchwork assembly of enzymes and regulators from different pathways and from different organisms.

These experiments confirm that experimental evolution of metabolic pathways is feasible and holds considerable potential for accelerating the evolution of microbes that will be able to degrade particularly recalcitrant and toxic compounds.

Although we have focused largely on the manipulation of genes of enzymes and regulators, it is evident that other targets for experimental intervention will become relevant in the near future. The recruitment of appropriate membrane transport systems for unusual growth or transformation substrates may, in some cases, be important, as will the isolation of mutants resistant to the toxicity of certain compound(s). In addition, however, there may be applications in which the efficacy of evolved activities can be considerably increased if the manipulated bacterium is able to undertake vectorial movement towards a nondiffusible or poorly diffusible target (for example, plant root, hydrophobic chemical). Thus, experimental manipulation of bacterial taxis and motility should receive increasing attention during the next few years.

Acknowledgments

The authors acknowledge the many fruitful and stimulating discussions with our colleagues, H.-J. Knackmuss and his group at the University of Stuttgart, S. Harayama at the University of Geneva, and the excellent secretarial assistance of H. Brink and I. James.

References

1. D.T. Gibson, *Microbial Degradation of Organic Compounds, Microbiology Series, Vol.13*, (Marcel Dekker, Inc., New York, 1984).
2. J.M. Pemberton, B. Corney, and R.H. Don, in *Plasmids of Medical, Environmental and Commercial Importance*, K.N. Timmis and A. Puhler, Eds. (Elsevier/North-Holland Biomedical Press, Amsterdam, 1979), pp. 287-299.
3. P.H. Clarke, in *The Bacteria, Vol. 4*, L.N. Ornston and J.R. Sokatch, Eds. (Academic Press, New York, 1978), pp. 137-218.

4. G.T. Cocks, J. Aguilar, and E.C.C. Lin, *J. Bacteriol.* **118**,83 (1974).
5. S. Harayama, J.L. Ramos, and K.N. Timmis, in *Antibiotic Resistance Genes: Ecology, Transfer and Expression, Banbury Report 24*, S.B. Levy and R.P. Novick, Eds. (Cold Spring Harbor Laboratory, Cold Spring Harbor, New York, 1986), pp. 389-402.
6. R.P. Mortlock, *Ann. Rev. Microbiol.* **36**, 259 (1982).
7. J.L. Ramos and K.N. Timmis, *Microbiol. Sci.* **4**, 228 (1987).
8. E. Dorn *et al.*, *Arch. Microbiol.* **99**, 61 (1974).
9. W. Reineke and H.-J. Knackmuss, *Nature* **277**, 385 (1979).
10. S. Harayama and R.H. Don, in *Genetic Engineering: Principles and Methods, Vol. 7*, J.K. Setlow and A. Hollaender, Eds. (Plenum Publishing Corporation, New York, 1985) pp. 283-307.
11. K.N. Timmis *et al.*, *J. Antimicrob. Chemother.* **18**, (Suppl. C), 1 (1986).
12. P.R. Lehrbach *et al.*, *J. Bacteriol.* **158**, 1025 (1984).
13. J.L. Ramos *et al.*, *Proc. Natl. Acad. Sci., U.S.A*. **83**, 8467 (1986).
14. J.L. Ramos *et al.*, *Science* **235**, 593 (1987).
15. J.H. Campbell, J.A. Lengyel, and J. Langridge, *Proc. Natl. Acad. Sci., U.S.A.* **70**, 1841 (1973).
16. N. Mermod, S. Harayama, and K.N. Timmis, *Bio/Technology* **4**,321 (1986).
17. K.N. Timmis *et al.*, in *Plasmids in Bacteria*, D.R. Helinski *et al.*, Eds. (Plenum Publishing Corporation, New York, 1985), pp. 719-739.
18. F. Rojo *et al.*, *Science* **235**, 1395 (1987).
19. M.J. Worsey and P.A. Williams, *J. Bacteriol.* **127**, 7 (1975).
20. J.L. Ramos, N. Mermod, and K.N. Timmis, *Molec. Microbiol.*, **1**, 293 (1987).
21. I. Bartels, H.-J. Knackmuss, and W. Reineke, *Appl. Environ. Microbiol.* **47**,500 (1984).
22. H.-J. Knackmuss, in *Biotechnology, Biochemical Society Symposium No. 48*, C.F. Phelps and P.H. Clarke, Eds. (Biochemical Society, London, 1983), pp. 173-190.
23. E. Schmid, I. Bartels, and H.-J. Knackmuss, *FEMS Microbiol. Ecol.* **31**, 381 (1985).
24. D.H. Pieper *et al.*, *FEMS Microbiol Lett.* **29**, 63 (1985).
25. H.-J. Knackmuss and M. Hellwig, *Arch. Microbiol.* **117**, 1 (1978).

Discussion

Ribbons: Ken, I thoroughly enjoyed your presentation. What you also have with the construction of some of these pathways is a whole new family of chiral intermediates in these butenolides (methylbutenolides, fluorobutenolides, chlorobutenolides, and so forth), which are valuable compounds for synthesis chemists. Furthermore, you should be able to provide these with both antipodes because some are available synthetically; by that way you can kinetically resolve them, apart from producing the "natural" enantiomers. So you have lots of beautiful compounds there. If I could just have two minutes in which to show a transparency that you stimulated me to construct during your talk; the slide is going to show exactly the opposite acquisition of new metabolic function that you have just described.

Ken, anyone must be impressed with the rational and systematic genetic alterations you and your colleagues have made to allow the TOL gene products to accommodate the 4-ethyl substituent of toluenes or benzoates so that they exert control of gene expression and then allow growth of *P. Putida* (TOL) on, say, 4-ethyltoluene, which the parent strains do not recognize as a growth supporting nutrient. There is clearly an interesting natural evolutionary process that has occurred to accommodate methyl versus higher alkyl (or aryl) 4-substituents of toluene or benzoate. I mention this because of natural enrichment experiments performed in 1970 by my colleagues Wendy Berg and Alison Smith. They, along with others, demonstrated unequivocally with more than 30 bacterial strains isolated with *p*-xylene or *p*-toluate that none of them could grow with *p*-ethyl or *p*-isopropyl analogues. All of these strains used *meta*-cleavage pathways for catechols, as typified by the TOL gene sequences.

By contrast, bacterial strains (>20) that we easily isolated with toluenes or benzoates with 4-substituents larger than methyl (for example, ethyl, isopropyl, phenyl) universally used *p*-cymene-like pathways for catabolism and growth (see Ribbons *et al.*, Chapter 13 in this volume, Figure 16). Neither *p*-xylene nor *p*-toluate could support growth of these strains (*P. putida, P. cepacia, P. aeruginosa*) (Smith, Wigmore, and Ribbons, 1977 PK 188, *Microbiol. Proc. ASM Ann. Meet.*). However, most of these strains grown with *p*-cymene readily oxidized *p*-xylene, *p*-toluate, and 2,3-dihydroxy-4-methyl-benzoate to pyruvate, but not 4-methylcatechol. A relevant nutritional spectrum of one strain of *P. putida* JT810 (Wigmore and Ribbons, 1980) is shown in the following chapter with examples of derivative mutants obtained that have been selected for growth with *p*-toluate. Alison Smith and Graham Wigmore found that it was not possible to acquire *p*-toluate (*p*-tol⁺) growing strains directly from wild type strain JT810, which had been isolated on 4-ethylbenzoate. At least two genetic events were required; this was possible because *p*-toluate is an excellent substrate for the *p*-cymene pathway enzymes. Two different pairs of sequential selections led to the *p*-tol⁺ phenotype in strains JT812 and JT814. First, strain JT810 was plated on *p*-phenylbenzoate, and strain JT811 was isolated (amongst many others). Strain JT811 was constitutive for the *p*-cymene pathway but still could not grow with p-toluate. *p*-Toluate was still an inhibitor of growth with *p*-cumate (an inhibitor of expression). However, secondary mutants that were *p*-tol⁺, for example, strain JT812, could be derived from JT811 (but not from JT810) and were easily obtained.

The *p*-tol⁺ phenotype was also derived in two steps from strain JT810 by different selections. First, strain JT813 was selected for resistance to *p*-toluate inhibition of growth with *p*-cumate. This mutant could not grow with *p*-toluate even though it was readily oxidized by cells grown with *p*-cumate. Strain JT814 was isolated as an example of a *p*-tol⁺ phenotype from strain JT813. The relevant nutritional characteristics of these strains are shown in Chapter 13.

Gunsalus: What do you know about the cymene pathway after you get started?

Timmis: I thank Doug for his nice analysis of the *p*-cymene pathway. I think the message should be that there is an enormous amount of evolutionary flexibility in these pathways provided one has the right selection procedures; one can generally get the phenotypes one wants. In so getting them, we find out quite a bit about biochemical strategies in these organisms.

Young: I also enjoyed your very lucid presentation. I have a question of a very different nature. Tthe strains that you have developed, can they or have they been used in treatment and also are they competitive once you put them back into the environment or once you put them back into the treatment plant?

Timmis: Yours is the kind of question that speakers dream about. This is the data you saw: if you take the organism that we constructed and do the same experiment with 4-methylbenzoate, you see that the more chlorobenzoate or chlorophenol you add, the better they grow. There is no killing, there is no anarchy, they grow well; we are talking here about shock loads. In fact, they tolerate shock loads very well, which are usually the problem in an industrial stream. They are degrading these compounds simultaneously; both compounds are there and both are being degraded simultaneously.

To the question, these are genetically engineered organisms so they are not going to be put into uncontained systems for the moment; but they have been looked at a little bit in a contained system. This is an activated sewage microcosm (transparency) and what we do is we put the GEMS into this microcosm to the level of 50 percent of the total microbial population and look to see what happens. This is the normal microbial population oscillating; there are predators there, as the bugs come up the predators come up and eat the bugs down. The bugs go down and the predators go down; it is an oscillating system and everything is there. The organism we constructed, as you see, drops as you might imagine. This is a laboratory strain; We expected that it would just go out of the system within a very short period of time and it dropped as we expected, but you will notice it then stabilizes at a concentration of approximately 10^5 per ml. If you add here 4-methylbenzoate, you see that the population really drops dramatically; down to this point, after which you see that the constructed strain actually starts to come up. As it comes up, then the normal population also comes up, and that tells you this organism is buffering the system against the toxic effects of the compound. Here we see the addition of a shock load of 4-methyl- and 4-chlorobenzoate together and you see that this has a drastic effect on the population; this corresponds to the collapse of the sewage treatment plant. Here you see the more drastic this total population falls, the more drastic the GEM rises; we have the engineered organism coming up, and as soon as it reaches a certain point, what it does is bring the level of the toxic mixture down to the threshhold level where it can be tolerated by the microbial community and again, the population comes up. To summarize my answer to your question, in this one system that we have looked at rather superficially, the organism survives over the time of the experiment; it functions in the sense that if the toxic mixture for which it was made is present, it deals with it, buffering the system against any major perturbation.

6

Engineering Bacteria For Environmental Pollution Control and Agriculture

John Davison
Transgène s.a.
11, rue de Molsheim
67,000, Strasbourg, France

Françoise Brunel
Angelika Phanopoulos
Koné Kaniga
European Patent Office,
Erhardstrabe, 27,
D8000, München 2, F.R.G.

The ability to use genetically modified Pseudomonads as pollution control or cleanup agents depends on the solution of the technical problems in genetic engineering: the ability to identify and clone degradative genes, and the ability to stably incorporate these degradative genes into suitable *Pseudomonas* strains. This publication reviews progress, in our laboratory, on both these subjects. Methods to isolate and characterize degradative genes have been evolved and two examples, the genes coding for the degradation of vanillate and sodium dodecyl sulphate, are described. Vanillate, in its chlorinated form, is a pollutant of the pulp and paper industry and sodium dodecyl sulphate is a component of many household and industrial detergents. For the insertion of cloned genes into suitable *Pseudomonas,* the currently used plasmid vectors are not sufficiently stable and we have constructed transposon vectors, carrying multiple cloning sites, that enable stable insertion of cloned DNA into the *Pseudomonas* chromosome.

Introduction

Genetic engineering using recombinant DNA molecules generated *in vitro* has existed for approximately 16 years. The new technology has generated considerable debate, fear, and even hysteria, about whether it was beneficial or detrimental to mankind. Some of these fears were real and others imaginary, but they represented a hesitation before the unknown. The debate culminated in the Asilomar Conference in 1975 and by 1979, prudent assessment of the nature of the risks involved led to the relaxation of the National Institutes of Health guidelines. Recombinant DNA technology then entered a rapid expansion phase during which it became applicable to a wide range of viruses, bacteria, fungi, plants, and animals.

As the technology evolved to soil bacteria such as *Pseudomonas* and *Rhizobium*, it was realized that recombinant DNA was useful not only for the analysis of interesting genes but also for their modification and improvement. In this way, new bacterial strains having desirable environmental properties could be created. Some potential benefits of such an approach are outlined in Table 1.

In many respects, the technical problems associated with the genetic improvement of soil bacteria for pollution control and for agricultural purposes are similar, and we will discuss examples of both.

The use of bacteria in the environment is not new; *Rhizobium* has been used for many years as seed inoculum (4 million kilograms of *Rhizobium* were used in the United States in 1980)[12] and *Bacillus thuringiensis* has been used in similar huge amounts for insect control. Neither has caused health or environmental problems. However, the proposed use of *genetically engineered* microorganisms for this purpose has reopened the recombinant DNA debate regarding the hypothetical risks involved.[12,13] Much discussion of the pros and cons of deliberate environmental release has been published in the scientific literature and will not be repeated here. However, instructive reviews have been written by Alexander[14] on pollution control and by Brill[15] on genetic engineering in agriculture. Although the hypothetical hazards are largely undefined, the problem of deliberate environmental release is complicated by the enormous numbers of bacteria required. It has been estimated that even a small agricultural field trial would require the liberation of a minimum

Table 1
Some Potential Environmental Benefits of
Genetically Engineered Bacteria*

Bacterium	Potential Environmental Use*
Rhizobium meliloti	Enhanced nitrogen fixation[1]
Azospirillium brazilense	Plant hormone production[2]
P. syringae	Reduced ice crystalization
P. putida	Antagonism of phytopathogens[3]
P. fluorescens	Antagonism of phytopathogens[3]
Bacillus thuringiensis	Insect toxins[4]
P. putida	Camphor degradation[5]
P. oleovorans	Alkane degradation
P. cepacea	2,4,5-Trichlorophenoxyacetic acid degradation[7]
P. mendocina	Trichloroethylene degradation[8]
P. sp. ATCC 19151	Sodium dodecyl sulfate degradation[9]
P. diminuata	Parathion (pesticide) degradation[10]
Bacillus ferrooxidans	Metal extraction[11]

*This table is intended to be illustrative rather than a comprehensive list. Other examples can be found in the references indicated.

of 10^{12} bacteria.[16] Such numbers are large compared to mutation rates and increase the possibility that horizontal transfer to other bacterial species or genera will occur, even though this may be the product of two or more independent events taking place at very low frequency.

The use of bacteria for pollution control or cleanup is fraught with difficulties such as substrate concentration, substrate accessibility, bacterial survival competition, and establishment. These have been discussed elsewhere[14] and will not be dealt with here. Instead, only the genetic engineering aspects will be treated. These include the choice and construction of recombinant DNA vectors and the cloning of the genes of biodegradative interest, which can serve as model systems for advancement of the technology and for risk assessment.

Table 2
Properties of an Ideal Cloning Vector for Environmental Release

Completely stable
No antibiotic resistance genes or other possibly deleterious genes
Efficient selective marker not possessed by soil bacteria
No selective disadvantage to host
No horizontal transmission
Suicide and fail-safe properties
Bank of useful cloning sites

Cloning Vectors for Environmental Release

Gene cloning in gram-negative bacteria invariably uses small plasmid vectors because these have a high copy number which facilitates the isolation of their DNA. For genetic engineering in *Pseudomonas*, wide host range vectors, based on plasmids such as RSF1010 and RK2 are used.[17-19] These plasmids are able to replicate in most, or all, gram-negative bacteria. They carry antibiotic resistance markers permitting selection of recombinant bacteria and multiple restriction sites to facilitate cloning. The plasmids carry mobilization functions and can be efficiently transferred to other bacteria in the presence of self-transmissible plasmids, such as RP4. This can be an efficient process and facilitates transfer of recombinant DNA to bacteria not susceptible to transformation by naked DNA. Similarly, it can be used for the identification of genes cloned, in a shotgun experiment, by conjugation to bacteria defective in the gene of interest.[20,21]

In Table 2, the properties of vectors needed for the improvement of bacteria for environmental and agricultural purposes are listed. It is immediately apparent that the plasmid vectors constructed for laboratory manipulations are unsuitable for environmental purposes. First, all presently used plasmid vectors show structural and segregative instability in the absence of continuous selection for their antibiotic markers. In an environmental release program, such selection could not be maintained and the plasmids would be rapidly lost.

Second, the use of antibiotic markers in bacteria to be liberated in large numbers into the environment is inadvisable; thus alternative selection methods must be used. Such selective markers should be without conceivable risk and should be rare in naturally occurring bacteria so that they can be used for the reisolation and quantitation of the released bacteria. However, the selective markers should not cripple the recombinant bacteria to the point where they become laboratory artifacts, unable to compete with the natural bacteria populations.

Third, the advantage of conjugal transfer with wide host range plasmid vectors becomes a handicap when present on vectors to be used for environmental purposes, where it is desirable to eliminate horizontal transfer of genes to other bacteria in the environment. It is clear that the inclusion of mobilization functions on a wide host range replicative plasmid could facilitate undesirable horizontal transfer and should be avoided.

Transposon Vectors for Stable Recombinants

A ideal vector having all of the characteristics outlined in Table 2 does not exist and, given the instability and mobilization properties of wide host range plasmid vectors, could not easily be constructed. As an alternative, we have designed vectors based on the transposon Tn5. This transposon is able to jump from one DNA molecule to another (for example from a plasmid to the chromosome) at low frequencies (10^{-5}-10^{-6} per recipient cell).[22] Once integrated into the host chromosome, Tn5 is very stable in the absence of any selection for the antibiotic resistance markers it contains. Tn5 has been used previously as a cloning vector to clone the *Bacillus thuringiensis* toxin gene in constructing insecticidal root colonizing pseudomonads.[4] However, Tn5 contains only *Bam*HI as a useful unique restriction site for gene cloning and so is cumbersome to use, particularly when multistep gene insertions are needed. This problem is further complicated by the fact that, being unable to replicate by itself, Tn5 must be carried by a plasmid or phage delivery vehicle, which further contributes to the physical and genetic complexity.

We have improved a modified tetracycline resistant (Tc^R) Tn5 (Tn5-Tcl)[23] as a cloning vehicle by adding a bank of unique restriction sites to the interior of the transposon and by constructing a small simplified plasmid delivery vehicle from which most useful restriction sites have been removed. One such transposon vector is shown in Figure 1 where a bank of restriction sites has been incorporated into a unique *Xba*I site of Tn5-Tcl . Cloning into this *Xba*I site does not inactivate tetracycline resistance nor interfere with transposition functions. The new transposon vector contains unique cloning sites for 13 different restriction enzymes.[24]

The transposon cloning vector is carried by small (2.7 kb) plasmid vector pIC20H[25] and the cloning strategy was chosen so that most unique restriction sites are removed by the construction method (Figure 1). This vector is based on a pMB9 type replicon and is unable to function in *Pseudomonas*. Thus, when transferred into *Pseudomonas*, the nonreplicating molecule is lost, and tetracycline resistance is only acquired by transposition to the chromosome. In order to effect transfer to *Pseudomonas*, use is made of strain S17-1 of *E. coli*, which contains a modified integrated RP4 plasmid containing the complete transfer region necessary to mobilize the vector.[26] Finally, it is necessary to equip the pIC20H plasmid with the mobilization functions of RP4[27] to permit its conjugal transfer. The strategy for cloning in transposon vectors and transposition to *Pseudomonas* is outlined in Figure 2.

The transposon vectors have two major disadvantages compared with plasmid vectors. First, the transposon is present only as a single copy in the chromosome so that the enhanced gene expression due to high copy number is lost. Nonetheless, high gene expression has been observed from chromosomally integrated, single copy genes when these have suitably strong promoters and ribosome binding sites.[28] Second, once integrated, the recombinant cannot easily be recovered from the chromosome. On the other hand, transposon vectors have the advantages of stability. We have shown that pseudomonads subcultured each day for one week in the absence of antibiotic selection showed 100 percent retention of transposon markers. Similarly,

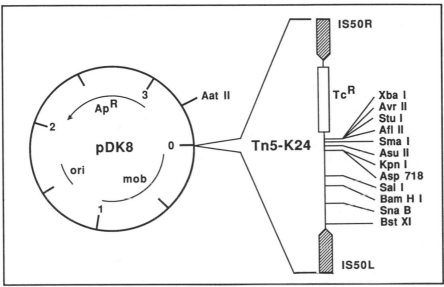

Figure 1. A Tn5 based transposon vector Tn5-Tc24A. Transposon cloning (shown on the right) is derived from Tn5-Tcl[23] by insertion of the restriction site bank carried by the *Xba*I-*Nhe*I fragment of pJRD184[20] into the unique *Xba*I site of Tn5-Tcl. Hatched boxes represent terminal repeats (1.5kb), and the open box represents the gene for resistance to tetracycline. Only restriction sites are shown. Unique restriction sites within the Tc[R] gene are not shown because they cannot be used for gene cloning without inactivation of the Tc[R] selective marker. Transposon vector is carried by a derivative (pDK8) of pIC20H[25] that carries the mobilization region (*mob*) of plasmid RK2.[27] Plasmid pDK8 acts as a suicide vehicle when transferred to Pseudomonads, where it is unable to replicate.

horizontal transmission would be greatly reduced compared with plasmid vectors, because this would require an independent event such as receiving a conjugative plasmid or infection by a phage to be coupled to the already low transposition frequency.

Our transposon vectors are still in a state of development and, like the plasmid vectors, still contain one or more antibiotic gene. Two lines of research are directed at solving this problem. The first would substitute the antibiotic genes by a catabolic function enabling the use of a rare carbon source not typically found among soil bacteria. The genes for the degradation of sodium dodecyl sulfate (SDS) and vanillate (3-methoxy-4-hydroxy benzoic acid)[21,29] are being investigated for this purpose (see following sections). An alternative possibility would be to locate a positive control gene on the trans-

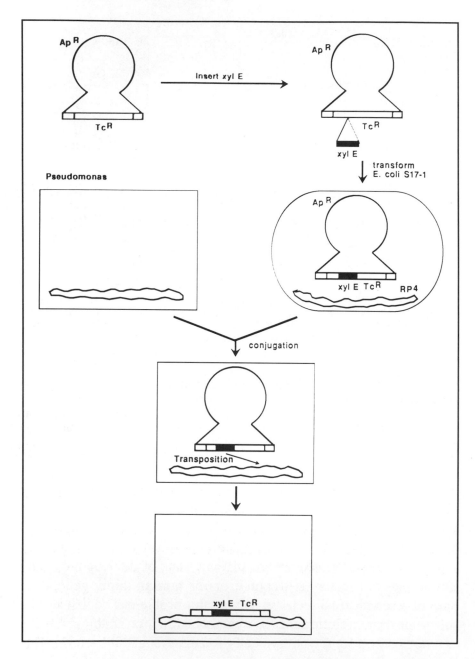

poson such that the presence of the transposon would activate transcription of an antibiotic resistance gene located on a plasmid.

Figure 2. (Left) Strategy for delivery of a Tn5-Tc24A containing a cloned gene. Plasmid pDK24A is cleaved with a unique restriction enzyme, and the *xyl*E gene, for example, is inserted. *E. coli* S17-1 is then transformed with the resulting hybrid plasmid. *E. coli* S17-1 has conjugative properties by virtue of the chromosomally integrated RP4 plasmid it contains,[26] and can then transfer the hybrid plasmid to *Pseudomonas* where it is usable to replicate. Transposition occurs to the chromosome and the resulting bacterium can be selected by virtue of the tetracycline-resistant marker. Activity of the *xyl*E gene is detected by spraying the plates with catechol or by enzyme assay (see Table 3).

Relaxation of antibiotic selection would then lead to loss of the plasmid, leaving a bacterium free of antibiotic resistance genes and containing an integrated transposon containing a harmless positive control gene.

Fail-safe or suicide markers may be useful for incorporation into vectors for environmental release (see Table 2). For example, we have constructed in *E. coli* a plasmid containing the lysis genes S, R, and Rz of phage λ under negative control by the thermolabile λcI_{857} repressor. In the laboratory, such bacteria lyse within 10 minutes at temperatures above 37°C and may have some value against the possibility of human ingestion. Changing the nature of the control mechanism could make such suicide mechanisms either sensitive to environmental stimuli or host dependent so that death would follow horizontal transfer. However, such methods may turn out to be clever genetical tricks that work well in the laboratory but have little practical importance in the field. There are three reasons for this. First, bacteria having such lethal genes may be at a selective disadvantage leading to instability of the recombinant. Second, the mutation frequency of the lethal genes is insufficiently low compared with the huge numbers of bacteria to be released. Third, as more cloned DNA is introduced into the vector, it becomes increasingly difficult to add subsequent DNA (for example, for environmental purposes) due to elimination of unique restriction.

Verification of the Utility of the Transposon Vectors

To check the efficiency of the transposon vectors for cloning into

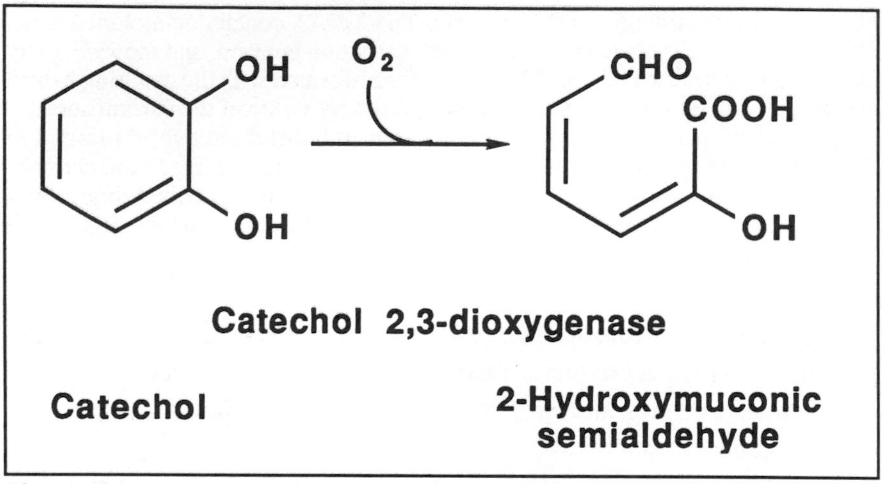

Catechol 2,3-dioxygenase

Catechol   **2-Hydroxymuconic semialdehyde**

Figure 3. Ring fission of catechol by catechol 2,3-dioxygenase.

Pseudomonas , several types of experiments were performed. The easiest first check was to use the internal bank of restriction sites to clone easily verified antibiotic-resistance genes such as kanamycin or streptomycin. In this way, selection could be performed in the recipient pseudomonads for the Tc^R marker and then verified by the unselected presence of the second resistance gene.

For the identification and quantitation of bacteria reisolated from agricultural or pollution cleanup trials, it is useful to have a chromogenic indicator marker. For example, it was possible to introduce the *lac*YZ genes into *Pseudomonas fluorescens*, which does not naturally possess these genes.[30] On plates containing the chromogenic indicator Xgal, such *Pseudomonas* produce a blue color that permits ready identification. We have used a different   approach cloning the *xyl*E gene into our transposon vectors. The *xyl*E gene codes for catechol 2,3-dioxygenase from the TOL plasmid responsible for the degradation of toluene. This enzyme cleaves catechol by the meta cleavage pathway (Figure 3) and it differs from the chromosomally coded ortho-cleavage enzyme.[31] Expression of catechol 2,3-dioxygenase in the absence of the rest of the degra-dation pathway, results in bright yellow colonies due to the pro-duction of 2-hydroxymuconic semial-dehyde when the plates are sprayed with the enzyme substrate catechol.[32] The presence of *xyl*E permits ready identification of cells containing the transposon and has been shown to be functional in several different species of gram-negative bacteria. Although the absolute amount of enzyme produced varies considerably (Table 3), the yellow colony color is easily detectable in all cases.

Cloning of Degradative Genes

Pseudomonads are remarkable in their catabolic ability; they are able to utilize a wide range of aliphatic and aromatic compounds as carbon source.[31] More surprising is the rapid evolution of these organisms to degrade man-made compounds not previously seen in nature.[7] These properties make pseudomonads the prime choice as pollution clean-up bacteria. Similarly, pseudomonads have interesting properties as biocontrol agents for the antagonism of phytopathogens.[3]

Advances in the cloning technology for pseudomonads has made the isolation of individual degradative genes a relatively simple, although still laborious task.[20] Similarly, vectors for the overexpression cloned genes in *Pseudomonas* have been constructed.[17-19]

Our first step was to study two model systems for degradation: (1) the conversion of vanillate (3-methoxy-4-hydroxybenzoic acid) to protocatechuate and (2) the conversion of sodium dodecyl sulfate to dodecanol. Both reactions are carried out by *Pseudomonas* sp. ATCC19151, which was originally isolated by Hsu[9] from the Baltimore Back River Sewage Treatment Plant, according to its ability to use the detergent sodium dodecyl sulfate as sole source of carbon and sulfur. The genes coding for these enzymatic activities were cloned by construction of a cosmid gene bank in a wide host range plasmid vector and identified by their ability to complement mutants unable to catalyze one or the other of the enzyme reaction.[20,21]

The Vanillate Degradation Genes

Vanillate is a degradation product of lignin and is liberated by ligninolytic fungi that degrade the lignin in order to attack the

Table 3
Activity of *xyl*E transposon in *Pseudomonas*.

Strains*	Catechol 2,3 dioxygenase*	
	No transposon	*xyl*E transposon
P. putida WCS 358	0	503
Pseudomonas ATCC 19151	0	510
P. putida KT2442	0	1100
Pseudomonas P07111	0	1481
P. methanolica ATCC 21968	0	2611
P. insueta ATCC 21276	0	3538

[†]Expressed in milliunits. One milliunit is the amount of catechol 2,3-dioxygenase necessary to convert one nanomole of catechol in 2-hydroxymuconic semialdehyde per minute per mg of protein at 32°C.

[*]Bacteria used have the following properties: *P. putida* WCS358, siderophore biosynthesis; *Pseudomonas* ATCC 19151, sodium dodecyl sulfate and vanillate degradation; *Pseudomonas* P07111, aspartate degradation, *P. methanolica* and *P. insueta*, methanol degradation.

cellulose.[33] Vanillate in its chlorinated form is also liberated in vast quantities by the bleaching of wood pulp and is an environmental pollutant. Finally, vanillate is a plant root exudate and may be used as a carbon source by some rhizosphere bacteria. The enzyme reaction catalyzing the conversion of vanillate to protocatechuate is a nicotinamide adenine dinucleotide (NADH) mediated oxidative demethylation (Figure 4). The vanillate degradation genes have been cloned and localized on the corresponding DNA fragment by deletion analysis and nucleotide sequence analysis.[21] Two genes are involved in the reaction, *van*A and *van*B. (Figure 5). The former is probably the monooxygenase responsible for the demethylation. Comparison of the *van*B gene to the NBRF Protein Identification Resource sequence bank reveals that the *van*B gene has strong similarities to various ferredoxins. Specific association of a ferredoxin type protein with a monoxygenase is frequently seen in degradative reactions to facilitate electron transport.[5,31] The cloned *van*AB operon, when transferred to *Pseudomonas oleovorans* (which contains all of the genes necessary for the degradation of protocatechuate), confers the ability to grow on vanillate as sole carbon source.

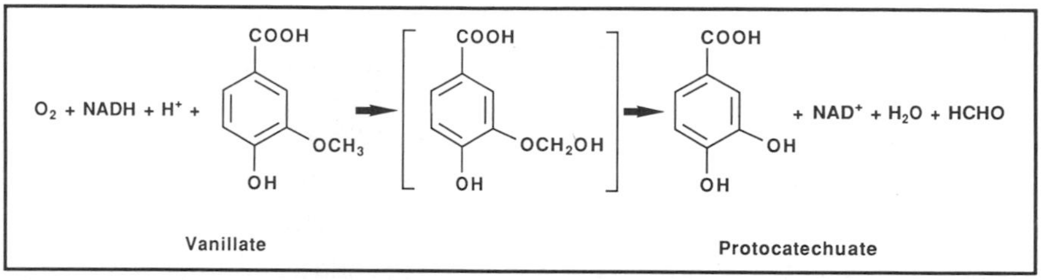

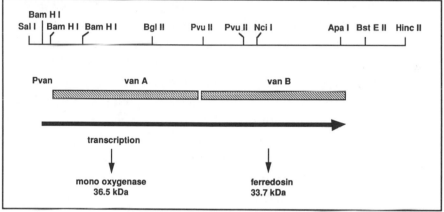

Figure 4. Oxidative demethylation of vanillate by *Pseudomonas.*

Figure 5. Physical and genetic maps of vanillate operon of *Pseudomonas* ATCC19151. Open reading frames identified by nucleotide sequence analysis and confirmed by expression in *E. coli*, using phage T7 RNA polymerase system.[21]

Gene fusion experiments with the *E. coli* gal k gene show that the *van*AB gene cluster is induced about sixfold by the presence of vanillate in the medium. At this time, we are unclear about the mechanism of induction. It remains possible that there is a third *van* gene coding for a repressor protein or for a positive activator function (as with the sodium dodecyl sulphate (*sds*)genes described in the following section).

It is also worth noticing that both the *van* and the *sds* genes are chromosomally located (like, for example, the genes for the degradation of catechol by the *ortho* pathway and the *alc* genes for degradation of alkanols). This is in contrast to many degradative pathways (for example for toluene, naphthalene and camphor) that are plasmid-borne.[5,6] Chromosomal genes of *Pseudomonas* are highly rich in guanine cytosine (GC) and the percentage utilization of GC in the third base of the coding triplet can exceed 90 percent.[21,29]

The Sodium Dodecyl Sulfate Genes

Alkyl sulfates are anionic surfactants present in many domestic and industrial laundry detergents and also in cosmetic preparations. Approximately 200 million tons are produced each year. They seem to show no hazardous effects on human health and are rapidly degraded in the environment by alkyl sulfatases in bacteria such as *Pseudomonas*.[34,35]

The *sds* genes were identified from the same cosmid gene bank of *Pseudomonas* sp. ATCC19151 as the *van* genes (previously described) by their ability to complement *sds* mutants of ATCC19151. These mutants are able to grow on dodecanol but not on sodium dodecyl sulfate as carbon source, because they lack alkyl sulfatase activity (Figure 6). Deletion analysis of the recombinant clones enabled the mutants to be classified into two complementation groups, and these groups were named *sds*A and *sds*B. Nucleotide sequence analysis of the region revealed two open reading frames corresponding in location to the *sds*A and *sds*B genes but coded by opposite strands of the DNA (Figure 7).[29]

Expression of the *sds*A and *sds*B genes in *E. coli* and *Pseudomonas* from the phage T7ϕ10 promoter[36] showed the synthesis and specific labeling of polypeptides of the same size as those predicted by the nucleotide sequence analysis, which confirmed the reality of the predicted open reading frames. The physical and genetic maps of the *sds* region is indicated in Figure 7.

Computer comparison of the predicted amino acid sequences of *sds*A with all of the known sequences in the NBRF Protein Identification Resource sequence bank gave no significant homologies. This is perhaps not surprising because this seems to be the first alkyl sulphatase gene to be cloned and sequenced. However, in the case of *sds*B, the comparison was highly informative because significant homologies were found with several proteins, all of which are positive transcriptional control functions in Gram-negative bacteria. In fact, a family of such proteins has now been detected (Table 4).[37,38] These share the properties listed in Table 5. These positive control elements facilitate transcription by binding to activator regions

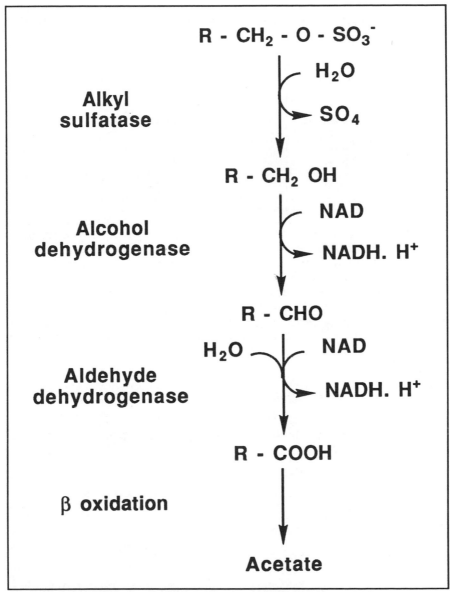

Figure 6. Degradation of Sodium Dodecyl Sulphate by *Pseudomonas*.

upstream of the transcriptional start sites near to the site of binding of RNA polymerase. In addition, like *sds*B, the positive control gene is often transcribed in the opposite direction to the gene(s) it controls.[37-39]

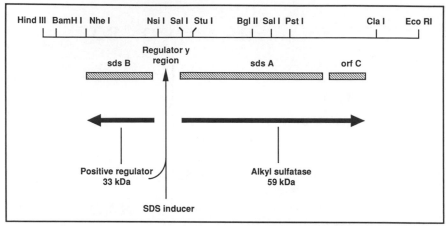

Figure 7. Physical and genetic maps of the *sds* genes of *Pseudomonas*. The open reading frames, *sds* A and B, were identified by nucleotide sequence analysis and confirmed by *in vivo* expression in *E. coli* and *Pseudomonas* using the phage T7RNA polymerase system.[21] The *orf*C open reading frame is indicated because its product can be expressed in the T7RNA polymerase system and because it has a high GC content in the third base of each triplet, characteristic of most *Pseudomonas* chromosomal genes. However, no mutants have been obtained that can be complemented by the *orf*C region, and we have no evidence for or against its involvement in SDS biodegradation.

The computer comparison was interesting in that it gave the first clue to the function of the *sds*B gene and enabled experiments to be performed to verify the function of *sds*B as a positive regulator protein. Thus, for example, it was possible to clone the *sds*A gene under control of the T7φ10 promoter and to clone this in a *Pseudomonas sds*B mutant. When the T7RNA polymerase was provided in trans by another plasmid, pT7pol[36] the strain was able to produce alkyl sulfatase and to grow on SDS as sole carbon source. In this case, replacement of the *sds*B positive control function by a different positive regulation factor (T7RNA polymerase) gave phenotypic complementation of the *sds*B mutant, indicating that *ds*B has no function in SDS degradation other than the activation of *sds*A transcription. Preliminary experiments using *xyl*E transcription fusions to the *sds*A promoter confirm the positive control action of *sds*B.

These results suggest that *sds*B is concerned with the positive control of transcription, presumably by binding to sequences

Table 4
Members of the *lys*R Family of Activator Proteins

Organism	Gene	Function
Escherichia. coli	*lys* R	Activator
E. cloacae	*amp* R	Activator
A. eutrophus	*tdf* O	ORF
S. typhimurium	*leu* O	ORF
E. coli	*ilv* Y	Activator
E. coli	*leu* O	ORF
E. coli	*cys* B	Activator
E. coli	*ant* O	ORF
E. coli	*oxy* R	Activator
Rhizobium meliloti	*nod* D	Activator
R. leguminosarum	*nod* D	Activator
R. trifolii	*nod* D	Activator
Bradyrhizobium sp.	*nod* D	Activator
Rhizobium sp.	*nod* Dl	Activator
S. typhimurium	*cys* B	Activator
Pseudomonas aeruginosa	*trp* I	Activator
P. putida	*trp* I	Activator
P. putida	*cat* M	Repressor
P. putida	*nah* R	Activator
Lactococcus lactis	*mle* R	Activator

Table 5
Characteristics of the *lys*R Family

Positive activators of transcription
DNA binding proteins (helix-turn-helix domain)
Homologous to each other at N-terminus
Often autogenously regulated
Often divergently transcribed from the gene they control

located in the intergenic regulatory region. The nature of these binding sites of *sds*B product is not yet defined but will be investigated by DNA binding experiments using gel retardation and footprinting experiments. However, in the case of *nod*D (the positive control gene for nodulation in *Rhizobium* sp.), a specific

SDS	ATCCA	CAACAACAACGAGCCGACC		
VAN	ATCCAATACAACAACAACGAG GACC			

n1	ATCCAA	ACAAT	CAA	TTTTACCAATC
n6	TCCCAA	ACAAT	CGA	TTTTCACACTC
n2	ATCCAA	ACAAT	CGA	TTTTACCAATC
n3	ATAAAA	ACAAT	CGA	TTTTACCAATC
n4	ATCCTC	ATAAT	CGA	TTTTACCAATC
n5	GTCCAA	ACAAT	CGA	TTTTACTAATC

Figure 8. Comparison of the 5' flanking region of *sds*A with those of *van*AB[21] and *nod*D.[39]

region known as the *nod* box is required for binding and regulation by nodD product.[39]

In fact, sequence comparison of the *sds* intergenic region with that of *nod* indicates a strong similarity at the left end but not the right end, of the *nod* box (Figure 8). Remarkably, similar sequences are seen in the 5' non coding region of the vanillate operon.[21] A model showing our present hypothesis of the control of alkyl sulfatase biosynthesis is shown in Figure 7. The *sds*B gene product is believed to bind to a regulatory region upstream of the *sds*A gene and, in the presence of inducer SDS, facilitates transcription of the *sds*A gene. This model is presently being tested together with the possibility that *sds*B, like several other members of the *lys*R family, is able to negatively control its own synthesis.

Conclusions

The work described in this article represents only initial steps in the engineering of bacteria for pollution control and agricultural purposes. The transposon vectors represent a real advance towards the construction of stable recombinants for environmental and agricultural purposes. The examples, vanillate and SDS utilization, are chosen as model degradative systems because of the relative simplicity of the enzyme reactions catalyzed. Each represents an extension of a degradation pathway that can be performed by many soil bacteria (that is, the degradation of protocatechuate in the case of vanillate or of dodecanol in the case of SDS). Small gene clusters such as *sds* and *van* can thus be easily isolated and transferred to suitable bacteria for environmental purposes.

However, it is clear that for many xenobiotics this may not be the case. Although evolution has managed to gather together on a single plasmid all of the genes coding for extremely complex degradation pathways,[5,6] it may be much more difficult, using present technology, for the genetic engineer to deal with such very large DNA fragments. Thus, it will be necessary to concentrate on a few key genes coding for enzymes catalyzing important rate-limiting steps. However, in many cases, the biochemistry of the system is unknown. For example, the degradation of 2,4,5-T[7], the production of antibiotics and siderophores by *Pseudomonas* able to antagonize phytopathogenic fungi,[3] and the process of nodulation by *Rhizobium*[39] are ill-defined biochemically, and this may hinder strain improvement.

Ecological factors will be important and the bacteria would need to be tailor-made to deal not only with a particular pollutant but with a particular environment. For example, a bacterium able to degrade in an oil spill in soil would not be adapted to dealing with an oil spill at sea. Similar consideration applies to bacteria engineered for agricultural purposes. For example, plant-beneficial bacteria able to antagonize phytopathogenic fungi in the rhizosphere of a potato plant may not be equally effective on corn. In the case of nitrogen fixing bacteria, nodulation (the process whereby the initial steps of the symbiosis are established), is known to be a highly specific interaction between particular species of leguminous plants and particular species of *Rhizobium* Furthermore, soil type, pH, and humidity are likely to make a large contribution to whether engineered bacteria are able to become established in the face of competition by the endogenous population. Our present state of knowledge in many of these areas is poor and should be given more attention. However, it may be useful to isolate bacteria from a particular ecological niche and to return them to that niche following strain improvement.

Despite many problems remaining unsolved, it is evident that initial progress has already been made in the technology for genetically improving bacteria for environmental purposes. However, like genetic engineering 10 years ago, the area of deliberate environmental release of genetically manipulated microorganisms is surrounded by suspicion and controversy. At present, it remains unclear whether this area will be used for the betterment of mankind or legislated out of existence by the regulating authorities.

Acknowledgments

This research was carried out under research contracts BAP-0048-B and BAP-0358 (GBF) of the Commission of the European Communities. A. Phanopoulos is grateful for a CEC-BAP training fellowship. We are grateful for extensive discussions with A. M. Chakrabarty during the tenure of a North Atlantic Treaty Organization travel grant (n° 0177/87).

References

1. G.N. Gussin, C.W. Ronson, and F.M. Ausubel, *Annu. Rev. Genet.* **20**, 567 (1986).
2. C. Elmerich, *Bio/Technology* **2**, 967 (1984).
3. J. Davison, *Bio/Technology* **6**, 282 (1988).
4. M.G. Obukowicz *et al., J. Bacteriol.* **168**, 982 (1986).
5. B.P. Unger, S.G. Sligar, and I.C. Gunsalus, in *The Biology of Pseudomonas,* J.R. Sokatch, Ed. (Academic Press Inc., Orlando, FL, 1986) pp. 557-589.
6. B. Frantz and A.M. Chakrabarty, in *The Biology of Pseudomonas*, J.R. Sokatch, Ed. (Academic Press Inc., Orlando, FL, 1986) pp. 295-323.
7. J.S. Karns *et al.*, in *Genetic Control of Environmental Pollutants*, G.S. Omenn and A. Hollaender, Eds. (Plenum Press, New York, 1984), pp 3-21.
8. R.B. Winter, K.M. Yen, and B.D. Ensley, *Bio/Technology* **7**, 282 (1989).
9. Y.C. Hsu, *Nature* **207**, 385 (1965).
10. C.M. Serdar and D.T. Gibson, *Bio/Technology* **3**, 567 (1985).
11. M. E. Curtin, *Bio/Technology* **1**, 228 (1983).
12. B. Dixon, summary of the First International Conference on the Release of Genetically Engineered Microorganisms (Regem Ltd., Cardiff, U.K., 1989).
13. M.A. Levin *et al., Bio/Technology* **5**, 38 (1987).

14. M. Alexander, in *Genetic Control of Environmental Pollutants*, G.S. Omenn and A. Hollaender, Eds. (Plenum Press, New York, 1984), 151-169.
15. W.J. Brill, *Science* **227**, 381 (1985).
16. H.S. Strauss, *Bio/Technology* **5**, 232 (1987).
17. J. Davison *et al.*, *Gene* **51**, 275 (1987).
18. J. Davison *et al.*, *Gene* **60**, 227 (1987)
19. V. Deretic *et al.*, *Gene* **57**, 61 (1987).
20. J. Davison, M. Heusterspreute, and F. Brunel, in *Recombinant DNA*, Part D, R. Wu, Ed. (Academic Press, San Diego, 1987) **153**, 34 (1987) pp. 34-54.
21. D. Brunel and J. Davison, *J. Bacteriol.* **170**,4924 (1988).
22. E. Berg and C.M Berg, *Bio/Technology* **1**, 417 (1983).
23. C. Sasakawa and M. Yoshikawa, *Gene* **56**, 283 (1987).
24. K. Kaniga, F. Brunel, and J. Davison, in preparation .
25. J.L. Marsh, M. Erfle, and E.J. Wykes, *Gene* **32**, 481 (1984).
26. R. Simon, U. Priefer, and A. Pühler, *Bio/Technology* **1**, 784 (1983).
27. G. Selvaraj, Y.C. Fong, and V.N. Iyer, *Gene* **32**, 235 (1984).
28. J. Davison, W.J. Brammar, and F. Brunel, *Mol. Gen. Genet.* **130**, 9 (1974).
29. A. Phanopoulos *et al.*, in preparation (1989).
30. D.J. Drahos, B.C. Hemming, and S. McPherson, *Bio/Technology* **4**, 439 (1986).
31. S. Dagley, in *The Biology of Pseudomonas*, J.R. Sokatch, Ed. (Academic Press Inc., Orlando, FL, 1986) pp. 527-555.
32. M. M. Zukowski *et al.*, *Proc. Natl. Acad. Sci. USA* **80**, 1101 (1983).
33. T.K. Kirk and R. Farrell, *Ann. Rev. Microbiol.* **41**, 465 (1987).
34. R.B. Cain, in *FEMS Symposium n°12*, T. Leisinger *et al.*, Eds. (Academic Press, London, 1981) pp. 325-370.
35. K.S. Dodgson and G.F. White, in *Sulfatases of Microbial Origin*, (CRC Press Inc., Boca Raton, FL, 1982) pp 9-48.
36. J. Davison, N. Chevalier, and F. Brunel, *Gene*, in press (1989).
37. S. Henikoff *et al.*, *Proc. Natl. Acad. Sci. USA* **85**, 6602 (1988).
38. M. Chang, A. Hadero, and I.P. Crawford, *J. Bacteriol.* **171**, 172 (1989).
39. K. Rostas *et al.*, *Proc. Natl. Acad. Sci. USA* **83**, 1757 (1986).

Discussion

Schink: Do you have any idea what the function of this SDS cleaving enzyme is with any kind of natural substrates. You know it has not been made just for SDS degradation. Is it a general unspecific esterase or is it specific to sulfate esters?

Davison: It is specific to sulfate esters. There was a lot of work done in the old days by Kennneth Dodgson, and he has published a lot of data on the range of enzyme substrates. These must be sulfate esters, and the size of the alkane chain must not be too big. I think it can be in the range of approximately 6 to 12, not larger than that.

Schink: There are not too many sulfate derivatives of that kind in nature. Most of them are polysacuritatives.

Davison: I have asked the question myself. Apparently there are some similar natural compounds produced by algae, although I do not know much about this. Wherever this activity does come from, it is not as uncommon in bacteria. This *Pseudomonas* ATCC19151 was isolated from the Baltimore Back River Sewage Treatment Plant in 1960, by Hsu. However, *P. aeruginosa* also produces an alkyl sulfatase.

7

Hydrolytic and Oxidative Degradation of Chlorinated Aliphatic Compounds by Aerobic Microorganisms

correspondence

Dick B. Janssen
Roelof Oldenhuis
Arjan J. van den Wijngaard
Department of Biochemistry
Biotechnology Center
University of Groningen
Nÿenborgh 16
9747 AG
Groningen
The Netherlands

Halogenated aliphatic hydrocarbons are an important class of environmental pollutants. Many of the haloaliphatics are susceptible to biodegradation under aerobic conditions, and much insight into the biochemistry of their degradation has been obtained from pure culture studies. The key steps in the microbial degradation and detoxification of these compounds are dehalogenation reactions. In aerobic microorganisms that can utilize halogenated compounds as a carbon source for growth, dehalogenation often proceeds by nucleophilic displacement reactions. This holds for compounds such as dichloromethane, 1,2-dichloroethane, and epichlorohydrin. As an alternative, oxidative formation of labile intermediates that undergo chemical decomposition may occur, especially in cases where only cometabolic conversions take place such as with trichloroethylene degradation by methanotrophic bacteria. Some of the properties of the enzyme systems that catalyze dehalogenation under aerobic conditions and the relevance to practical application of microorganisms for decontamination purposes are discussed.

Table 1.
Production and Use of Some Chlorinated Aliphatic Hydrocarbons

Compound	Production (10^6 tons/yr)	Use
1,2-Dichloroethane	13.0	Vinylchloride, gasoline
Vinylchloride	12.0	Polyvinylchloride
Perchloroethylene	1.1	Solvent
Trichloroethylene	1.0	Solvent
Carbon tetrachloride	1.0	Solvent, CHC
1,1,1-Trichloroethane	0.45	Solvent
Methylene chloride	0.4	Solvent
Methylchloride	0.35	Solvent, blowing agent
2-Chlorobutadiene	0.3	Polymers
Chloroform	0.24	Solvent, CHC
1,1-Dichloroethylene	0.1	Solvents, polymers

Introduction

Chlorinated aliphatic hydrocarbons are industrially produced in large amounts for use as solvents, cleaning agents, intermediates for further chemical synthesis, pesticides, and so forth (Table 1). Many cases of pollution of aquifers, surface waters, and soils have been reported.[1] Furthermore, applications of these chemicals are a cause of increased concentrations of volatile halogenated compounds in some industrial areas, partly due to emission of exhaust gases. Contamination of drinking water by chlorinated methanes, ethylenes, and propanes has also occurred.

Biological treatment of waste streams and soil or water contaminated with these compounds would be very attractive. For this, it is essential that efficient biodegradation of chloroaliphatics to harmless products can be achieved. This could be troublesome because of the reported persistence of many xenobiotic chemicals in the environment. Under suitable conditions, however, a number of microbial conversions of chlorinated aliphatic hydrocarbons have been found,

Table 2.
Bacterial Degradation of Chlorinated Aliphatic Hydrocarbons Under Aerobic Conditions

Hydrocarbon Reference	Degradation	Culture	Dechlorininating mechanism
Methylchloride[4]	+	P	
1-Chloro-n-alkanes[5-9,56]	+	P, E	H
α,ω-Dihalo-n-alkanes[5,6]	+	P, E	H, O
2-Chloroethanol[5,13]	+	P	H
Dichloromethane[11,12,52,55]	+	P, E, M	G
Chloroform[24,28,34]	+	M	O
Carbon tetrachloride	-		
1,2-Dichloroethane[5,13,34]	+	P, E, M	H, O
1,1,1-Trichloroethane[34]	-	M	O
Vinylchloride[14]	+	P, M	O
t-1,2-Dichloroethylene[23-25]	+	P, M	O
Trichloroethylene[23,24,26,27,34,53]	+	P, M, T, N	O
Tetrachloroethylene	-		
Allylchloride[3]	+	E	H
Epichlorohydrin[3,40]	+	P, E	I
1,3-Dichloro-2-propanol[40]	+	P, E	
1,2-Dichloropropane[3]	-		
1,3-Dichloropropene[18,34]	+	E, M	H, A
Chlorofluorocarbons	-		

Abbreviations:

+, (partial) degradation possible;
-, recalcitrant behavior described or likely;
A, addition of water to an unsaturated bond;
E, microbial enzyme capable of degradation known;
G, nucleophilic substitution by glutathione transferase;
H, hydrolysis by dehalogenases;
I, intramolecular nucleophilic displacement;
M, cometabolic conversion by methanotrophic bacteria;
N, cometabolic conversion by an ammonium oxidizing bacterium;
O, oxidative conversion by monooxygenase producing organisms;
P, pure culture uses compound for growth;
T, cometabolic conversion by toluene utilizing organisms.

both with mixed cultures that simulate aquifers or sewage treatment systems and with pure cultures (Table 2,3).[2]

During the last several years, much attention has been paid to determining what type of microbial activity yields optimal degrada-

Table 3.
Pure Bacterial Cultures That Use Haloaliphatics for Growth

Strain	Isolated on	Growth rate (h^{-1})	reference
Hyphomicrobium	Methylchloride	0.09	4
Pseudomonas DM1	Dichloromethane	0.11	52
Hyphomicrobium DM2	Dichloromethane	0.07	55
Methylobacterium DM4	Dichloromethane	0.22	12
Xanthobacter GJ10	1,2-Dichloroethane	0.12	5
Pseudomonas CE1	2-Chloroethanol	0.09	13
Arthrobacter HA1	1-Chlorohexane	0.14	8
Mycobacterium m15-3	1-Chlorobutane	–	9
Pseudomonas	1,6-Dichlorohexane	–	7
Strain GJ70	1,6-Dichlorohexane	–	6
Mycobacterium L1	Vinylchloride	0.05	14
Pseudomonas AD1	Epichlorohydrin	0.20	40

tion of various compounds. Studies toward the character of the microorganisms that carry out degradation and the enzymes that catalyze dehalogenation have made it possible to understand why some compounds are more difficult to degrade than others. An understanding of the biochemical pathways and genetics of chlorinated hydrocarbon degradation will be useful for designing experiments for further adaptation. Furthermore, a detailed insight into the possibilities for biotransformation and the products formed will be essential for the development of optimal biological treatment systems for the removal of xenobiotic compounds.

Utilization of Chlorinated Aliphatics as a Growth Substrate

Several pure bacterial cultures that use chlorinated aliphatics such as (di)chlorinated alkanes and halohydrins as a growth substrate have been isolated and studied. Table 3 illustrates this with a list of organisms isolated by different researchers who used enrichment with chloroaliphatics as sole carbon source.

When a series of inocula is tested, often only a small number of enrichments are positive, dependent on the compound tested and the nature of the inoculum. Not all chloroaliphatics are difficult to degrade, however. Chloroacetate utilizing bacteria, for example, can easily be isolated from samples of soil with no history of chemical pollution. Dichloromethane degraders seem to be more seldom isolated. The distribution of 1,2-dichloroethane degrading bacteria is even more limited, because we observed that most enrichments with nonpolluted inocula do not give growth.[3]

All 1-monochloro-n-alkanes (C1-C12) appeared to be degradable by pure bacterial cultures that could use these chemicals as a carbon and energy source for growth.[4-9] In general, generation times of bacteria were in the order of five to 10 hours (see Table 3). Quantitative dechlorination occurred, which points to complete detoxification. Pure cultures have also been obtained for dichloromethane[10-12] and the α,ω-dihaloalkanes (C2, C3, C4, C6, C9); (see Table 3).[5,6,13] Terminally halogenated alkanes are in general easier to degrade than secondary alkylchlorides.[3] The presence of two or three chlorines bound to the same carbon atom seems to prevent aerobic degradation, because attempts to isolate cultures utilizing 1,1-dichloroethane, 1,1,1-trichloroethane, and 1,1,2-trichloroethane were unsuccessful.[3] The same was found with trihalomethanes and carbon tetrachloride. From the chlorinated ethylenes, only the isolation of a vinylchloride utilizing *Mycobacterium* strain has been reported.[14] In general, the lower the number of halogen substituents, the better the chances for degradation by organisms utilizing the compound for growth under aerobic conditions.

Under anaerobic conditions, several conversions of highly chlorinated aliphatic hydrocarbons to lesser chlorinated compounds that may serve as a growth substrate for aerobic organisms have been found,[2] but these will not be further discussed here.

A critical step in the microbial metabolism of chlorinated compounds are the dehalogenation reactions. The enzymes that catalyze these conversions must have an unusual activity because they have to act on carbon-halogen bonds in compounds that do not or only at very low concentrations occur in natural evironments. As an alternative, dehalogenation may be caused by enzymes that do not directly cleave carbon-halogen bonds but produce unstable intermediates by incorporation of oxygen atoms. During dehalogenation the organochlorine character of the compounds, which is the actual cause of toxicity, is lost. This makes dehalogenation a key step in the bacterial metabolism of chlorinated compounds.

Five dehalogenation mechanisms have been found in aerobic bacteria (Figure 1). From the obtained insight in these degradation mechanisms, their substrate range, the products which are formed, and the properties of the enzymes, it is possible to understand why some compounds are recalcitrant and what remedies could lead to improved degradation. Not all mechanisms have been characterized in detail, but in some cases the enzymes have been purified and studied.

Glutathione Transferase

A role for glutathione transferases in detoxification is clearly established in mammals where these enzymes mediate conversion of several compounds to mercapturic acids that are excreted in urine. Leisinger and co-workers have shown that a glutathione transferase is also present in bacteria that grow with dichloromethane as sole carbon source. Degradation of dichloromethane has been found with obligatory methylotrophs such as *Hyphomicrobium* and with facultative methylotrophs of the genus *Methylobacterium*.[11,12,52,55] The dichloromethane dehalogenating glutathione transferase probably produces the unstable intermediate chloromethylglutathione, which is converted chemically to formaldehyde with regeneration of glutathione. The enzyme does not have a high V_{max} (1 µmol/mg of protein·min) and is induced to very high levels in dichloromethane degrading methylotrophs.[10,12]

The enzyme has been purified from several different isolates and was found to be a hexameric protein of subunit molecular weight 33kD.[10] Recently, a faster growing dichloromethane utilizer (μ=0.22 h^{-1}) that produced a dehalogenase with 5.6–fold higher activity has

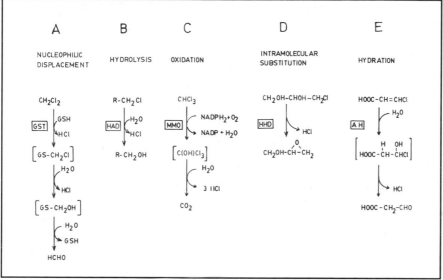

Figure 1. Mechanisms for the dehalogenation of chlorinated hydrocarbons by bacterial cultures. (A), nucleophilic displacement catalyzed by glutathione transferase in methylene chloride–utilizing bacteria; (B), hydrolysis catalyzed by dehalogenases. Substrates converted in this way are 2-halocarboxylic acids, 1-halo-n-alkanes, α,ω-dihalo-n-alkanes, α,ω-halohydrins, and some related compounds; (C), oxidative conversion by a monooxygenase yielding an unstable intermediate, as illustrated here for chloroform; (D), intramolecular nucleophilic substitution yielding epoxides, a mechanism involved in *vic*-halohydrin metabolism; (E), hydration of 3-chloroacrylic acid, yielding malonic acid semialdehyde. See Table 2 and text.

been described.[12] This enzyme has a very different amino acid sequence and is immunologically only weakly cross-reactive with the dehalogenases from earlier isolates of dichloromethane degraders. The higher catalytic activity of the enzyme is caused by its higher V_{max} and cooperative binding of glutathione, possibly making the enzyme much more efficient at low glutathione concentrations.

Hydrolytic Dehalogenases

Hydrolytic dehalogenation has been well documented for the conversion of 2-halocarboxylic acids by bacteria that utilize chloropropionate or chloroacetate for growth. Most of these dehalogenases

Figure 2. Catabolic route for 1,2-dichloroethane by *Xanthobacter autotrophicus*.[5,17] Two different hydrolytic dehalogenases, produced constitutively, cause dechlorination. The inducible dehydrogenases are usual enzymes of *Xanthobacter* and play a role in the metabolism of natural alcohols. The final product, glycolic acid, is a normal intermediate in bacterial metabolism. The organism can also convert the structural analogue 1,2-dibromoethane, but this yields a toxic product, presumably bromoacetaldehyde, that is not further converted and completely blocks growth.

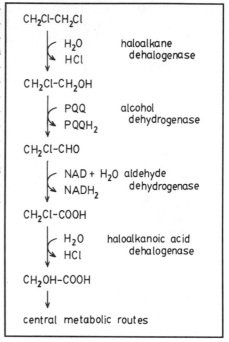

are small proteins, with molecular weights in the range of 17 to 68kD.[15,16] The dehalogenases seem to form a rather heterogeneous class of enzymes, because they show different dehalogenation mechanisms and are immunologically distinguishable.

Direct hydrolytic dehalogenation of a chlorinated hydrocarbon was first found with the haloalkane dehalogenase from *Xanthobacter autotrophicus* GJ10, an organism obtained in our laboratory using enrichment with 1,2-dichloroethane as sole carbon source (Figure 2).[5,17] Other 1,2-dichloroethane degrading bacteria have been isolated by us and other groups.[3,51] Most of these are facultative methylotrophs, which can partly be explained by the involvement of the quinoprotein methanol dehydrogenase in chloroethanol oxidation (Figure 2). Some chloroethanol-utilizing *Pseudomonas* strains also produce an inducible Phenazine methosulfate coupled alcohol dehydrogenase for chloroethanol oxidation.

The hydrolytic dehalogenase from *X. autotrophicus* GJ10 has been purified, characterized,[18] and crystallized.[19] The three-dimen-

Table 4.
Characteristics of Haloalkane Dehalogenases

Organism (Reference)	Molecular Weight	Substrates
Xanthobacter autotrophicus[3,18]	35,143D	C1-C4 1-Chloroalkanes C1-C12 1-Bromoalkanes epichlorohydrin
Strain GJ70[21]	28kD	C3-C6 1-Chloroalkanes C4-C9 α,ω-Dichloroalkanes bis(2-chloroethyl)ether
Arthrobacter HA1[20]	36kD	C2-C9 1-Chloroalkanes C3-C6 Dichloroalkanes
Corynebacterium m15-3[22]	36kD	C3-C9 1-Chloroalkanes C3-C9 α,ω-Dichloroalkanes C3-C4 α-Chloro-ω-alkanols

sional structure of the protein is currently resolved.[19] Furthermore, we have cloned and sequenced the gene encoding this enzyme. The gene appeared to encode a 310 amino acid polypeptide of molecular weight 35,143D and is preceded by two *E. coli* consensus promotor sequences, which explains the high expression observed in *Xanthobacter* and other gram-negative bacteria.

Three other dehalogenases that convert haloalkanes to their corresponding alcohols have been found in gram-positive bacteria (Table 4).[20-22] These proteins have an activity toward the environmentally less important long chain chloroalkanes but do not convert 1,2-dichloroethane. All enzymes found are composed of a single polypeptide chain of molecular weight 28 to 36kD. The haloalkane dehalogenases seem to form a distinct class of enzymes because no overlap in substrate range with other hydrolytic dehalogenases has been found, and the enzymes are not immunologically cross-reactive with halocarboxylic acid dehalogenases in tests so far. We found that antiserum against the haloalkane dehalogenase from *X. autotrophicus* GJ10 does not react with the halocarboxylic acid dehalogenase from a 2-chloroethanol–utilizing *Pseudomonas*, *Pseudomonas* 113, *Moraxella*, or with haloalkane dehalogenases from other organisms.[3,16]

Hydrolytic dehalogenations are particularly attractive for the conversion of chlorinated aliphatics because the enzymes do not need oxygen or cofactors for activity and catalyze simple dechlorination with water as the nucleophile, yielding alcohols as products. A limitation of the dehalogenases is that they are not active with halogens bound to unsaturated carbon atoms, because vinylic halogens are very resistant to nucleophilic displacement reactions. Other compounds that are not converted in this manner are trihalomethanes and alkanes with more than one chlorine bound to the same carbon atom. Furthermore, the enzymes have a relatively low affinity for their substrates. It is not yet clear whether this is directly related to the affinity of the microorganisms for their substrates, which causes high Monod constants.

Oxidative Conversions

Compounds with vinylic halogens, trihalomethanes, and several other highly chlorinated aliphatics may be degraded by oxidative conversion mediated by monooxygenases that are produced by methanotrophic bacteria.[23-29] Monooxygenases require a reduced cofactor or cytochrome for activity and incorporate one oxygen atom of molecular oxygen in the substrate; another oxygen atom ends up incorporated into water (see Figure 1C).[30] Monooxygenase reactions are electrophilic in nature instead of nucleophilic, and therefore oxidation provides an alternative for degradation of various compounds that are structurally insensitive to nucleophilic substitution reactions.

The methane monooxygenases are very aspecific[30,31] and are proposed to oxidize many halogenated methanes, ethanes, and ethylenes.[23-25] Oxidation can lead to dehalogenation as a result of the formation of chemically labile products (Figure 3) such as *gem*-halohydrins or chloroepoxides. Typical half-lives of chlorinated epoxides in neutral buffers are 30 hours (*trans*-1,2-dichloroethylene oxide), 5 hours (*trans*-1,3-dichloropropene oxide), 1.5 minutes (vinyl chloride oxide), and 12 seconds (trichloroethylene oxide).[25,32,33]

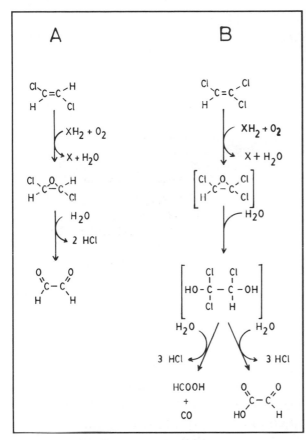

Figure 3. Proposed routes for the degradation of *trans*-1,2-dichloroethylene (A) and trichloroethylene (B) by methanotrophic bacteria.[21,34]

Initial observations on trichloroethylene degradation were made with soil columns[29] and with mixed enrichments of methanotrophs.[23] Pure cultures also showed degradation of trihalomethanes and chlorinated ethylenes.[3,25,26,34] Chloroform and chloroethylenes have been found to be converted in soil exposed to methane.[3,24,28]

Methanotrophs can, for example, efficiently degrade *trans*-1,2-dichloroethylene.[25] This cometabolic process required the presence of 16 moles of methane per mole of dichloroethylene and produced *trans*-1,2-dichloroethylene oxide as a chemically unstable intermediate. The metabolism of other chlorinated ethylenes by a strain of *Methylomonas* was found to be hindered by the toxicity of primary products of the methane monooxygenase. Conceivably, the unstable *gem*-halohydrins, epoxides, or reactive aldehydes that are produced

Table 5.
Degradation of Chloroaliphatics by *Methylosinus Trichosporium* OB3b[34]

Compound	Chlorinated product(s)[a]
Dichloromethane	Chloride
Chloroform	Chloride
Carbon tetrachloride	No conversion
1,1-Dichloroethane	Chloride
1,2-Dichloroethane	Chloride
1,1,1-Trichloroethane	2,2,2-Trichloroethanol
trans-1,2-Dichloroethylene	Chloride, epoxide
cis-1,2-Dichloroethylene	Chloride, epoxide
Trichloroethylene	Chloride, 2,2,2-Trichloroethanol
Tetrachloroethylene	No conversion
1,2-Dichloropropane	1,2-Dichloro-3-propanol

[a] Incubations were done at 30°C with resting cells from chemostat cultures grown in medium containing no added copper. Compounds were added at 0.2mM, and formate was used as electron donor.

from the substrates are toxic to the cells or inhibit methane monooxygenase. As a result, compounds such as chloroform and trichloroethylene, which are relatively inert and of low toxicity to cultures that grow with methanol, caused inhibition of growth at concentrations above 100μM when methane was supplied as carbon source.[25]

We have found that very efficient degradation of trichloroethylene and several other chloroaliphatics can be achieved by a culture of *Methylosinus trichosporium*, which can produce a soluble type of methane monooxygenase[35] that converts several chlorinated compounds[34] (Table 5). Only when cultivated under copper limitation, which caused expression of the soluble type methane monooxygenase, were cells able to degrade trichloroethylene. Dechlorination of the compound was achieved, with only traces of 2,2,2-trichloroethanol and trichloroacetaldehyde being formed. The methane monooxygenase seems to have a low affinity for trichloroethylene because degradation proceeded according to first order kinetics at concentrations below 0.1mM, with a rate constant of $2ml \cdot min^{-1} \cdot (mg\ cells)^{-1}$. Higher concentrations were toxic and inhibited degradation. In these experiments, formate was used as the electron-donating agent. Besides trichloroethylene, other chloroaliphatics were degraded by *M. trichosporium*, including dichloromethane, chloroform, dichloroethanes, 1,1,1-trichloroethane, and dichloroethylenes, but formation of chlorinated organic products occurred in some cases (see Table 5). The perchlorinated compounds tested, carbon tetrachloride and tetrachloroethylene, were not converted.

The biochemical characteristics of soluble methane monooxygenase from *M. trichosporium* OB3b and *Methylococcus capsulatus* (Bath) are very similar and have been studied in detail.[30,36] The enzyme is a three-component complex. The hydroxylase component A has a molecular weight of 210kD containing 2.3 non-heme iron atoms/molecule.[36]

The rates that we have observed with cells of *M. trichosporium* expressing soluble monooxygenase are much higher than the rates found with either the same organism expressing particulate monooxygenase[34] or with a Type I methanotroph that was grown in the presence of copper (and thus presumably also expressed a particulate type of enzyme).[26]

Catabolism of trichloroethylene and dichloroethylenes has been found with toluene utilizing strains of *Pseudomonas putida*.[37,38] Degradation has been concluded to be mediated by toluene dioxygenase encoded by the *todC* gene,[38] and induction of the degradative activity with aromatic compounds was necessary. First order kinetics with a rate of 1.8nmol/min·mg of protein at 80μM trichloroethylene was found. These data on toluene utilizing strains of *P. putida* indicate that the rate of trichloroethylene conversion proceeds faster than it does with methanotrophs producing particulate monooxygenase but approximately 100 times slower than it does with *M. trichosporium* expressing the soluble enzyme.[34]

Recently, a DNA fragment that harbors genes for toluene oxidation in *Pseudomonas mendocina* was expressed in *E. coli* and found to enable this organism to degrade toluene at a rate of 1 to 2nmol/mg of protein·min⁻¹.[57] Although this rate is rather low when compared with the velocity of trichloroethylene catabolism in *M. trichosporium*, degradation was found not to require the presence of an inducer, which is, in the case of toluene, an important advantage compared with the *P. mendocina* strain when practical application is considered.

Oxidative conversions seem of primary importance in organisms that convert chloroaliphatics cometabolically, that is, the organisms do not use these compounds as a sole carbon source and need a second oxidizable electron donor for growth and for supplying reducing equivalents. The involvement of oxidative conversion as the mechanism for dehalogenation in organisms growing with chloroalkanes such as methylchloride, 1,2-dichloroethane, and 1-chlorobutane has been suggested (see Table 3), but no biochemical experiments with cell-free extracts to support this have yet been reported.

Halohydrin Dehalogenases

Another alternative for dehalogenation is intramolecular nucleophilic substitution. This reaction was discovered by Castro and Bartnicki[39] in bacteria growing with 1-bromo-2,3-propanediol as a carbon source. The enzyme catalyzed formation of epoxides from a number of *vicinal* halohydrins, yielding epoxides as the product of dehalogenation (see Figure 1D). The enzyme from a *Flavobacterium* also converted bromohydrins to chlorohydrins and vice versa.[39]

Recently, we discovered enzymes catalyzing the same reaction but with a different substrate range in organisms utilizing epichlorohydrin as a carbon source.[40] Epichlorohydrin, an important industrial chemical that spontaneously hydrolyzes at a low rate, appeared to be used as a sole carbon source by different bacterial cultures (*Pseudomonas, Arthrobacter*) isolated form freshwater sediment. The substrate range of these dehalogenases differed from the *Flavobacterium* enzyme and included chloroacetone, which has no free hydroxyl group *vicinal* to the chlorine substituent.

Preliminary characterization of a purified epoxide forming halohydrin dehalogenase indicates that this enzyme is a dimer of molecular weight 68,000 daltons.[3]

Hydration

Hydration of unsaturated bonds could yield dechlorination of vinylic compounds, such as 3-chloroacrylic acid, which is an intermediate in the degradation of 1,3-dichloropropene.[41] Hydration may also be the cause for dechlorination of Coenzyme A derivatives formed during the metabolism of b-chlorocarboxylic acids in a strain of *Alcaligenes*.[42] No biochemical details about the enzyme(s) involved in these dehalogenations have been reported.

Causes of Recalcitrance

For some chlorinated aliphatics, attempts to isolate pure bacterial cultures that use these compounds as a growth substrate have repeatedly been unsuccessful. Thus, no cultures have been isolated that use 1,1,1- or 1,1,2-trichloroethane; trichloroethylene; 1,2-dichloropropane; and tri- or tetrahalomethanes for growth.

Highly chlorinated aliphatics obviously do not serve as an energy source under aerobic conditions because oxidation does not provide a net yield of reducing equivalents (Figures 1 and 3), and hydrolysis directly produces carbon dioxide. This holds for compounds such as chloroform, carbon tetrachloride, and tri- and perchloroethylene.

In other cases, there seems not to be a biochemical factor that makes utilization as a carbon and energy source impossible. Compounds such as 1,1,1-trichloroethane and 1,2-dichloropropane could theoretically be converted by hydrolysis to acetic acid and 1-chloro-2-propanol, respectively, which support growth of pure cultures. Hydrolytic dehalogenases (mechanism B in Figure 1) that carry out these conversions have never been found, however. We thus propose that the recalcitrant behavior is due to a lack of activity of enzymes that carry out hydrolytic dehalogenations with these substrates. Of course, it is well possible that further evolved enzymes that can hydrolyze these compounds will be found in the future or will be selected in the laboratory.

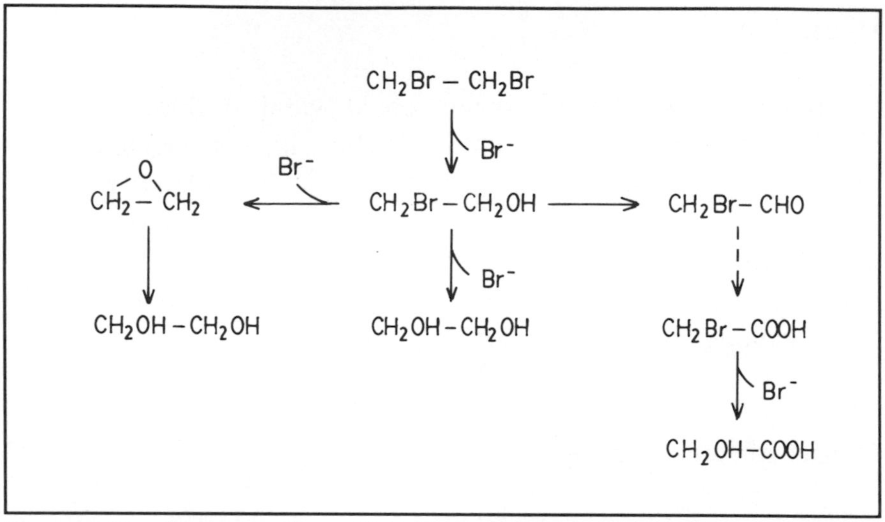

$$CH_2Br - CH_2Br$$

$$\downarrow Br^-$$

$$CH_2 \overset{O}{-} CH_2 \quad \xleftarrow{\;Br^-\;} \quad CH_2Br - CH_2OH \longrightarrow CH_2Br - CHO$$

$$\downarrow \qquad\qquad\qquad\qquad \downarrow Br^- \qquad\qquad\qquad \vdots$$

$$CH_2OH - CH_2OH \qquad CH_2OH - CH_2OH \qquad CH_2Br - COOH$$

$$\downarrow Br^-$$

$$CH_2OH - COOH$$

Figure 4. Possible conversions of 1,2-dibromoethane in different bacterial cultures. Several theoretical steps enabling dehalogenation and utilization of this compound are shown. The necessary combination of these activities that yields a complete catabolic route, however, has not yet been found.[3,6,40]

The same compounds can be converted to, respectively, trichloroethanol and 1,2-dichloro-3-propanol by oxidation, but the methanotrophs that carry out these reactions are unable to derive carbon and energy from the products. Recalcitrance is thus caused in part by the absence of the right combination of a set of catabolic enzymes. A similar situation has been described with bacteria that degrade aromatic compounds, and assembly of new catabolic routes for chlorinated aromatics metabolism was proposed.[54]

Accumulation of toxic intermediates also appeared to be a cause of poor degradation of some haloaliphatics. The soil fumigant 1,2-dibromoethane, for example, can be converted by dehalogenase to 2-bromoethanol and ethylene glycol (Figure 4).[6] Furthermore, 2-bromoethanol was a substrate for the halohydrin dehalogenase of another organism, which produced ethylene oxide. Although several reactions were possible, 1,2-dibromoethane was found to be very resistant to degradation. We propose that this was caused by the accumulation of toxic bromoacetaldehyde (formed by alcohol dehydrogenase activity), which is lethal to organisms that carry out the initial dehalogenation. Mutant strains lacking alcohol dehydrogenase still do not utilize 1,2-dibromoethane due to the fact that they could not grow with ethylene glycol. *X. autotrophicus* GJ10 was also very sensitive to the toxic effects of 1,2-dibromoethane (2μM), possibly due to accumulation of aldehyde. Thus, recalcitrance behavior was again caused by the absence of the right combination of metabolic activities in a single organism.

Assembly of new catabolic routes using recombinant DNA techniques for combining catabolic genes from different organisms, as suggested for the degradation of substituted aromatic compounds,[54] could become feasible for the construction of organisms with enhanced catabolic potential.[57] Hydrolytic dehalogenases and monooxygenases would be good targets for such an approach because the substrate ranges of these enzymes generally include several environmentally important compounds that do not support growth of the organisms that produce the enzymes.

Biological Treatment of Chlorinated Hydrocarbons:Prospects

Specialized cultures as described here will become increasingly important for the application of biological techniques for environmental protection and cleanup. Main fields of application include: treatment of industrial waste gases, soil and aquifer decontamination, and elimination of chloroaliphatics from wastewater and groundwater. For slowly growing organisms, immobilization can help to obtain a high steady state level of biomass in the reactor used. With compounds that support growth of microorganisms that perform catabolic reactions, the approach seems straightforward. Only problems related to volatilization are expected. Fluidized bed reactors[43] and trickling filters[44] have been investigated for the elimination of, respectively, dichloromethane and 1,2-dichloroethane from contaminated water. Furthermore, the development of treatment systems for removing chlorinated hydrocarbons from waste gas is under way.[45,46]

An important goal will be to achieve biological removal of chlorinated hydrocarbons by microorganisms that rely on cometabolic conversion. The applicability of methanotrophs for the removal of trichloroethylene and related compounds will be complicated by three factors. First, degradation is cometabolic and requires the availability of another carbon source for stimulating growth of the desired population. Selective growth of the organisms that exhibit the desirable catabolic feat cannot always be achieved simply by adding a growth supporting substrate such as methane or toluene, since this often will not be selective for the required species. This is caused by the fact that cometabolism is very strain-specific.[35,37,38] Thus, only specific cultures of methanotrophs and only certain toluene catabolizing bacteria rapidly degrade trichloroethylene. For the application of such cultures, a detailed insight into the ecophysiology of the organisms will be necessary. The development of recombinant DNA techniques as a tool for studying the distribution of catabolic trates may be very useful to tackle this problem.

A second complicating factor is that oxidative cometabolic conversion requires the presence of a second substrate for supplying reducing equivalents needed by the monooxygenase system. Methane may, because of competition, not be optimal for this purpose. Finally, the first order kinetics, as observed with trichloroethylene, may cause degradation to proceed to sufficiently low levels only after long residence times.

Applicability of methanotrophs has now been studied for aquifer decontamination in the field[47] and with laboratory scale simulation systems for *in situ* biorestoration.[48] A laboratory scale bioreactor for the removal of trichloroethylene and *trans*-1,2-dichloroethylene from contaminated water has also been tested.[49] In general, the observations made indicate that *trans*-1,2-dichloroethylene conversion proceeds more rapidly than trichloroethylene removal. It is well possible that the population of methanotrophs used in these systems was far from optimal.

So far, no aerobic transformation has been found with perchlorinated compounds, although there seems to be no reason why this is impossible *per se*. Anaerobic conversions that cause dechlorination have been described for several highly chlorinated compounds such as carbon tetrachloride, perchloroethylene, and 1,1,1-trichloroethane. These conversions could become very important for removing chlorinated aliphatics at low redox potential, for example, in anaerobic subsurface environments. The rates are generally in the order of 0.1 to 10nmol/min·mg protein,[50] which is rather low compared with what can be achieved with cometabolic trichloroethylene oxidation or with aerobic organisms that use chloroaliphatics as a carbon source.

An interesting option might be to combine anaerobic treatment steps for initial dechlorination of highly chlorinated compounds such as perchloroethylene to trichloroethylenes and dichloroethylenes, with oxidative treatment to give complete mineralization.

Acknowledgments

Our studies have been financed in part by the Werkgroep Milieubiotechnologie and the Dutch Ministry for Housing, Physical Planning and Environment. The work of Dr. Janssen has been made possible by a fellowship from the Royal Netherlands Academy of Sciences.

References

1. J.J. Westerick, J.W. Mello, and R.F. Thomas, *J. Am. Water Works Assoc.* **76**, 52 (1984).
2. T.M. Vogel, C.S. Criddle, and P.L. McCarty, *Environ. Sci. Technol.* **21**, 722 (1987).
3. D.B. Janssen, R. Oldenhuis, A.J. van den Wijngaard, and S. Keuning, unpublished experiments.
4. S. Hartmans *et al.*, *J. Gen. Microbiol.* **132**, 1139 (1986).
5. D.B. Janssen *et al.*, *Appl. Environ. Microbiol.* **163**, 635 (1985).
6. D.B. Janssen, D. Jager, and B. Witholt. *Appl. Environ. Microbiol.* **53**, 561 (1987).
7. T. Omori and M. Alexander, *Appl. Environ. Microbiol.* **35**, 867 (1978).
8. R. Scholtz *et al.*, *J. Gen. Microbiol.* **133**, 267 (1987).
9. T. Yokota *et al.*, *Agric. Biol. Chem.* **50**, 453 (1986).
10. D. Kohler-Staub and T. Leisinger, *J. Bacteriol.* **162**, 676 (1985).
11. D. Kohler-Staub *et al.*, *J. Gen. Microbiol.* **132**, 2837 (1986).
12. R. Scholtz *et al.*, *J. Bacteriol.* **170**, 5698 (1988).
13. G. Stucki and T. Leisinger, *FEMS Microbiol. Lett.* **16**, 123 (1983).
14. S. Hartmans *et al.*, *Biotechnol. Lett.* **7**, 383 (1985).

15. D.J. Hardman and J.H. Slater. *J. Gen. Microbiol.* **123**, 117 (1981).
16. K. Motosugi and K. Soda. *Experientia* **39**, 1214 (1983).
17. D.B. Janssen, S. Keuning, and B. Witholt. *J. Gen. Microbiol.* **133**, 85 (1987).
18. S. Keuning, D.B. Janssen, and B. Witholt. *J. Bacteriol.* **163**, 635 (1985).
19. H.J. Rozeboom *et al.*, *J. Mol. Biol.* **200**, 611 (1988).
20. R. Scholtz *et al.*, *J. Bacteriol.* **169**, 5016 (1987).
21. D.B. Janssen *et al.*, *Eur. J. Biochem.* **171**, 67 (1988).
22. T. Yokota, T. Omori, and T. Kodama. *J. Bacteriol.* **169**, 4049 (1987).
23. M.M. Fogel, A. R. Taddeo, and S. Fogel. *Appl. Environ. Microbiol.* **51**, 720 (1986).
24. J.M. Henson *et al.*, *FEMS Microbiol. Ecol.* **53**, 193 (1988).
25. D.B. Janssen *et al.*, *Appl. Microbiol. Biotechnol.* **29**, 392 (1988).
26. C.D. Little *et al.*, *Appl. Environ. Microbiol.* **54**, 951 (1988).
27. D. Arciero *et al.*, *Biochem. Biophys. Res. Commun.* **159**, 640 (1989).
28. S.E. Strand and L. Shippert. *Appl. Environ. Microbiol.* **52**, 203 (1986).
29. J.T. Wilson and B.H. Wilson. *Appl. Environ. Microbiol.* **49**, 242 (1985).
30. C. Anthony, *Adv. Microbiol. Physiol.* **27**, 113 (1986).
31. J. Colby, D.I. Stirling, and H. Dalton. *Biochem. J.* **165**, 395 (1977).
32. S.A. Kline and B.L. Van Duuren. *J. Org. Chem.* **43**, 3597 (1978).
33. R.E. Miller and F.P. Guengerich. *Biochemistry* **21**, 1090 (1982).
34. R. Oldenhuis *et al.*, *Appl. Environ. Microbiol.*, (1989) in press.
35. K.J. Burrows, *J. Gen. Microbiol.* **130**, 3327 (1984).
36. B.G. Fox and J.D. Lipscomb, *Biochem. Biophys. Res. Commun.* **154**, 165 (1988).
37. M.J.K. Nelson, *Appl. Environ. Microbiol.* **52**, 383 (1987).
38. L.P. Wackett and D. T. Gibson, *Appl. Environ. Microbiol.* **54**, 1703 (1988).
39. C.E. Castro and E.W. Bartnicki, *Biochemistry* **7**, 3213 (1968).
40. A.J. van den Wijngaard, D.B. Janssen, and B. Witholt, *J. Gen. Microbiol.*, (1989), in press.
41. N.O. Belser and C.E. Castro, *J. Agric. Fd. Chem.* **19**, 23 (1971).
42. D. Kohler-Staub and H.-P.E. Kohler, *J. Bacteriol.* **171**, 1428 (1989).
43. R. Gälli, *Appl. Microbiol. Biotechnol.* **27**, 206 (1987).
44. D.D. Friday and R.J. Portier, *Evaluation of a packed bed immobilized microbe bioreactor for the continuous biodegradation of halocarbon-contaminated groundwater.* (AWMA/EPA International Symposium on Biosystems for Pollution Control, Cincinnati, 1989).
45. S.P.P. Ottengraf, *Trends in Biotechn.* **5**, 132 (1987).
46. S.P.P. Ottengraf *et al.*, *Bioproc. Engineering* **1**, 61 (1986).
47. P.L. McCarty, L. Semprini, and P.V. Roberts, *Methodologies for evaluating the feasibility of in-situ biodegradation of halogenated aliphatic groundwater contaminants by methanotrophs.* (Proceedings AWMA/EPA International Symposium on Biosystems for Pollution Control, Cincinnati, 1989).
48. A.T. Moore, A. Vira, and S. Fogel, *Environ. Sci. Technol.* **23**, 403 (1989).
49. G.W. Strandberg, T.L. Donaldson, and L.L. Bolla, *Environ. Sci. Technol.*, (1989) in press.
50. R. Gälli and P.L. McCarty, *Appl. Environ. Microbiol.* **55**, 845 (1989)
51. G. Stucki, U. Krebser, and T. Leisinger, *Experientia* **39**, 1271 (1983).
52. W. Brunner, D. Staub, and T. Leisinger, *Appl. Environ. Microbiol.* **40**, 950 (1980).

53. C.B. Fliermans *et al.*, *Appl. Environ. Microbiol.* **54**, 1709 (1988).
54. F. Rojo *et al.*, *Science* **238**, 1395 (1987).
55. G. Stucki *et al.*, *Arch. Microbiol.* **130**, 366 (1981).
56. R. Scholtz *et al.*, *Appl. Environ. Microbiol.* **54**, 3034 (1988).
57. R.B. Winter, K.-M. Yen, and B.D. Ensley, *Biotechnology* **7**, 282 (1989).

Methods and Applications in Biodegradation

8

Principles of and Assay Systems for Biodegradation

J.P.E. Anderson

Bayer A.G.
Crop Protection Research
Chemical Product Development
and Environmental Biology
Institute For
Ecological Biology
D-5090 Leverkusen,
Bayerwerk
Federal Republic of Germany

The biodegradation of organic substrates in liquid, moist solid, or flooded solid matrices is regulated by the structure of the substrate, the availability of the substrate to reactive sites, the quantities and distribution of the reactive sites, and if the substrate is being degraded by living cells, the activity level of the cells. This paper describes five systems for assaying biodegradation. Four systems are for the assay of aerobic biodegradation, and one is for the assay of anaerobic biodegradation. One system for aerobic biodegradation can be used conveniently with radiolabeled substrates.

Introduction

This paper deals with the selection of assay systems for biodegradation. Biodegradation is a catabolic process in which biologically formed entities convert substrates into less complex intermediates or end products. The entities mediating degradation can be as simple as cell-free enzyme preparations or as complex as intact microbial populations in soils. The process of biodegradation can be a single-step conversion in the catabolism of a substrate or a chain of conversions in which a substrate is reduced to its basic components.

The system chosen for assaying biodegradation can also be simple or complex. Here, the degree of complexity will depend on the biodegradation process under study and the needs of the investigator.

No single assay system will fit all needs. Because selection of an effective assay system is aided by a basic understanding of the principles of biodegradation, the first section of this paper will briefly discuss variables known to influence both the rates and the extent of substrate degradation. The second section will discuss a series of questions that will aid in the selection of an appropriate system. The final section will describe four assays for aerobic and one for anaerobic biodegradation. The principles discussed will apply to biodegradation in any matrix in any assay system; the assay systems discussed were selected on the basis of analytical simplicity and broadness in their range of application. For more extensive reviews of special assay systems and special analytical methods, the reader is referred to other publications.[1,7]

A number of terms will be repeatedly used in this paper: "substrate" means the material subjected to biodegradation; "bioreactive sites" or "reactive sites" are enzymes, enzyme systems, intact cells, microorganisms, or combinations of these that have the capacity to degrade the substrate; "matrix" means the liquids, moist solids, or flooded solids in which biodegradation is being investigated; and "system" or "assay system" means the container (and its parts) that encloses or holds the matrix during biodegradation.

Variables Regulating Biodegradation Rates

In any matrix, be it liquid nutrient medium, natural water, a soil, a soil slurry, a compost, a sediment or a sludge, four major variables determine the rates and extent of substrate biodegradation. These are the structure of the substrate, the availability of the substrate to bioreactive sites, the quantities of bioreactive sites, and the activity levels of the bioreactive sites.[8,9] Interacting with these variables to speed or slow biodegradation are the temperature, moisture content, aeration, and pH of the matrix.

Structure of Substrate

The structure of a substrate determines whether or not it is bio-degradable. If a substrate is biodegradable, the chemical bonds that hold it together determine how much energy is needed to start and maintain degradation reactions, and, if intact cells are responsible for biodegradation, the amount of energy that can be won by the cells by breaking the bonds.

The initial steps in degradation of water-soluble, energy-rich substrates (for example, glucose) by most intact cells or microorganisms requires energy for transport of the substance through the cell membrane. This expended energy can first be regained when the cells metabolize the substrate. Biodegradation of hydrophilic but water-insoluble substrates (for example, cellulose) initially costs cells both energy and cell substance. Enzymes must be synthesized and then released into the solution that wets the substrate. After extracellular degradation starts, cells must expend further energy to take up the degradation products and transport these into the cytoplasm. Only there can the products be metabolized with a gain of energy and building materials. Some substrates require a high and constant input of energy for their biodegradation that can only be obtained through the cometabolism of a second, readily degradable substrate. Without energy input, degradation proceeds at low rates, which make accurate measurement quite difficult. Examples of such substrates are some of the humus fractions of soil and some synthetic organic compounds such as DDT.

The elemental composition of a substrate determines its nutrient value and can thereby determine both the speed and extent of its biodegradation. If substances of otherwise equal stability and physical characteristics enter matrices in which essential elements are limiting (for example, groundwater, soils, or subsoils), the materials with the highest nutrient value (for example, with the most favorable C/N, C/P, and C/S ratios) will be degraded most rapidly and most extensively.

The physical behavior of a substrate is determined by its structure. The structure determines whether or not the substrate will volatilize from the matrix, whether or not it is water-soluble or wettable, whether or not it will clump, and whether or not it will be adsorbed or bind to solids in the matrix.

Substances whose structures make them water-repellent (for example oils, waxes) usually resist biodegradation. The enzymatic attack and subsequent degradation of these materials occur best if cells produce and secrete their own emulsifiers. In such cases, biodegradation occurs at the water-solvent interfaces.[10]

Availability of Substrate to Bioreactive Sites

In any matrix, biodegradation can only take place when the substrate and the bioreactive sites come into contact. This obvious geometric fact is often forgotten or ignored when data on the kinetics of biodegradation or even on the biodegradability of substrates are interpreted. Assay systems containing liquid matrices without suspended solids (for example, aqueous solutions containing water-soluble substrates and soluble enzymes) are the simplest in their geometry; they allow the greatest freedom of movement and provide the greatest opportunity for contact between substrate and reactive sites. In liquid matrices, the geometry of contact increases in complexity when slightly soluble or insoluble substances clump together or crystallize out of solution. This retards the movement of these materials and exposes less surface area to attack. The geometry in liquid matrices is even further complicated when the system contains suspended solids. In water-sediment systems, both the substrates and the bioreactive sites, be these extracellular enzymes or intact microbial cells, can be adsorbed or chemically bound to solids. In moist solid matrices (soils, composts) with their tricompartmental structure (that is, liquid, solid, and air spaces), the geometry is most complex, and biodegradation is most difficult to regulate or predict. In such matrices, the rates of desorption of one or both parties and the diffusion patterns that result from repeated adsorption/desorption determine the rates of degradation. With some substrates, binding can be so avid that transport and biodegradation stop.

In matrices where substrates partition between aqueous and solid phases, as in soils containing small quantities of plant protection chemicals, the total amount added to the matrix determines the total concentration in solution. This directly influences the total amount degraded per unit time. In such systems, the highest nontoxic quantity of substrate usually gives the maximum amount of degradation product(s). Similarly, in any matrix, the amounts of free water (solvent) and the temperature influence the amount of substrate in solution and, thereby, the amount of product formed per unit time.

Quantity of Active Sites

The quantities of bioreactive sites in a matrix, measured as enzyme titers or as cell mass, directly influence the rates of biodegradation of most substrates. This can be readily seen when substrates that are degraded by specialized cells (for example, cellulose, chitin, keratin, some plant protection chemicals) are repeatedly added to matrices such as natural waters, sediments, or soils. In such cases, each renewed addition increases the rates of degradation, and this continues until an essential element becomes limiting or the degradation products poison the system. Such accelerations of degradation can have two causes: the specialists responsible for degradation use the substrate for production of new biomass or the cell mass at large is induced to produce greater quantities of degradative enzymes. To maintain or further increase degradation rates, enzyme titers or cell mass must be maintained or further produced.

Activity Level of Active Sites

One of the most important variables regulating biodegradation rates is the activity level of the bioreactive sites. This determines the quantity of substrate degraded per unit bioreactive site (enzyme titer or biomass) per unit time. The activity level is influenced by variables that can often be readily manipulated; these include the temperature of the system, the pH, the amount of available moisture in the matrix, and the amounts of oxygen or other electron acceptors available to the bioreactive sites.

Brief Survey of Assay Systems

No single assay system will fit all needs. To select the most effective system, several points must be considered:

1. Will biodegradation take place under aerobic or anaerobic conditions? The answer determines whether or not an airtight assay system is needed.
2. Which type of bioreactive sites will be involved in biodegradation? If purified enzymes or pure cultures of plant, animal, or microbial cells are to be used, the parts of the assay system that come in contact with the matrix must be able to withstand sterilization, and the system must be closed to foreign infections during biodegradation.
3. How will biodegradation be measured? This is the most complex question, and the answer will depend on the needs and the resources of the investigator. Measurement can be as simple as monitoring the uptake or production of respiratory gases, or as complex as bioassay, and chemical or radiochemical analysis of matrix extracts for substrate residues and/or metabolite production.

During aerobic biodegradation of most substances, oxygen is consumed and carbon dioxide is released. During anaerobic degradation, mainly carbon dioxide and methane are released. This uptake or release of gases during metabolism has been utilized by many researchers and has led to development of a battery of technically simple but highly effective assay systems. This paper describes five such systems. The systems were selected to present various degrees of technical sophistication; they range in complexity from handmade, manually operated respirometers to technically advanced, fully automated systems. Regardless of which system is selected, it is obvious that biodegradation can be and often is assayed by methods other than gas exchange. A system that has been used extensively to study the biodegradation of radiolabeled plant protection chemicals in soils has been included as an example of the combination of gas exchange analysis and other means.

Simple System for Assay of Oxygen Consumption

A simple, low-cost assay system for measurement of oxygen consumption in short term-experiments is shown in Figure 1. The unit can be used with all matrices but is best used with moist solids (soils, composts). To use the unit, the matrix and a small quantity of alkali solution (1N KOH) are sealed in the chamber, and the manometer is filled to a calibration mark with water. During incubation, oxygen is consumed, and carbon dioxide is released. Because the carbon dioxide is adsorbed in the alkali, it does not add to the gas volume in the chamber; the net result is a decrease in gas volume within the chamber. This decrease is measured as a change in height of the fluid in the manometer; from this change, the volume of oxygen consumed can be determined. Because one arm of the manometer is open to the ambient air, atmospheric pressure changes must be corrected for by use of a thermobarometer (a unit containing a nonreactive solid having the same volume as that of the matrix).

The advantages of this system are its simplicity and its low costs. The unit can be constructed from components available in most laboratories, and no special training is required for its use. If needed, the quantities of carbon dioxide released during biodegradation can be determined by titration analysis of the alkali solution. The system is best used with grams per kilogram quantities of substrate. The assay system has several disadvantages. Oxygen consumption readings are manual; after each reading, the system should be briefly ventilated (stopcock opened) to allow the partial pressure of oxygen in the flask to return to that in the ambient atmosphere. Further, for the calculation of results, a "flask constant" must be established for each unit. The construction and use of such units are described in detail elsewhere.[1]

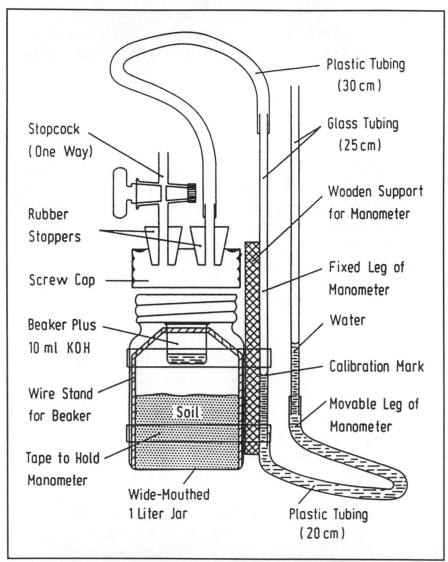

Figure 1. Large volume incubation unit for manometric assay of oxygen consumption during biodegradation.[1]

Automated System for Assay of Oxygen Consumption

An automated, commercially available system for measurement of oxygen consumption is shown in Figure 2 (Sapromat from

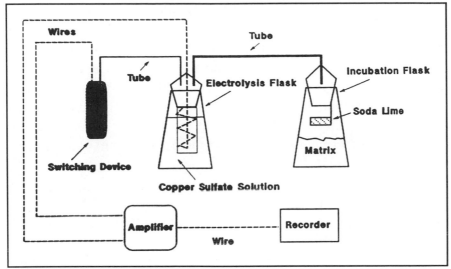

Figure 2. Automated system for assay of oxygen consumption during aerobic degradation of substrates in liquid, moist solid, or flooded solid matrices.[1]

Voith Inc., D-7920, Heidenheim, Germany). This unit can be used with all matrices and comes with either six or twelve 500-ml capacity sample flasks as standard equipment. Liquid matrices can be agitated with magnetic stirrers. The reaction flasks of the instrument are connected by tubing to two further containers, one of which holds an electrolyte and two platinum wires and serves as a switching device, and one of which contains a saturated solution of copper sulfate and serves as an electrolytic cell. During use, the air spaces of the three flasks are united as a closed system. As carbon dioxide is produced, it is adsorbed by granular soda lime, which is held in a small container in the flask containing the matrix and thus does not contribute to the volume of gas in the system. As oxygen is consumed, pressure within the system is reduced; this reduction draws an electrolyte solution in the switching device into a capillary containing a platinum wire. Contact between the wire and the salt solution closes a circuit; after amplification, current is sent through the electrolysis cell. The resulting electrolytic decomposition of copper sulfate releases oxygen, which increases the pressure in the system and forces the electrolyte out of contact with the wire. This breaks the circuit, and electrolysis ceases. The volume of oxygen produced, which is equal to the volume consumed during biodegradation of the substrate, is computed from the current used. The results are registered either as a numerical printout or as a cumulative curve on a strip chart. The unit is well designed, uses rugged glassware, and provides reliable service. The unit does, however, require several hours to stabilize and requires special attention for use in short-term (one to four hours) experiments. It is effectively used with grams per kilogram quantities of substrate.

Simple System for Assay of Carbon Dioxide Production

A flow-through system for monitoring the release of carbon dioxide in long-term biodegradation studies is shown in Figure 3. The system is best used with moist solid matrices (soils or composts) and grams per kilogram quantities of substrate. The reaction flask consists of a screw-capped jar with a volume of either 350 or 700ml. The center of the plastic screw cap is bored with a 3-cm diameter hole. Beneath the cap, the jar is sealed with a 2-mm thick rubber membrane through which two holes have been punched. One hole holds a capillary flow regulator that serves as an air inlet; the other hole holds a teflon tube that serves as an outlet. The flask is swept with approximately 30ml of carbon dioxide-free air per minute. Carbon dioxide-free air is prepared by drawing ambient air first through a series of 500-ml wash flasks containing 250ml each of 1N NaOH and then drawing the air through a cylinder that contains about 250g of soda lime. The dried "carbon dioxide-free" air (that can contain traces of carbon dioxide) is forced through an aquarium pump into a manifold that is connected by small pieces of tubing to the capillary inlets of 50 such reaction flasks. The inlets of the flasks contain matched pieces (2cm long) of thick-walled capillary glass that act as fine regulators for the flow of gas through the units. To regulate the pressure in the manifold and therefore the flow of gas to the capillary inlets, the exit of the manifold is fitted with an adjustable needle valve. By means of this valve, the

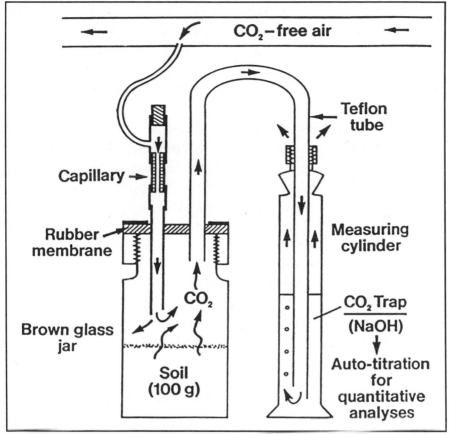

Figure 3. Incubation unit for assaying release of carbon dioxide during aerobic biodegradation of substrates in moist solid matrices.

overall flow rates in all of the units can be roughly adjusted. The fine regulation of air flow, which gives roughly equal flow rates (for example, 30 ± 5ml/min) through each flask, is determined by the matched capillary units. When carbon dioxide is released from the matrix, it is carried with the stream of air from the jar into a 50ml glass cylinder containing 40ml of 1N NaOH. To prevent saturation of the NaOH trap with carbon dioxide from the atmosphere, the exit of the cylinder, which is fitted with a stopper, is reduced to the size of a pinhole which lets the air in the trap out but prevents a backwash of atmospheric air into the cylinder. The carbon dioxide content of the alkali solution can be quantitatively analyzed by titration.

This system has several advantages. It is readily constructed from simple materials and can accommodate large numbers of respiration units. Through the use of matched capillaries, the flow rates through the units are almost identical, and variations between respirometers are minimal. A leak in any of the units has no effect on any other unit because the air is forced into each flask via a capillary; hence, the pressure in the system is at the entrances of the capillaries. Leaks in individual flasks influence those flasks only. In systems that pull air through the respirometers, a leak in any part of the system stops the air flow through all units. The major disadvantage of this system is the need to analyze the alkali solution by titration. For large numbers of samples, this problem is readily solved by use of a computer controlled autotitrator (double end-point titration) equipped with a sample changer. If the titrator and sample changer are enclosed in a chamber that is continuously flushed with carbon dioxide-free air, large numbers of samples can be analyzed conveniently and rapidly.

System for use With Radiolabelled Substrates

An assay system for measurement of the biodegradation of radiolabeled substances is shown in Figure 4. The system consists of an incubation chamber plus a cartridge for trapping radioactive carbon dioxide. Oxygen moves into the flasks by diffusion. This takes place through a layer of granulated soda lime and a cotton plug held in a glass column, which serves as an elongated neck of the incubation chamber. Gas chromatographic analyses of the atmosphere in the flasks during incubation have shown that the concentration of oxygen in the flask is equal to that of the ambient atmosphere. Figure 4 shows that the lower layer of soda lime in the neck of the flask serves as the trap for radioactive carbon dioxide. For long-term experiments, it is advisable to use an upper layer of soda lime to protect the lower layer from saturation with atmospheric carbon dioxide.

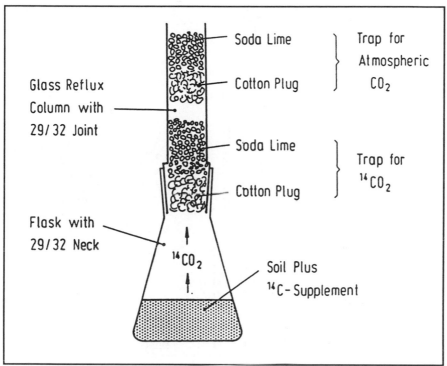

Figure 4. Incubation unit for assaying release of radiolabeled carbon dioxide during aerobic degradation of ^{14}C-labeled substrates in liquid, moist solid, or flooded solid matrices.[1,11]

This system is quite versatile and has been used for assaying the degradation of radiolabeled substrates in liquid matrices (shake cultures of plant cells, pure cultures of microorganisms); moist solids (soils, compost); and flooded solids (sediments).[1,11] It has been extensively used for studying the biodegradation of milligrams per kilogram quantities of radiolabeled plant protection chemicals in soils. By extraction and analysis of the matrices, distribution of the parent materials and their degradation products can be readily followed. By replacing the glass wool plug in the cartridge beneath the soda lime with an oil-coated glass wool plug, volatile radioactive products other than carbon dioxide can also be investigated. A full description of this assay system, the chamber used for transferring radiolabeled carbon dioxide from the soda lime to an alkaline solution

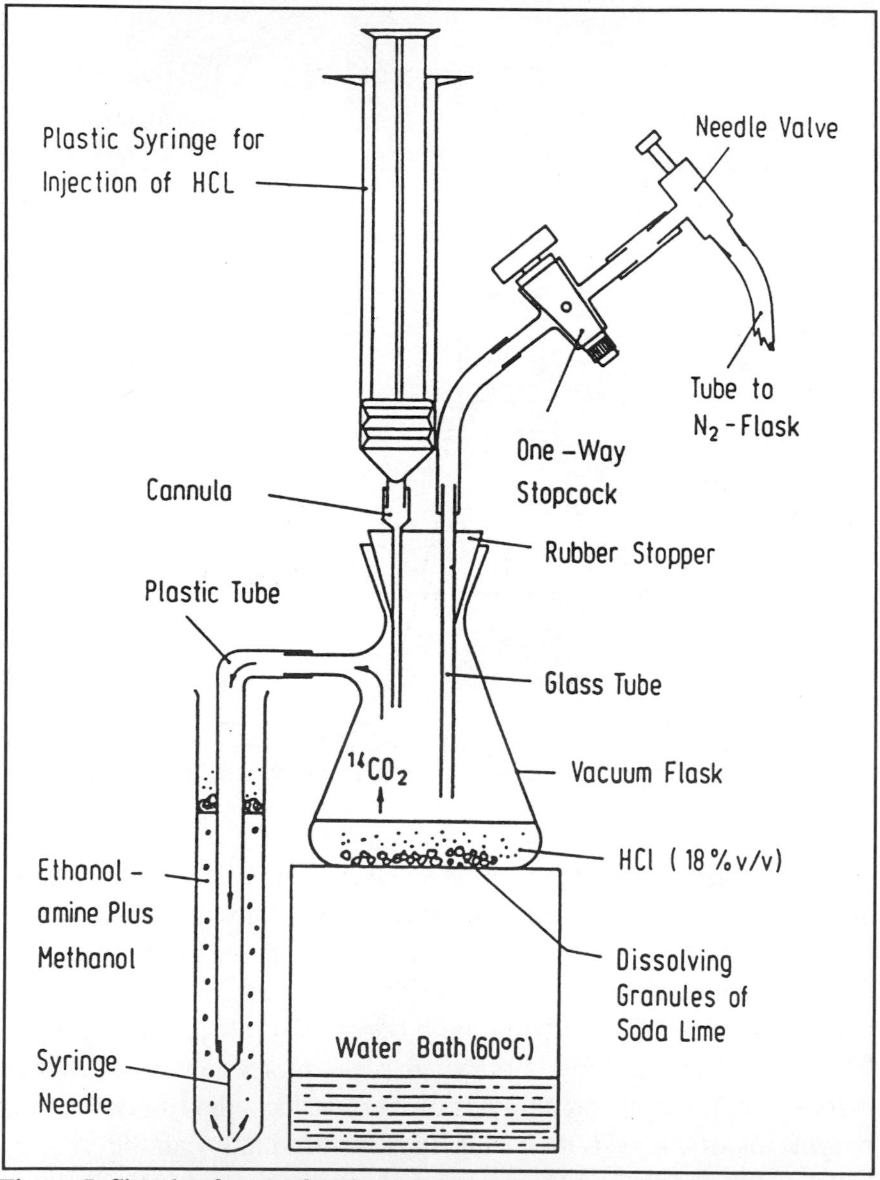

Figure 5. Chamber for transfer of radiolabeled carbon dioxide to alkaline solution for scintillation counting.[1]

(for example, ethanolamine plus methanol, 1N NaOH) for scintillation counting (Figure 5), and the variety of uses of the system is given elsewhere.[1,8,9]

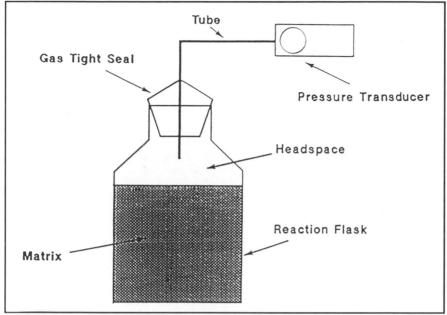

Figure 6. Incubation unit for assaying release of gases (mainly carbon dioxide and methane) during biodegradation of substrates in liquid, moist solid, or flooded solid matrices.[14]

System for Assay of Anaerobic Biodegradation

Figure 6 shows a simple vessel for assaying anaerobic biodegradation. The method of assay is based on the release of carbon dioxide and methane as the two main gaseous end products of anaerobic biodegradation. The exact design of the apparatus is not critical. The system must be airtight and must have a means of measurement of the amounts of gas produced. For measurement of gas volumes, a hand-held pressure meter (John Watson and Smith, Ltd., Leeds, England) attached to a three-way inlet valve can be used conveniently.[12,13] For calculation of results, the total volume of the container, the volume of the matrix, and the volume of the gas phase must be known. For effective use, the volume of the matrix phase should not be less than 40 percent of the total vessel volume.[14] The system is best used with grams per kilogram quantities of substrate.

This assay system is very simple; because of the solubility of carbon dioxide and methane in the aqueous phase, the system is not particularly accurate. It can be used for rough estimations of biodegradation activity. For precise measurements, analyses of matrices for substrate loss or metabolite production are usually necessary. Using parallel samples, it is possible to differentiate between the amounts of carbon dioxide and methane produced by adsorption of the carbon dioxide. For precise analyses, however, work with radiolabeled substances is most convenient.

References

1. J.P.E. Anderson, *Methods of Soil Analysis, Part 2. Chemical and Microbiological Properties – Agronomy Monograph No. 9 (2nd Ed.)* 831, (1982).
2. Amtsblatt der Europ. Gemeinschaft, *Biologische Abbaubarkeit, Nr. L 133/99 - L 133/ 127* (1988).
3. W.C. Evans, *Nature* **207**, 17 (1977).
4. J.A. Guth, *Process Pesticide Biochemi* .**2**, 85 (1981).
5. Organisation for Economic Cooperation and Development, *Guidelines for Testing Chemicals, Section 3*, Paris (1981).
6. R.J. Shimp and R.L. Young, *Ecotox. Eviron. Safety* **14**, 223 (1987).
7. D.F. Toerien and W.H.J. Hattingh, *Water Res.* **3**, 385 (1969).
8. J.P.E. Anderson, *Pflanzenproduktion* **6**, in press.
9. H. Frehse and J.P.E. Anderson, International Union of Pure and Applied Chemistry Pesticide Chem., *Human Welfare and the Environment* **2**, 23 (1983).
10. R.S. Boething, *Environ. Toxicol. Chem.* **3**, 5 (1984).
11. K. Scholz et al., *Pests and Diseases*, (Brighton Corp Protection Conference, 3B-4, Brighton, 1988), p. 149.
12. N.S. Battersby and V. Wilson, *Chemosphere* **17**, 2441 (1988).
13. D.R. Sheldon and J.M. Tiedje, *Appl. Environ. Microbiol.* **47**, 850 (1984).
14. European Chemical Industry Ecology and Toxicology Centre, Technical Report No. 28 (1988).

Discussion

Salkinoja-Salonen: I found it very interesting that you were trying to set the framework for studying biodegradation in natural ecosystems. Did you observe correlation between toxicity and the moisture content of the soil? Some chemicals are more toxic depending on the pH because they are sometimes phenols or acids and sometimes ionized, but would the moisture influence the toxicity? Also, how long does the soil preserve its biodegradation capacity for a given chemical?

Anderson: The moisture in the soil has a definite influence on both the toxicity and degradation of compounds. Usually, increasing the water content of the soil increases degradation. However, if you increase to the point of flooding you exclude air from the soil, which slows degradation. If a soil containing a compound gets too dry, the toxicity usually decreases. If the same soil is dampened, the toxic potential returns. We work in our laboratory with freshly collected soils. This gives us reasonably reproducible results. You can look at the soil and see how fast the total microbial biomass degenerates. For example, we studied biomass degeneration in moist, stored soils at 20 to 22°C for 3 months; approximately 50 different soils from different parts of the world were studied. Under these conditions, between 30 percent and 50 percent of the total biomass is lost; both bacteria and fungi die or go into resting conditions in the soil. In general, storage of moist soils at room temperature not only causes a loss of microbial biomass but also decreases the general degradation potential of the soil.

Bedard: You commented that you did not like the method that Tiedje uses with the pressure transducer. Could you elaborate?

Anderson: When working with this system, one knows that carbon dioxide and methane are produced, but one cannot quantify how much of each is present in the gaseous mixture, or how much is dissolved in the liquid phase of the matrix.

Bedard: They can be quantified by gas chromatography.

Anderson: Yes, they can. We can work in all of our systems with gas chromatography as an analytical tool, but we want a simple method of analysis for the first steps of our screening, one where the carbon dioxide can be separated from the methane. For example, we are considering setting up parallel flasks to absorb the carbon dioxide. Then you could estimate the quantity of methane.

Bedard: But you are not saying that it is an invalid measurement?

Anderson: By no means.

Young: You can measure gas volume as you do with the CO_2 anaerobically, and if you have gas volume over background, that would be a very good indication of anaerobic decomposition. It is as simple as your previously described systems other than to have to keep oxygen out of it.

Anderson: Could you suggest how you separate the amounts of carbon dioxide from those of methane?

Young: I was responding to your answer to Dr. Bedard's question. If you want a first-cut that is very simple, gas volume itself would do it. Then for those samples that are interesting, you could proceed with either gas chromatography analysis or, as you suggested, absorbing the CO_2 and looking at the methane.

9

Military Applications of Biodegradation

F. Prescott Ward

U.S. Army Chemical Research, Development and Engineering Center
Aberdeen Proving Ground, MD 21010-5423

The molecular processes involved in microbial and enzymatic degradation are being exploited by agencies of the U.S. Department of Defense in diverse ways. Biodegradation often provides an attractive alternative or adjunct to conventional methods of restoring contaminated soils or groundwater. On the battlefield, enzymatic catalysis could provide significant operational gains in decontaminating chemical and biological warfare agents and could offer novel modes of medical protection and therapy for the same agents. Denitrification of propellant grains has been accomplished experimentally at ambient temperatures, and the prospect of enzyme-based biosensors heralds a bright future for detecting and monitoring xenobiotics and other compounds in industrial, environmental, and medical settings.

Introduction

In this paper, biodegradation refers to the use of microorganisms or enzymes to break down chemical compounds. Applications include detoxification and bioreclamation of toxic waste sites, battlefield decontamination of chemical and biological warfare agents, and injectable enzymes. Microbial and enzymatic degradative processes are yielding novel products useful in the propellants field. Finally, enzymes coupled to miniature electrical or optical devices can be used as rapid and sensitive biosensors. Each of these applications has significant military utility.

Bioreclamation of military toxic waste sites. This is the topic of a broad U.S. Department of Defense (DOD) proposal submitted last year for funding. In 1980, Congress enacted legislation (unofficially called "Superfund") to identify, finance, and monitor cleanup of the nation's most serious hazardous waste dumps. Currently, DOD has 739 sites in need of remediation, and cleanup costs are estimated at five to 10 billion U.S. dollars. The number of U.S. military bases on the Superfund list has recently been expanded from 38 to 53, with 32 on the National Priorities List.

The primary hazardous wastes found on military installations are fuels and cleaning solvents. Other major contaminants include pesticides, heavy metals, industrial chemicals, propellants and explosives, acids, radium, and uranium.

Virtually all conventional technologies for land reclamation have proved to be unsatisfactory. For example, landfilling is not a permanent solution, and costs are increasing dramatically (in the United States, from US$10 to US$250 per ton in the last five years). Incineration produces toxic air pollutants, and many organic compounds are difficult to burn. *In situ* solidification (chemical fixation), capping, and vitrification are largely unproved, costly, and aesthetically objectionable technologies. Volatile organics in groundwater have been removed via strategically located slotted wells and by airstripping where contaminated groundwater is pumped through large, packed-bed towers; both are costly, labor-intensive solutions.

In contrast, bioprocessing or biodegradation often provides a low-technology, permanent, inexpensive, effective, nonpolluting alternative for land reclamation and treatment of industrial effluents.[1] Microbes have evolved or can be genetically altered to degrade virtually any toxic organic chemical. Hydrocarbons, a major class of military wastes, are particularly susceptible to biodegradation. Detoxification using microbes or enzyme systems can often be accomplished on site without excavation or elaborate containment procedures. When excavation is required, decomposition can be achieved using simple composting procedures. Biodegradation is effective over a range of environmental conditions and for a wide variety of contaminants. Often, bioprocesses can be integrated with conventional technologies, resulting in efficient, multicomponent systems. In addition to degrading organic chemicals, microbes that actively sequester heavy metals can be used for leaching soils contaminated with toxic or radioactive metals. (Such biosequestering processes have been applied successfully in commercial mining operations.)

The biodegradation program developed by the U.S. Department of Defense has three broad categories: *in situ* degradation, treatment and processing of excavated landfills, and purification of groundwater and aquifers. Specific program areas include:

1. Determining factors to optimize biodegradation under laboratory and field conditions,
2. Use of immobilized microbes and enzymes for biodegradation, and development of field bioreactors,
3. Adapting existing technologies to produce, distribute, and apply large batches of microbes,
4. Studying mechanisms of biodegradation including metabolic pathways; identification, isolation and characterization of degradative enzymes; oxidative versus reductive catabolism; symbiotic relationships among organisms; nutrient requirements; and location and sequences of important genes,
5. Genetic engineering of detoxifying microbes,
6. Strategies for degrading adsorbed contaminants, and novel technologies for purifying groundwater.

Battlefield decontamination of chemical and biological warfare agents. Battlefield decontamination is a rather specific application of biodetoxification. Currently, fielded military decontaminants have many disadvantages. They are bulk liquids; thus the logistical burden of transporting them on the battlefield is immense. They are toxic, caustic (one formulation is an excellent paint remover), and must be used at full strength. Special equipment must be used to disperse them, a rinse is required, and they are quite expensive. Their major advantage is that they decontaminate all chemical and biological agents.

On the other hand, catalytic enzymes could be fielded in concentrated or powdered formulations; they are mild reagents, cheap, one-step, and easy to use. Their major liability is that they are class-specific; for example, many different enzymes would have to be developed to assure comprehensive decontamination capabilities for all classes of chemical and biological warfare agents.

Current U.S. military doctrine identifies three levels of decontamination:

1. Basic soldier skills involve a personal wipe-down of body and equipment, and spraying of frequently touched surfaces.
2. Hasty decontamination permits a unit to fight longer by removing gross contamination and limiting its spread. Superficial vehicle wash-down and change of protective clothing are accomplished as soon as practical.
3. Deliberate decontamination is normally performed behind the lines by a special unit, with assistance from contaminated soldiers. The goal is to reduce contamination to negligible levels; this requires considerable effort, large quantities of decontamination solution and other supplies, and much coordination.

Enzymes in reconstitutable form could provide significant operational gains in the basic and hasty scenarios but, because of the volumes required and other factors, would probably not offer any advantage over conventional solutions in deliberate decontamination. Enzymes would obviously be quite useful as skin decontaminants and as ingredients in protective skin creams. Other applications could involve incorporation into materials such as fibers, fabrics, filters, and paints to provide for self-decontamination.

Of most interest in agent decontamination is recently published work on enzyme activity in organic solvents.[2] Many enzymes in solvents not only continue to catalyze reactions but can also be heated to quite high temperatures without denaturing and with catalytic activity increased proportionately. Scientists at the U.S. Army Chemical Research, Development and Engineering Center have discovered many enzymes from diverse sources that degrade several classes of threat agents. Incorporation of enzymes with inert solvents in an aerosol can could provide for a type of decon that is currently impossible: vehicle interiors, aircraft cockpits, electrical equipment, and the like.

Another type of military decontamination is called demilitarization: the detoxification of obsolete stocks of chemical warfare agents. Microbial and enzymatic approaches were recently considered but were rejected for a variety of reasons. Enzymes (or microbes) are not currently available for all types of agents to be destroyed. This type of demilitarization would require draining agents from munitions and containers; fermenters could detoxify agents, but furnaces would still be needed to destroy explosives and to decontaminate munition bodies. The nature of a biological demilitarization process would be quite similar to the much simpler chemical neutralization, but in the former, agents would not be completely destroyed, and the process would generate a great amount of solid wastes. Biodetoxification would require dilution of drained agents by a factor of approximately 5,000 before destruction; this would require huge fermenters. High aeration rates from large fermenters would dictate use of large scrubbers. Fermentation would be slow compared with incineration, requiring at least 25 hours for 99 percent destruction of the agent, and fermenters would require significant inputs of energy, nutrients, and other resources. Finally, biodemilitarization would not be possible for munitions containing unidentified chemical agents.

Injectable enzymes. These enzymes comprise the final category of biodetoxification (biodegradation). Until recently, parenteral enzyme therapy in humans was generally not feasible because enzymes, as foreign proteins, elicit immune responses (for example, anaphylactic shock). However, the attachment of polyethylene glycol (PEG) "hairs" to an enzyme molecule's surface confers several desirable attributes: the protein is rendered nonantigenic; the half-life in the blood stream is markedly extended in most cases; the enzyme's active site is not sterically occluded, and catalysis proceeds normally.[3-5] There is considerable military interest in using PEG-treated, agent-degrading enzymes as protective and therapeutic agents in the event of exposure to chemical or biological agents.

Novel propellants. Propellants are currently being produced experimentally using microbial-enzymatic degradative processes. For example, nitrocellulose is a polymer commonly used as a propellant for small-arms ammunition. When fully nitrated, there are three energetic nitrate ester groups per polymeric repeating unit; when ignited, the fully nitrated polymer burns at a maximum rate and generates the most gas.

Deterrents are materials that are diffused into nitrocellulose propellant grains (for example, gunpowder) to remove nitrate groups near the surface and thus slow the initial burn rate. For various physical reasons, maximum ballistics performance is attained if gas (pressure) is generated evenly in the gun tube during a burn cycle. Early in the cycle when the propellant-bed surface area is at its maximum, a diminished burn rate produces pressure equivalent to a full burn of the spherical central specks of propellant left at the end of the cycle.

Conventional methods of diffusing chemical deterrents into propellant grains involve raising the process temperature to approximately 70°C; powder plants have sometimes exploded as a result. Other disadvantages include lot-to-lot ballistic variations, plus the possibility that deterrent migration can occur under extreme storage conditions.

Recently, scientists at the U.S. Army Armament Research, Development and Engineering Center have demonstrated that denitrating microbes, such as *Aspergillus fumigatus*[6] and denitrating enzymes can perform the deterrence function at ambient temperatures. Furthermore, the process can be terminated at any time (kill the microbes, denature the enzymes), thus controlling batch variations and obviating subsequent deterrent migration.

Enzyme-based biosensors. The only commercialized examples of a family of emerging detectors that marry biological materials to miniature electrical or optical devices are the enzyme-based biosensors.[7] In enzyme-based configurations, a redox reaction occurring on the surface of a probe transduces an electrochemical signal. An example is immobilization of glucose oxidase on the surface of a tiny probe to provide real-time monitoring of levels of blood glucose.

Military interest and development are focused on the use of antibodies and neuroreceptors on capacitance chips (electrical) and fiberoptic waveguides (optical) to detect chemical and biological warfare agents. However, there is burgeoning interest in using immobilized enzymes for detection and monitoring in the workplace, for environmental use, and for medical applications.

In summary, processes involved in microbial and enzymatic biodegradation are being exploited in innovative ways by agencies of the U.S. Department of Defense. Examples include reclamation and restoration of contaminated lands, treatment of industrial effluents, battlefield decontamination, medical prophylaxis and therapy, novel propellants, and enzyme-based biosensors.

References

1. K. Gold and B.W. Brodman, U.S. Patent No. 4, 756, 832 (July 12, 1988).
2. A. Zaks and A. Klibanov, *Science* **224**, 1249 (1984).
3. F.F. Davis *et al.*, *Enzyme Eng.* **4**, 169 (1978).
4. K.J. Wieder, *Diss. Abstr. Int.* **39**, 5368 (1979).
5. F.F. Davis and A. Abuchowski, *Polymer. Prep.* **27**, 5 (1986).
6. B.W. Brodman and M.P. Devine, *J. Appl. Polym. Sci.* **26**, 997 (1981).
7. P. Knight, *Bio/Technol.* **7**, 175 (1989).

Discussion

Eveleigh: Why not compost residues of explosives? The stuff has been sitting there for 10 years anyway; why not take a little more time now and simply let it go through a low-cost treatment?

Ward: Where biological remediation is not expected to be effective by itself, it should be considered for use with conventional treatments, including composting. I agree with you.

Timmis: The whole idea of chemical warfare surely is to slow down the opposition and to knock them out for a while. I cannot imagine that enzymes would be as rapid as chemical means of decontamination. If a platoon has been hit by a chemical weapon, I would think it would be much more effective in terms of response time to use chemical decontamination, especially if the opposition was advancing.

Ward: The decontamination kit currently fielded for personal use by troops consists of little "handy-wipe" towelettes. Each soldier opens a foil packet and pulls out a towel that has phenol and other chemicals on it. These do not cover an awful lot of surface area. To be able to decontaminate significant areas not only of yourself but also of your rifle and other pieces of equipment that you need to sustain combat, the unit has to carry relatively large amounts of the liquids that I mentioned before. The philosophy in the U.S. Army right now is that we are moving away from a 19,000-man division, which is extremely heavy in armor (lots of Abrams M1 tanks, lots of Bradley fighting vehicles), because we simply do not have the airlift or sealift capacity to get that stuff rapidly where we might need it (in Africa or Central America or other trouble spots). The emerging philosophy favors the so-called light division of 10,000 men; everybody up to rank of company commander would walk and would be able to sustain combat for 72 hours with nothing more than he carries. Combat scenarios are evolving so that they will not resemble grand football-like skirmishes where two lines get down, the ball is hiked, and two lines bash into each other. Combat in the future will be more like a soccer match: a skirmish here, then a skirmish there. The point is that soldiers in a mobile light division must have decontamination options other than carting gallons of chemical decontamination solution with them. Many of the enzymes that Joe DeFrank and his colleagues are discovering would very well fit the bill for rapid decontamination. They are approaching the 10-half-lives-in-10-minutes baseline criterion. They work very quickly.

Timmis: You already articulated the problems of enzymatic decontamination. They are problems of specificity. So I believe you about half lives, but then you still face the variability of the weapons and the variability of the enzymes needed.

Ward: I agree. We are not going to solve all the problems by using an enzymatic option. But we know, for example, that the Russians have got stockpiles of agent GD (soman); we know that it is in their armamentarium. We have enzymes that will detoxify GD rapidly. The choice is either nothing for mobile combat troops or an aerosol can that will do one category of agents. I think our troops would rather go into combat with a limited decontamination capability than with nothing.

10

Biotransformation Pathways of Hazardous Energetic Organo-Nitro Compounds

David L. Kaplan

U.S. Army Natick Research,
Development, and
Engineering Center
Science and Advanced
Technology Directorate
Natick, MA 01760-5020

Hazardous energetic organonitro compounds are found as contaminants in many environments. One option to ameliorate this contamination problem is the biological degradation of these compounds to nonhazardous products. A series of nitroaromatics, nitrate esters, and nitramines, all characteristic of this class of hazardous energetic organonitro compounds, has been studied for their susceptibility to biological transformation. Biotransformation pathways for each of these compounds have been identified and are summarized. The author discusses implications for these findings in light of current contamination issues.

Introduction

Hazardous energetic organonitro compounds may be defined as a class of synthetic chemicals characterized primarily by the presence of one of the following functional groups or moieties:[1-4] (1) nitro aromatic, (2) nitrate ester, (3) nitramine. The hazardous nature of these compounds arises from their high energy properties and their toxicity to biological systems. The capacity of these compounds to release large quantities of energy is of primary importance in the application and use of these classes of organic structures.

Wastewaters, soils, groundwater, and surface waters have become contaminated with a variety of energetic organonitro compounds arising from ordnance manufacture and processing. This contamination represents a significant environmental concern. Chemically analogous compounds can also be found as contaminants from pesticide and pharmaceutical manufacturing.

The presence of toxic organonitro compounds is not confined to synthetic manufacturing processes. A variety of naturally occurring organonitro compounds have been isolated and identified from biological systems, including higher plants, bacteria, and fungi.[5] Unlike the synthetic compounds, the naturally occurring compounds are generally not highly substituted with nitro-moieties. These naturally occurring compounds usually exhibit antibiotic activity or other toxicological effects. Examples include ß-nitro-propionic acid, isolated from higher plants and fungi; antibiotics such as chloramphenicol, which was probably the first naturally occurring organonitro compound identified; pyrrolnitrin, isolated from bacteria; 3-nitropropanol, isolated from plants; and a variety of other nitro-containing compounds, including 2-nitro-imidazole, *p*-nitrobenzylpenicillin, aristolochia acid, aureothin, 1-phenyl-2-nitroethane, miserotoxin, and *p*-methylnitroamino-benzaldehyde.

A variety of alternative treatments have been developed to reduce or eliminate environmental contamination due to hazardous organonitro compounds, including: (1) physical approaches, such as activated carbon absorption, air stripping, filtration, incineration; (2) chemical approaches, such as solvent extraction, surfactant precipitation, and neutralization; and (3) biological approaches, including denitrification and batch and continuous fermentation systems. Biological approaches, if appropriate, usually offer the most advantageous cost benefits and effectiveness in reducing contaminant burdens without additional insult to human health or the environment.

The three classes of energetic organonitro compounds can be biologically transformed through generic pathways as illustrated by the following:

(1) Nitro Aromatics[6]

$$>C\text{--}NO_2 \xrightarrow{\;\;H_2\;\;} >C\text{--}NO + H_2O$$

$$>C\text{--}NO \xrightarrow{\;\;H_2\;\;} >C\text{--}NHOH$$

$$>C\text{--}NHOH \xrightarrow{\;\;H_2\;\;} >C\text{--}NH_2 + H_2O$$

(2) Nitrate Esters

$$>C\text{--}O\text{--}NO_2 \xrightarrow{\;\;H_2O\;\;} >C\text{--}OH + HNO_3$$

(3) Nitramines

$$>N\text{--}NO_2 \xrightarrow{\;\;H_2\;\;} >N\text{--}NO + H_2O$$

$$>N\text{--}NO \xrightarrow{\;\;H_2\;\;} >N\text{--}NHOH$$

$$>N\text{--}NHOH \xrightarrow{\;\;H_2\;\;} >N\text{--}NH_2 + H_2O$$

For each nitro group (nitramine or nitroaromatic), three moles of hydrogen are required for reduction to the amino group. Mammalian, bacterial, and fungal systems are capable of catalyzing the stepwise reduction of the nitroaromatic groups through the nitroso and hydroxylamino to the amino.[6] The biological reduction of nitroaromatic compounds may modify toxicity. Anaerobic conditions are required for the enzymatic reduction of nitro to amino compounds because the hydroxylamino intermediates are reoxidized in air to the nitroso. Aside from mammalian nitroreductases (microsomal and soluble), a bacterial nitroreductase has been characterized. This system is nicotinamide-adenine dinucleotide (NAD)–dependent and requires a sulfhydryl donor such as glutathione or cysteine and Mn^{+2}.[7]

The intent of this paper is to summarize some of the data on the biotransformation pathways for these energetic organonitro compounds by microorganisms. Additional data on toxicity of microbial intermediates is included, because this is relevant to the consideration of the use of biological systems to reduce contamination problems. No attempt has been made to include all the data generated to date on the compounds reviewed or to provide all of the information on concentrations of parent compounds versus rates of biotransformation, minimal nutrient requirements, effects of temperature, influence of multiple compounds on rates of biotransformation, and other aspects important to consider for biological transformation systems. Much of this information still needs to be developed.

Nitroaromatic Compounds

2,4,6-Trinitrotoluene (TNT) [118-96-7] . The metabolic fate of TNT in mammalian and microbial systems has been extensively studied. TNT is biotransformed, but the aromatic ring is not cleaved; therefore, subsequent mineralization of the molecule does not occur.[8]

TNT toxicity to humans, including liver damage and anemia, has been reported.[9-11] Concentrations above 2 μg/ml are toxic to some fish,[12,13] and toxicity to rats, mice, unicellular green algae, copepods, and oyster larvae has been reported. TNT inhibits the growth of many fungi, yeasts, actinomycetes, and gram-positive bacteria and exhibits mutagenicity in the Ames screening test.[14,15] In feeding studies with rabbits, rats, and humans, TNT was excreted in the urine as transformation products 4-amino-2,6-dinitrotoluene (4A); 2,4-diamino-6-nitrotoluene (2,4-DA); and 2,2',6,6'-tetranitro-4,4'-azoxytoluene (4,4'Az); or as glucuronide conjugates.[10,16-18] *In vitro* studies have implicated a role for NAD and flavoproteins in the metabolism of TNT to 4A.[16,19-21]

Bacterial and fungal transformations of TNT have been reported, with 4A, 4-hydroxylamino-2,6-dinitrotoluene (4OHA), and 4,4'Az reported as products. Additional studies with several strains of *Pseudomonas* identified 2-amino-4,6-ditritrotoluene (2A) and 4,4',6,6'-tetranitro-2,2'-azoxytoluene (2,2'Az) as additional transformation

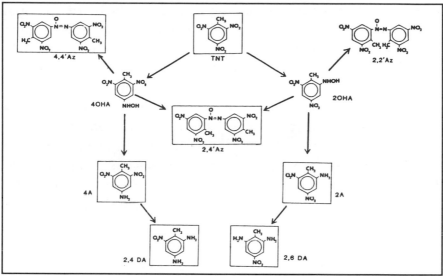

Figure 1. Proposed pathway for biotransformation of 2,4,6-trinitrotoluene. See text for compound identifications with the exception of the following: 2,6DA=2,6-diamino-4-nitrotoluene; 2OHA=2-hydroxylamino-4,6-dinitrotoluene; and 2,4Az=4,2',6,6'-tetranitro-2,4'-azoxytoluene.

products.[13,22] Cell-free extracts of the strict anaerobe *Veillonella alkalescens* catalyzed the reduction of nitro groups to amino groups for a number of nitroaromatic compounds.[23]

A substantive biotransformation pathway for TNT is shown in (Figure 1).[8] The formation of azoxy compounds appear to be due to the nonenzymatic oxidation of the reactive intermediate 4HA. The 4-nitro group is reduced preferentially to the 2-nitro group. These studies on the biotransformation pathway for TNT did not detect or isolate the proposed nitroso intermediate, but the hydroxylamino intermediate was identified. TNT and the biotransformation intermediates have been determined by a variety of analytical techniques, including high performance liquid chromatography.[24-26]

Anaerobic and aerobic bacterial transformation of TNT has been reported.[8] Cell-free extracts of anaerobic organisms, with hydrogen gas, reduced all three nitro groups to the corresponding amino groups (2,4,6-triaminotoluene). Addition of a hydrogen donor was required to achieve reduction of the third nitro group; without this addition, only two of the three nitro groups were reduced to the corresponding amino groups.[8] Organisms studied included *V. alkalescens*, *Escherichia coli*, and *Clostridium pasteurianum*.

Studies with a diversity of nitroaromatic compounds and their susceptibility to nitrogen group reduction indicate the nonspecificity of the nitroreductase system in microorganisms responsible for the biotransformation of TNT. The order of reduction rate of nitro compounds increased with increasing electron withdrawing power of the functional groups at the para position: $-NH_2 < -OH < -H < -CH_3 < -COOH < -NO_2$.[8] Preliminary attempts to isolate and characterize the nitroreductase system from microorganisms suggested the presence of a hydrogenase and ferredoxin-like molecules.[8] *V. alkalescens* was used in these studies, and extracts were partially purified by column chromatography and disc gel electrophoresis.

Complex condensation products arising from hydroxylamino intermediates were identified (for example, 2,2'Az, 4,4'Az).[8] There is reason to speculate that complex intermediates other than those that have been definitively identified may arise from condensation reactions, either with other biotransformation intermediates from TNT or from other compounds or components present (for example, pesticides, soil components).

Biotransformation pathways for TNT in soils and composting systems have also been reported.[27,28] In soil lysimeter systems, TNT at continuous feed concentrations of 70mg per liter was immobilized and retained in soil. A number of biotransformation products were identified in leachates from the soil systems, including 4A and 2A. Carbon supplementation was not required to achieve biotransformation in the soil columns studied. Interaction between TNT or TNT biotransformation products and soil components was evident.

Further studies to evaluate soil-TNT interaction were carried out in order to better define the potential for the formation of TNT-soil conjugates.[29] Aryl-amino biotransformation products (for example, 4A; 2A; 2,4-DA; 2,6-DA) interacted with soil humic acids to form conjugates, whereas the aryl-nitro TNT was relatively unreactive;

binding occurred after biotransformation of the TNT. The toxicity, long-term stability, and exact structures of these biotransformed TNT–humic acid conjugates were not identified. Support for TNT-soil interactions comes from a number of studies.[27-29] In composting studies, a significant percentage of TNT became unextractable with nonpolar and polar organic solvents; this percentage increased with compost age and stabilization. TNT-surfactant complexes were found strongly associated with soil,[14] and higher molecular weight insoluble TNT-conjugates were found during the biotransformation of TNT in water systems.[8] These conjugation reactions may play a significant role in influencing bioavailability, toxicity, leaching rates, and rates of biotransformation, as has been demonstrated for pesticides.

Under simulated composting conditions (55°C), a similar set of biotransformation products and a pathway for TNT were elucidated as described in Figure 1.[28] In addition, a significant percentage (>20 percent) of the original radiolabeled ^{14}C-TNT was found bound in soil fractions during the 91-day study. The similarity in biotransformation pathways under mesophilic and thermophilic conditions is significant in implicating a rather universal and nonspecific enzymatic and/or redox system.

The reduction of TNT contamination in the environment has been approached with a number of potential solutions, including carbon absorption, lagoon storage, photolysis, and chemical treatments. Treatment with amino surfactants under alkaline conditions, which results in complexation products that are water insoluble and nonexplosive,[30,31] was proposed as a potential solution to process water treatments and environmental restoration through immobilization and/or precipitation. These surfactant-TNT complexes, formed under alkaline conditions, were studied using soil lysimeters. Excessive concentrations of the surfactant were required to complex the TNT in soils, and TNT-biotransformation products were also detected in column leachates.[14] These complexes exhibited higher mutagenicity potential than the parent TNT, as determined by Ames testing.

The effects of a variety of environmental factors on the fate of

TNT in soils have been assessed.[32] The initial concentration of TNT was the most significant factor in affecting rates of appearance of TNT biotransformation products. In addition, conditions of high TNT concentration, reduced microbial populations, colder temperatures, and low moisture combined to provide the most stable conditions under which the concentration of TNT remained unchanged over extended incubation in soils.

Nitroaromatic compounds can be transformed by microbial systems by two different pathways: (1) the reduction of the nitro group to an amino group, followed by oxidative deamination to a phenol, with the release of ammonia, or (2) the release of a nitro group as nitrite and the corresponding formation of a phenol. Hydroxyl groups that are ortho or para to each other on an aromatic ring are required for ring cleavage enzymes such as dioxygenases to function.[33] For TNT to be converted to catechol, one of the nitro groups would have to be converted to a hydroxyl group, and also an adjacent unsubstituted ring position would have to be hydroxylated. Although the nitro groups of TNT are reduced by aerobic or anaerobic systems, no evidence has been found for the formation of diphenols. The reducing power of the system used to study the transformation of TNT determines whether one, two, or three of the nitro groups are reduced to amino groups.[8] Nitrite release, as an alternative pathway, does not appear to be significant in the organisms studied.

A related trinitro substituted aromatic, picric acid (2,4,6-trinitro-phenol), has been shown to be biotransformed under anaerobic conditions to 2-amino-4,6-dinitrophenol (picramic acid) but was resistant to complete degradation or ring cleavage under the conditions studied.[8,34] These findings implicate the absence of nitrite release as a significant pathway for these highly substituted nitro-aromatics.

2,4-Dinitrotoluene (2,4-DNT). Both nitro groups of 2,4-DNT can be enzymatically reduced to amino groups.[35] A biotransformation pathway has been proposed as shown in Figure 2.

Biotransformation products including 4,4'-dinitro-2,2'-azoxytolu-ene (2,2'Az); 2,2'-dinitro-4,4'-azoxytoluene (4,4'Az); 4-hydroxyl-amino-2-nitrotoluene (4HA); 4-acetamido-2-nitrotoluene (4Ac2NT); and 2-acetamido-4-nitrotoluene (2Ac4NT) were identified by thin

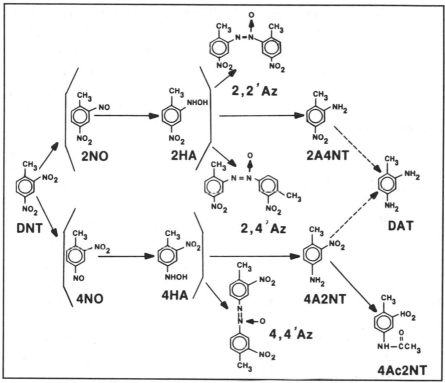

Figure 2. Proposed pathway for biotransformation of 2,4-dinitrotoluene. Hypothetical intermediates are in brackets, and the potential formation of 2,4-diaminotoluene (DAT) is indicated by dashed arrows. From reference 35. DNT=2,4-dinitrotoluene; 2NO=2-nitroso-4-nitrotoluene; 2HA=2-hydroxylamino-4-nitrotoluene; 4NO=4-nitroso-2-nitrotoluene; 2,4'Az=4,2'-dinitro-2,4'-azoxytoluene; 2A4NT=2-amino-4-nitrotoluene; 4A2NT=4-amino-2-nitrotoluene.

layer chromatography and gas chromatography–mass spectrometry (GCMS) run against standards. Biotransformation studies were conducted with supplemental carbon in the form of glucose. The 4HA was unstable, resulting in the formation of 4A2NT and 4,4'Az. This instability was responsible for the inability to detect hydroxylamino intermediates during the microbial transformation of 2,4-DNT and the increased concentration of other metabolites such as aminotoluidines and azoxy compounds. Under the aerobic conditions of this study, the hydroxylamino intermediates are sufficiently stable to undergo oxidative coupling to form azoxy compounds. Under anaerobic conditions, the nitro groups would be enzymatically reduced to amino groups through the hydroxylamino intermediate. The 2,4-diaminotoluene (DAT) was not detected under aerobic conditions; however, complete reduction of both nitro groups was found under anaerobic conditions.[35] The 4-nitro group is preferentially reduced prior to reduction of the 2-nitro group, as indicated by the absence of 2-amino-4-nitrotoluene during rate studies.[35]

Nitrate Esters

Nitroglycerin (glycerol trinitrate) [55-63-0]. The microbial degradation of glycerol trinitrate (GTN) has been reported.[36] The biodegradation process proceeds through a series of successive denitration steps through glycerol dinitrate and glycerol mononitrate isomers, with each succeeding step proceeding at a slower rate (Figure 3).

In addition to direct microbial degradation, chemical treatments of GTN have been developed in order to desensitize wastestreams, resulting in the disappearance of glycerol tri-, di-, and mononitrates, but with the corresponding formation of glycidol and glycidyl nitrate (Figure 4).[37] These products contain a highly reactive epoxide moiety that tends to confer mutagenic properties.

These chemical by-products, glycidol and glycidyl nitrate, have also been studied to determine their biodegradability. The pathway from glycidyl nitrate to glycerol 1-mononitrate to glycerol proceeds more slowly with each succeeding step. The steps from glycidol to glycerol and glycidyl nitrate to glycerol 1-mononitrate occur spontaneously in aqueous solutions but appear to be accelerated (directly or indirectly through secondary effects) by microbial activity.[37]

Glycidol and glycidyl nitrate tested positive in the Ames test screening for mutagenicity, whereas the transformation product glycerol-1-mononitrate tested negative.[37] Both glycerol trinitrate and glycerol 1-mononitrate have been shown to be toxic to mammals.[38]

Propylene glycol dinitrate (PGDN), diethylene glycol dinitrate (DEGN), triethylene glycol dinitrate (TEGDN), and trimethylolethane trinitrate (TMETN). PGDN, DEGN, TEGDN, and TMETN

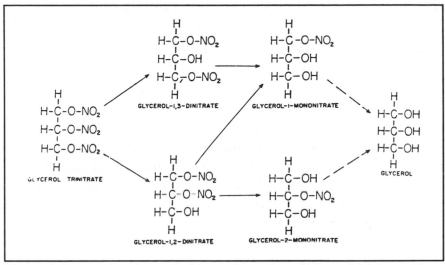

Figure 3. Proposed pathway for biotransformation of glycerol trinitrate. From reference 36.

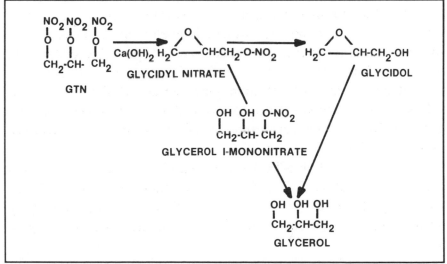

Figure 4. Proposed pathway for chemical and biological degradation of glycerol trinitrate. From reference 37.

undergo microbial transformation via successive denitration steps, leading to the formation of the corresponding glycols: propylene glycol (PG), diethylene glycol (DEG), triethylene glycol (TEG), and trimethylolethane glycol (TMEG) (Figure 5).[39]

The degradation of the resulting glycols at concentrations of

100mg per liter has also been assessed.[40] Rates of degradation were as follows: PG>DEG>TEG>TMEG, from high to low, although degradation appeared to be due to a combination of biological and nonbiological processes.

PG, DEG, and TEG present minimal toxicity and carcinogenic hazards. PG is the least toxic of the glycols and is commonly used in pharmaceutical, cosmetic, and food applications. DEG and TEG are slightly toxic; repeated large doses are needed for toxicity.[41] TMEG had negative test results in Ames test screening for mutagenicity.[40]

Hydroxylammonium nitrate (HAN), trimethylammonium nitrate (TMAN), isopropylammonium nitrate (IPAN), and triethanolammonium nitrate (TEAN). The biodegradation of four ammonium nitrate liquid monopropellants, HAN, IPAN, TMAN, and TEAN, has been determined (Figure 6).[42]

Under aerobic conditions, TMAN, IPAN, and TEAN were mineralized, whereas under anaerobic denitrification conditions, TMAN and TEAN were mineralized, and IPAN was incompletely degraded. Batch studies were conducted with radiolabeled substrates as the sole source of carbon and nitrogen in aerobic and anaerobic systems. In continuous flow denitrification systems, the ammonium nitrates were studied at concentrations of 100mg per liter and 1000mg per liter as sole sources or carbon and nitrogen or with supplemental carbon and nitrogen. No significant accumulation of intermediates was observed in these studies.

TMAN, IPAN, and TEAN were readily mineralized in soils at concentrations of 50, 500, and 5000mg per liter, and HAN was labile under slightly acidic and alkaline conditions. All four ammonium nitrates had negative test results in Ames test screening for mutagenicity.[42]

During the biotranformation studies, contamination of solutions of TMAN and TEAN with nitrosamines was identified. This problem was first identified with the appearance of N-nitrosodimethylamine (NDMA) in influent and effluent samples from continuous flow systems under study. The identification of this problem led to a study of the biodegradability of NDMA (Figure 7) by microbial systems.[43] These pathways had been proposed for mammalian systems.[44] NDMA

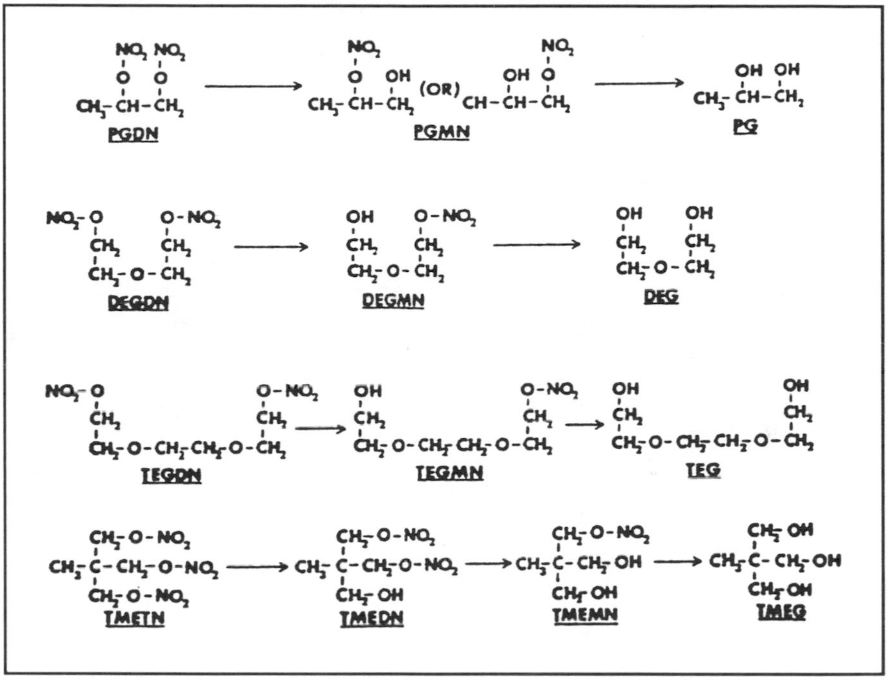

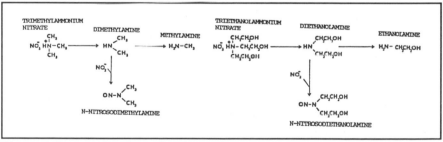

Figure 5. Proposed pathway for biotransformation of nitrate esters to the corresponding glycols. From reference 39.

Figure 6. Proposed pathway for biotransformation of trimethylammonium nitrate and triethanolammonium nitrate. From reference 42.

biotransformation was studied over a range of concentrations from ng per liter to mg per liter in aqueous systems and μg per liter to mg per liter in soil systems.[43]

The use of denitrification systems in these studies also led to research on alternate carbon sources for the continuous flow systems, where the degradation of nitrated species was desirable.[45] A

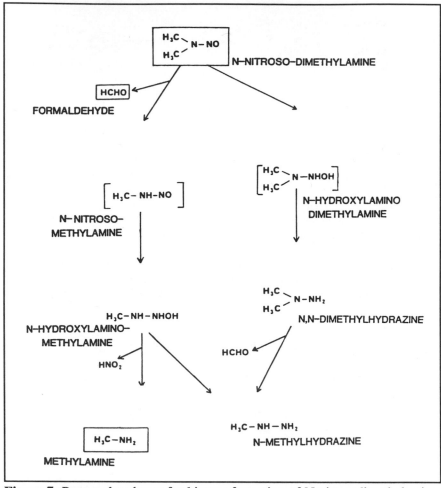

Figure 7. Proposed pathway for biotransformation of N-nitrosodimethylamine. From reference 43.

series of alternative carbon sources was studied to evaluate efficacy (Table 1).

Nitrocellulose. Nitrocellulose represents a highly substituted cellulose that is not subject to direct microbial attack.[46] In studies where growth of microorganisms on nitrocellulose has been observed, the growth may have been due to contaminants, the presence of unsubstituted cellulose, or the effects of secondary metabolites on the nitrocellulose structure. The biodegradability of nitrocellulose

Table 1
Efficiencies of Alternate Carbon Sources Evaluated in the Denitrification Process[45]

Carbon Source	C/N[a]
(1) *95 percent denitrification, 90 percent TOC[b] removal*	
Methanol	1·1
Sweet whey	1·4
Acid whey	1·4
Corn steep liquor	1·6
Soluble potato solids	1·7
(2) *95 percent denitrification, 80 percent TOC removal*	
Nutrient broth	1·7
Brewery spent grain	2·3
Sugar beet molasses	3·6
(3) *Others*	
Acid hydrolyzed sewage sludge digest	2·1[c]
Volatile fish condensate	2·5[d]
Sewage sludge digest	—[e]

[a]Ratio of grams of carbon to grams of nitrogen in media.
[b]Total organic carbon.
[c]At C/N ratios above 2·1 the percent TOC removal decreased from 87 percent.
[d]Insufficient medium to complete study.
[e]95 percent denitrification and 80 percent TOC removal never achieved.
[*]From reference 45.

has been studied in batch and continuous fermentation systems, and the polymer has been found to be resistant to direct microbial transformation. Chemical pretreatment of the insoluble nitrocellulose was required to generate a biologically susceptible substrate for degradation (Figure 8).[47,48] Alkaline hydrolysis with heating was used to denitrate the cellulose, followed by anaerobic denitrification of the susceptible residues with supplemental carbon. Nitrocellulose was found to be acceptably degraded in this chemical-biological system, with no toxic products, and nitrate and nitrite concentrations were maintained below drinking water standards.

Triaminoguanidine nitrate. Triaminoguanidine nitrate (Figure

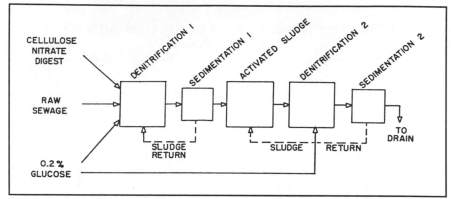

Figure 8. Flow diagram for biological treatment of alkali-digested nitrocellulose. From Reference 47.

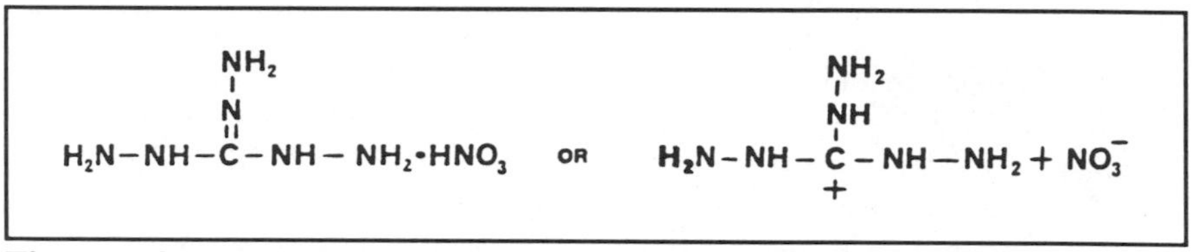

$$H_2N-NH-\underset{\overset{\displaystyle N}{\underset{\displaystyle NH_2}{\shortmid}}}{\overset{\displaystyle \|}{C}}-NH-NH_2\cdot HNO_3 \quad \text{OR} \quad H_2N-NH-\underset{\overset{\displaystyle NH}{\underset{\displaystyle NH_2}{\shortmid}}}{\overset{}{C}}-NH-NH_2 + NO_3^-$$

Figure 9. Structure of triaminoguanidine nitrate. From Reference 49.

9) was biodegraded under both aerobic and anaerobic conditions.[49] Supplemental carbon was required in most studies, particularly in denitrification systems. No evidence was found for the buildup of intermediates such as guanidine; hydrazine; urea carbohydrazide (1,3-diaminourea); cyanamide; or cyanoguanidine during batch or continuous studies. Nitrate formed during the degradation process was reduced in denitrification systems when sufficient alternative carbon was present.

Nitramines

Nitroguanidine [556-88-7]. Nitroguanidine is an aliphatic nitramine that exists in two tautomeric forms. The biodegradation of nitroguanidine has been studied in aqueous and soil systems.[50,51] In aqueous systems, nitroguanidine was not biotransformed under aerobic conditions but was cometabolized to nitrosoguanidine in anaero-

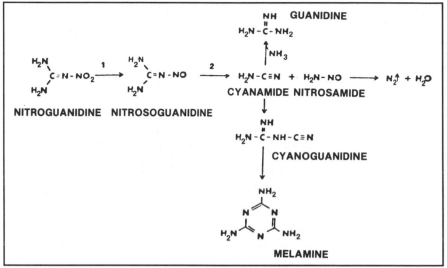

Figure 10. Proposed pathway for biotransformation of nitroguanidine in aqueous systems under anaerobic conditions. Step 1 is biologically mediated, whereas step 2 is chemically mediated. From reference 50.

bic incubations (Figure 10).[50] No evidence was found for further microbial reduction of nitrosoguanidine to hydrazine and urea or aminoguanidine and guanidine. An extended period of acclimation was observed before activity commenced. The nitrosoguanidine decomposed by nonbiological mechanisms to form cyanamide, cyanoguanidine, melamine, and guanidine as determined by thin layer chromatography and GCMS. Melamine represents the trimeric cyanamide product with a dimer cyanoguanidine intermediate. Cyanamide can also react with ammonia to form guanidine. The nitrosamide formed is transitory and decomposes to nitrogen gas and water.

Results from degradation studies in aqueous systems suggest that residual levels of nitrosoguanidine persist because of slow rates of decomposition under the mild ambient conditions necessary for biological activity. More stringent chemical conditions would presumably enhance the rate of decomposition of nitrosoguanidine.

Nitroguanidine and nitrosoguanidine had negative test results in Ames test screening for mutagenicity.[50] Nitroguanidine was reported to be a carcinogen in screening tests with Chinese hamster cells;

cyanamide is metabolized by plants to arginine through various guanidino compounds; calcium cyanamide is used as a plant fertilizer and root stimulator and is not carcinogenic; cyanamide is bacteriostatic at 1000mg per liter and toxic to mammals; melamine presents a low toxicity hazard; and nitrosoguanidine is a suspected carcinogen.[52-55]

In soil studies,[51] cometabolic biodegradation of nitroguanidine was demonstrated. Traces of nitrosoguanidine were detected (below 100µg/liter), and ammonia was the principal nitrogen product. No biotransformation of nitroguanidine occurred without supplemental carbon. Nitroguanidine was studied at a concentration of 150mg per liter with glucose as the supplemental carbon source. Between 1.0 percent and 0.5 percent glucose was required, representing a C/N ratio of approximately 68 to 1 to 34 to 1, to achieve complete degradation of nitroguanidine. The ammonia concentrations in leachates from continuous flow soil columns correlated directly with the rates of degradation of nitroguanidine, and nitrate and nitrite concentrations in column leachates were low throughout the study (usually in the µg per liter range). None of the other organic-nitrogen intermediates identified during degradation studies in aqueous systems was identified in these soil studies. Mass balance studies revealed an 85 percent conversion of the nitrogen bound in nitro-guanidine to ammonia nitrogen.

RDX [121-82-4] and AcRDX [14168-42-4]. RDX and AcRDX represent heterocyclic nitramines. The biotransformation of hexahydro-1,3,5-trinitro-1,3,5-triazine (RDX) and the corresponding N-acetylated derivative hexahydro-1-N-acetyl-3,5-dinitro-1,3,5-triazine (AcRDX) has been determined.[56-60] RDX was biotransformed only under anaerobic conditions (Figure 11) with supplemental carbon. Biotransformation products included mono-, di-, and trinitroso-derivatives arising from the sequential reductions of the nitro groups to nitroso groups, and formaldehyde and methanol. Traces of hydrazine; 1,1-dimethylhydrazine; and 1,2-dimethylhydrazine were detected, as confirmed by GCMS analysis.

AcRDX was also biotransformed under anaerobic conditions, with mono- and di-nitroso-AcRDX appearing in sequential reduction steps analogous to the biotransformation pathway for RDX, although

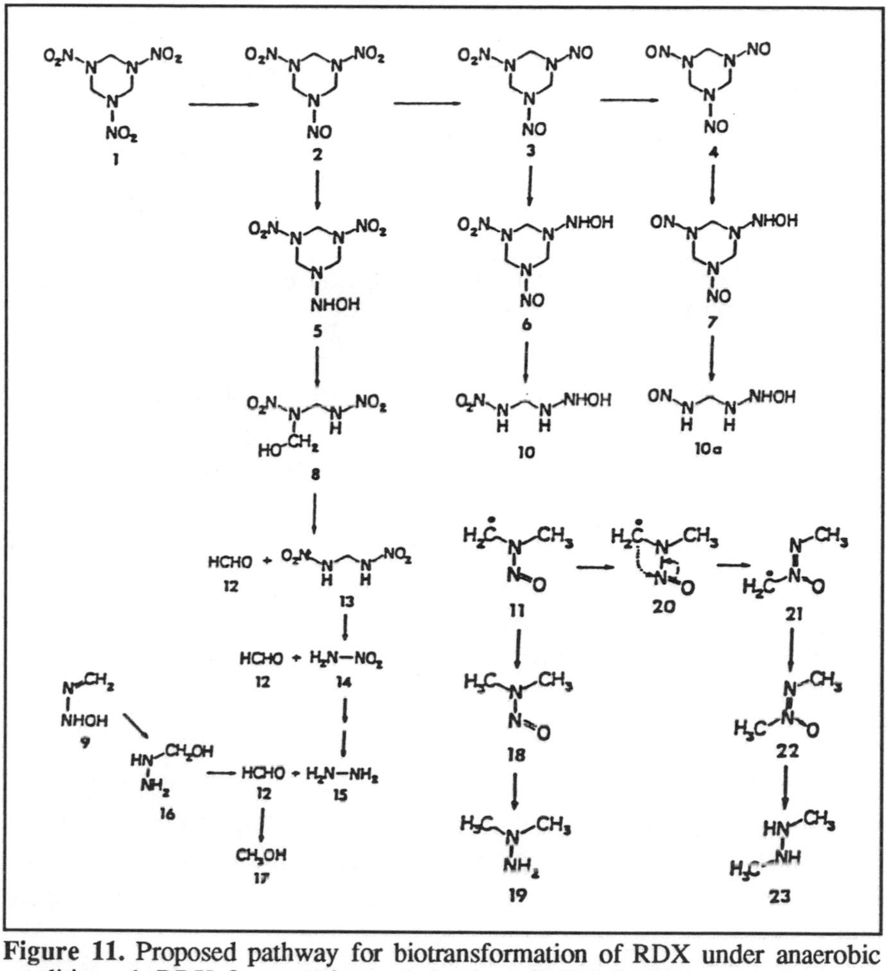

Figure 11. Proposed pathway for biotransformation of RDX under anaerobic conditions. 1=RDX; 2=mononitroso derivative of RDX; 3=dinitroso derivative of RDX; 4=trinitroso derivative of RDX; 5=1-hydroxylamino-3,5-dinitro-1,3,5-triazine; 6=1-hydroxylamino-3-nitroso-5-nitro-1,3,5-triazine; 7=1-hydroxylamino-3,5-dinitroso-1,3,5-triazine; 8=N-hydroxymethylethylenedinitramine; 9=N-hydroxymethylene hydrazone; 10=N-hydroxylamino–N'-nitromethylenediamine; and 11=dimethylnitrosamine. Cleavage of the hydroxylamino (5) yields products 8 and 9, and cleavage of compound 6 yields products 10 and 11. Compound 7 undergoes cleavage by either route. Additional compounds: 12=formaldehyde; 13=methylenedinitramine; 14=nitramide; 15=hydrazine; 16=hydroxymethylhydrazine; 17=methanol; 18=dimethylnitrosamine; 19=1,1-dimethylhydrazine; 20=hypothetical intermediate; 21=dimethyldiazene-1-oxide radical; 22=dimethyldiazene-1-oxide; 23=dimethylhydrazine.

no hydrazine or dimethylhydrazine was detected in concentrated culture extracts (Figure 12).[57]

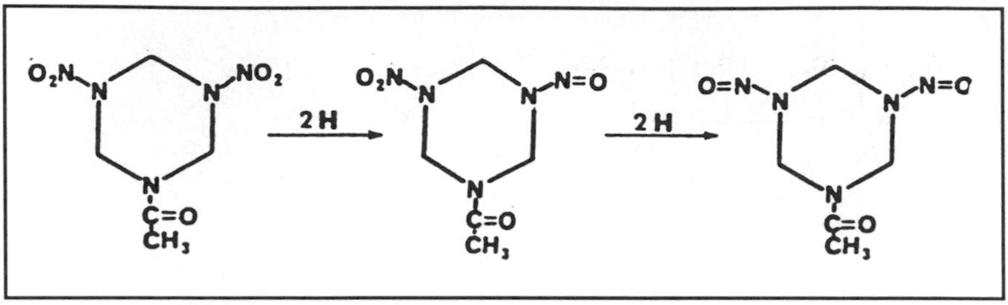

Figure 12. Stepwise reduction of nitro groups on hexahydro-1-N-acetyl-3,5-dinitro-1,3,5-triazine. From reference 57.

Under continuous culture anaerobic denitrification conditions with supplemental carbon, RDX was biodegraded, with no evidence for the intermediates identified in batch cultures just described.[60] Similar findings with AcRDX were noted.

HMX [2691-41-0] and AcHMX [13980-00-2]. HMX and AcHMX also represent heterocyclic nitramines. The biodegradation of octahydro-1,3,5,7-tetranitro-1,3,5,7-tetrazocine (HMX) and octahydro-1-N-acetyl-3,5,7-trinitro-1,3,5,7-tetrazocine (AcHMX) has been determined.[57,60] Under anaerobic conditions with 50 mg per liter HMX, slower rates of biotransformation were observed when compared with similar conditions for RDX. HMX was incompletely biotransformed under these conditions, with the appearance of mono- and di-nitroso intermediates (two isomers of the dinitroso) (Figure 13). As with RDX, these transformations required cometabolic carbon.

AcHMX was even more slowly biotransformed than HMX, with two isomers of dinitroso-AcHMX formed. No traces of hydrazine; 1,1-dimethylhydrazine; or 1,2-dimethylhydrazine were detected in culture concentrates when HMX or AcHMX were parent compounds. As in the case of RDX and AcRDX, HMX and AcHMX degraded more slowly in continuous culture anaerobic denitrification systems, and none of the intermediates identified during batch culture studies were detected (Figure 14).

As with RDX, these biotransformations occurred only under anaerobic conditions. No changes in concentration of HMX or AcHMX were noted under aerobic conditions over time. In all cases, under an-

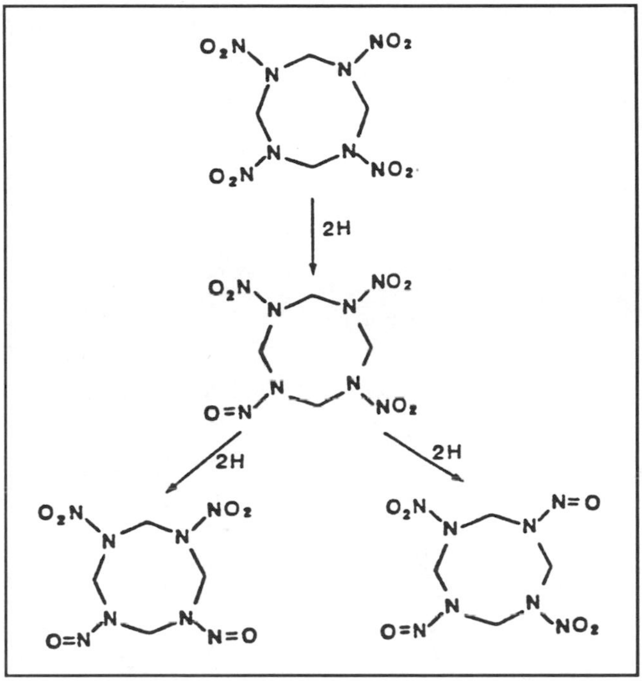

Figure 13. Stepwise reduction of nitro groups on octahydro - 1, 3, 5, 7 - tetranitro - 1, 3, 5, 7 - tetrazocine. From reference 57.

aerobic conditions the first step appears to be a reduction of a nitro group to a nitroso group, followed by the reduction of a second nitro group. The identities of the parent compounds and the nitro intermediates were confirmed by GCMS, infrared spectroscopy, high performance liquid chromatography, and nuclear magnetic resonance spectroscopy against synthesized standards.

Discussion

Biotransformation pathways for nitroaromatics, nitrate esters, and nitramines have been reviewed. In many cases, biological treatment to transform these hazardous energetic organonitro compounds is feasible. The organonitro compounds studied were susceptible to biotransformation either directly or after chemical pretreatment. In many cases, appropriate conditions must be established to foster the biotransformation process. For example, RDX and HMX will biode-

Figure 14. Stepwise reduction of nitro groups on octahydro - 1 - N - acetyl - 3, 5, 7 - trinitro - 1, 3, 5, 7 - tetrazocine. From reference 57.

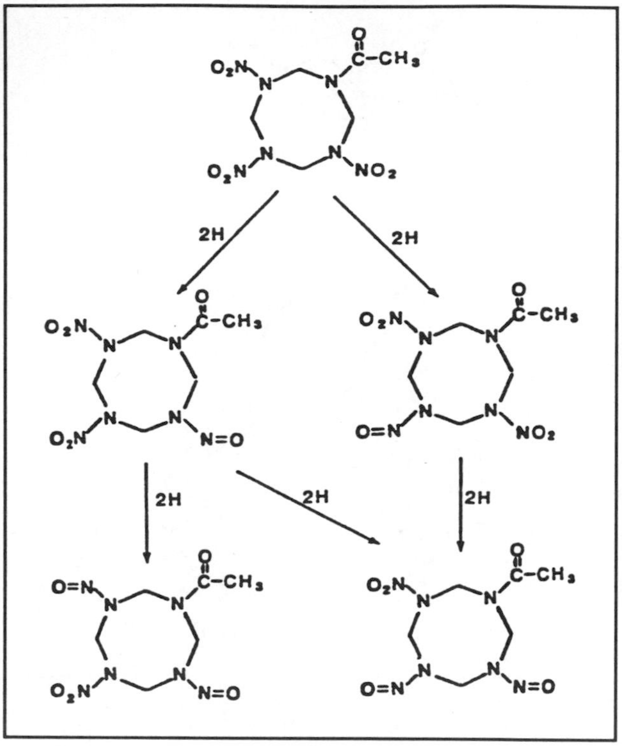

grade only under anaerobic conditions. Supplemental carbon for cometabolism is usually required for these transformations.

TNT was one of the most recalcitrant compounds studied, with the aromatic ring resistant to cleavage in all conditions studied. The reduction of TNT results in the formation of a variety of intermediates that also exhibit toxicity. In addition, higher molecular weight conjugates have been identified but have not been fully characterized. Nitrocellulose was also resistant to biotransformation unless an alkaline pretreatment was used.

Generally, alternative carbon sources are required in the biological systems described. The role of cometabolism in these pathways must be considered during the development of any biological treatment approach for these classes of compounds.

Additionally, denitrification systems are often beneficial in these processes due to the preponderance of nitro or nitrate functional groups that result in the formation of nitrates or nitrites under many environmental conditions. Denitrification systems not only promote the biotransformation of the hazardous energetic organonitro compounds under anaerobic conditions but also reduce the oxidized nitrogen species that form to more volatile products (for example, ammonia). In a sequential treatment system, an aerobic treatment step could follow the anaerobic denitrification process to serve as a final "polish" for the wastestream.

Generic Biological Treatment Concept for Wastewaters Contaminated With Hazardous Nitrate Esters or Nitramines:

Influent → Chemical → Anaerobic → Aerobic → Effluent
Pretreatment Denitrification Treatment
(if required) Treatment

Mixed cultures were used in many of the studies reported here. The ability of microorganisms to biotransform this class of compounds is apparently ubiquitous in nature. The use of acclimatized cultures from environments previously exposed to the compounds under study perhaps would have accelerated some of the initial rates of transformation observed; however, once acclimatized, random environmental microbial inocula were capable of transforming the compounds studied.

Aside from nitrates and nitrites, nitrosamines are key intermediates that have to be considered during biotransformations of the nitramines and nitroaromatics.

In soil systems, similar biotransformation intermediates were identified as those found in aqueous systems. Differences in recovery efficiencies of the parent and intermediate compounds were found. In addition, interactions with soil components (conjugates) appear to be significant in influencing the environmental fate and availability of biotransformation intermediates and deserve considerable attention.

Acknowledgments

The research reported on biotransformation pathways was conducted at the U. S. Army Natick Research, Development, and Engineering Center, Natick, Massachusetts. My deepest appreciation is given to Dr. John H. Cornell and Dr. Neil G. McCormick of this center for their support and guidance during much of the work reported here. In addition, the contributions of many students and technicians and the support of Dr. Arthur Kaplan are gratefully acknowledged. I also acknowledge the support of the U. S. Army Toxic and Hazardous Materials Agency for their foresight in funding most of the work described here.

References

1. T. Urbanski, *Chemistry and Technology of Explosives, Vol. 1* (Pergamon Press, New York, 1964).
2. T. Urbanski, *Chemistry and Technology of Explosives, Vol. 2* (Pergamon Press, Oxford, 1965).
3. T. Urbanski, *Chemistry and Technology of Explosives, Vol . 3* (Pergamon Press, Oxford, 1967).
4. T. Urbanski, *Chemistry and Technology of Explosives, Vol . 4* (Pergamon Press, Oxford, 1984).
5. J. Venulet and R.L. VanEtten, in *The Chemistry of the Nitro and Nitroso Groups*, H. Feuer, Ed. (Krieger Publishing Co., Melborne, FL, 1969), pp. 201-287.
6. I.Yamashina, S. Shikata, and F. Egami, *Bull. Chem. Soc. Japan* 27, 42 (1954).
7. M. Mitchard, *Xenobiotica* 1(4/5), 469 (1971).
8. N.G. McCormick, F.E. Feeherry, and H.S. Levinson, *Appl. Environ. Microbiol.* 31(6), 949 (1976).
9. J.E. Bridge *et al.*, *Proc. R. Soc. Med.* 35, 553 (1942).
10. H.H. Dale, *Med. Res. Counc. (G.B.) Spec. Rep. Ser.* 58, 53 (1921).
11. A. Hamilton, *J. Ind. Hyg.* 3,102 (1921).
12. M.W. Nay, Jr., *J. Water Poll. Control Fed.* 46, 485 (1974).
13. J.L. Osmon and R. E. Klausmeier, *Dev. Ind. Microbiol.* 14, 247 (1972).
14. D.L. Kaplan and A. M. Kaplan, *Environ. Sci. Tech.* 19(9), 566 (1982).
15. B.N. Ames, J. McCann, and E. Tamasaki, *Mut. Res.* 31, 347 (1975).
16. E. Bueding and N. Jolliffe, *J. Pharmacol. Exp. Ther.* 88, 300 (1946).
17. H.J. Channon, G.T. Mills, and R.T. Williams, *Biochem. J.* 38, 70 (1944).
18. R. Lemberg and J. P. Callaghan, *Nature* (London), 154, 768 (1944).
19. A.K. Saz and R.B. Slie, *Arch. Biochem. Biophys.* 51, 5 (1954).
20. B.B. Westfall, *J. Pharmacol. Exp. Ther.* 79, 23 (1954).

21. M. Zucker and A. Nason, in *Methods in Enzymology, Vol . 2*, S.P. Colwick and N.O. Kaplan, Eds. (Academic Press Inc., New York, 1955), pp. 406-411.
22. W.D. Won *et al., Appl. Microbiol.* 27, 513 (1974).
23. C.A. Woolfolk, Ph.D. Thesis, University of Washington, Seattle (1963).
24. D.L. Kaplan and A.M. Kaplan, *Anal. Chim. Acta* 136, 425 (1982).
25. T.F. Jenkins, P.H. Miyares, and M.E. Walsh, *An Improved RP-HPLC Method for Determining Nitroaromatics and Nitramines in Water*, Technical Report No. 88-23 (U. S. Army Corps of Engineers Cold Regions Research and Engineering Laboratory, Hanover, NH, 1988).
26. T.F. Jenkins *et al., Development of an Analytical Method for the Determination of Explosive Residues in Soil*, Technical Report No. 88-8 (U. S. Army Corps of Engineers Cold Regions Research and Engineering Laboratory, Hanover, NH, 1988).
27. B. Greene, D.L. Kaplan, and A.M. Kaplan, *Degradation of Pink Water Compounds in Soil–TNT, RDX, HMX*, Technical Report No. 85-046 (U. S. Army Natick Research, Development, and Engineering Center, Natick, MA, 1985).
28. D.L. Kaplan and A.M. Kaplan, *Appl. Environ. Microbiol.* 44(3), 757 (1982).
29. D.L. Kaplan and A.M. Kaplan, *Reactivity of TNT and TNT-Microbial Reduction Products With Soil Components*, Technical Report No. 83-041 (U.S. Army Natick Research, Development and Engineering Center, Natick, MA, 1983).
30. Y. Okamoto and J.Y. Wang, *J. Organ. Chem.* 42, 1261 (1977).
31. M. Croce and Y. Okamoto, *J. Organ. Chem.* 44, 2100 (1978).
32. D.L. Kaplan *et al., Effects of Environmental Factors on the Transformation of 2,4,6-Trinitrotoluene in Soils*, Technical Report No. 85-052 (U. S. Army Natick Research, Development, and Engineering Center, Natick, MA, 1985).
33. S. Dagley, *Am. Scientist* 63, 681 (1975).
34. J.F. Wyaman *et al., Appl. Environ. Microbiol.* 37(2), 222 (1979).
35. N.G. McCormick, J.H. Cornell, and A.M. Kaplan, *Appl. Environ. Microbiol.* 35(5), 945 (1978).
36. T.M. Wendt, J.H. Cornell, and A.M. Kaplan, *Appl. Environ. Microbiol.* 36, 693 (1978).
37. D.L. Kaplan, J.H. Cornell, and A.M. Kaplan, *Appl. Environ. Microbiol.* 43(1), 144 (1982).
38. L.V. Melinikova and A.M. Klyachkina, *Toksikol. Nov. Prom. Khim. Veshchestv.* 15, 97 (1979).
39. J.H. Cornell *et al., Biodegradation of Nitrate Esters Used as Military Propellants*, Technical Report No. 81-029 (U. S. Army Natick Research, Development, and Engineering Center, Natick, MA, 1981).
40. D.L. Kaplan, J.T. Walsh, and A.M. Kaplan, *Environ. Sci. Tech.* 16(10), 723 (1982).
41. R.E. Gosselin *et al., Chemical Toxicity of Commercial Products, 4th Edition* (Williams & Wilkins, Baltimore, MD, 1976).
42. D.L. Kaplan *et al., Environ. Sci. Tech.* 18(9), 694 (1984).
43. D.L. Kaplan and A.M. Kaplan, *Appl. Environ. Microbiol.* 50(4), 1077 (1985).
44. A. Grilli and G. Prodi, *Gann.* 66, 473 (1979).
45. D.L. Kaplan *et al., Inter. Biodeter.* 23, 233 (1987).
46. P.A. Riley, D. L. Kaplan, and A.M. Kaplan, *Stability of Nitrocellulose to Biological Degradation*, Technical Report No. 85-004 (U. S. Army Natick Research, Development, and Engineering Center, Natick, MA, 1984).
47. T.M. Wendt and A.M. Kaplan, *J. Water Poll. Control Fed.* 48(4), 660 (1976).

48. T.M. Wendt and A.M. Kaplan, *Process for Treating Waste Water Containing Cellulose Nitrate Particles*, United States Patent No. 3,939,068 (1976).
49. D.L. Kaplan and A.M. Kaplan, *Bioconversion of Nitramine Propellant Wastewaters—Triaminoguanidine Nitrate,* Technical Report No. 85-045 (U. S. Army Natick Research, Development, and Engineering Center, Natick, MA, 1985).
50. D.L. Kaplan, J.H. Cornell, and A.M. Kaplan, *Environ. Sci. Tech.* **16**(8), 488 (1982).
51. D.L. Kaplan and A.M. Kaplan, *Degradation of Nitroguanidine in Soils*, Technical Report No. 85-047 (U. S. Army Natick Research, Development, and Engineering Center, Natick, MA, 1985).
52. U. S. Army Medical Research and Development Command, *Mammalian Toxicity of Munition Compounds: Phase I. Acute Oral Toxicity, Primary Skin and Eye Irritation, Dermal Sensitization and Disposition and Metabolism*, Technical Report No. ADB011150 (U. S. Army Medical Research and Development Command, Washington, D.C., 1975).
53. M. Ishidate and S. Odashima, *Mut. Res.* **48**, 337 (1977).
54. National Cancer Institute, *Bioassay of Calcium Cyanamide for Possible Carcinogenicity*, (National Technical Information Service, PB-293625, 1979).
55. M.I. Sax, *Dangerous Properties of Industrial Materials* (Van Nostrand Reinhold, New York, 1975).
56. N.G. McCormick, J. H. Cornell, and A.M. Kaplan, *Appl. Environ. Microb.* **42**(5), 817 (1981).
57. N.G. McCormick, J.H. Cornell, and A.M. Kaplan, *The Anaerobic Biotransformation of RDX, HMX, and Their Acetylated Derivatives*, Technical Report No. 85-007 (U. S. Army Natick Research, Development, and Engineering Center, Natick, MA, 1985).
58. R.J. Spanggord *et al., Environmental Fate Studies on Certain Munition Waste Water Constituents. Final Report, Phase II—Laboratory Studies.* (SRI International, Menlo Park, CA, U. S. Army Medical Research and Development Command, Fort Detrick, MD, 1980).
59. H.C. Sikka *et al., Environmental Fate of RDX and TNT. Final Report* Syracuse Research Corporation, Syracuse, NY, 1980). U. S. Army Medical Research and Development Command, Fort Detrick, MD.
60. N.G. McCormick, J.H. Cornell, and A.M. Kaplan, *The Fate of Hexahydro-1,3,5-Trinitro-1,3,5-Triazine (RDX) and Related Compounds in Anaerobic Denitrifying Continuous Culture Systems Using Simulated Waste Water*, Technical Report No. 85-008 (U. S. Army Natick Research, Development, and Engineering Center, Natick, MA, 1985).

Discussion

Timmis: You did not give any details about what kind of soil you were using or what kind of conditions you were using to observe these biodegradation pathways, so it is difficult to interpret how general your conclusions are. For the nitrotoluenes, you end up with reactive compounds that will form polymers that are not biodegradable in the environment. Although it is not my area, I think that Hans

Knackmuss would argue that your scheme is the wrong strategy for the biodegradation of such compounds. What you really want is oxidative removal of the nitro groups so that you do not end up with reactive amines. I think he has proposed conditions where nitrogen is limiting, so you get the organisms to grow on those nitro groups and use them as nitrogen sources. You end up with denitrated compounds, which are then biodegradable by aerobic processes.

Kaplan: When I showed this scheme I indicated that it applies to the nitrate esters and nitramines, but I excluded the nitroaromatics for just the reason that you mentioned. I question, however, whether one can envision the highly substituted nitroaromatics, even under nitrogen-limiting conditions, undergoing ring cleavage. We have no evidence for that, if it happens, that would be terrific.

Gunsalus: Are these compounds very toxic to organisms?

Kaplan: Usually, the solubility of the nitroaromatics is low enough that you do not have to deal with toxicity to the microorganisms.

Gunsalus: Do you have any evidence of building up cultures that operate more quickly? These require weeks or more. What is your starting material?

Kaplan: We use mixed inocula from a number of sources to start our systems with a broad distribution of microorganisms, and allow the system to select what is going to utilize the compound. In the case of a compound like nitroguanidine, the system did not do anything for months. Then finally the system took off, and biotransformation started. I think you could accelerate these reaction pathways by selection of appropriate organisms, but we have not looked at that directly.

Gunsalus: After the long lag phase, would the inoculum that takes off be active if you put it back into your initial starting conditions?

Kaplan: Yes, once the inoculum is acclimated or selected, subsequent studies using this seed culture will show accelerated rates. This occurred in studies with nitroguanidine.

Gunsalus: There is some hope then of accelerating the rates of biotransformation?

Kaplan: Yes.

Eveleigh: Are you making nitrosoguanidine, one of the most active mutagens around?

Kaplan: This is not the same nitrosoguanidine [674-81-7] that is used in standard mutational biochemical work, which is N-methyl-N-nitro-N-nitrosoguanidine [70-25-7]. It is still a concern in terms of mutagenicity but not to the degree of the standard mutagen.

11

Enzymatic Hydrolysis of Toxic Organofluorophosphate Compounds

Wayne G. Landis
Joseph J. DeFrank
*U.S. Army Chemical Research
Development and
Engineering Center
Aberdeen Proving Ground,
Maryland 21010-5423*

Research in recent years has delineated a number of enzymes, now called organophosphorus acid (OPA) anhydrases, that are able to rapidly degrade organophosphate nerve agents and pesticides. Systems in bacteria, protozoa, mammals, and invertebrates have been identified. The best understood of the current systems are the *opd* gene product OPA anhydrase (parathion hydrolase) and the squid-type OPA anhydrase from the nervous tissue of squid. Several enzymes from the protozoan *Tetrahymena thermophila* and a variety of thermophilic and halophilic bacteria are promising for their potential activity under a variety of environmental conditions.

Background

Organofluorophosphate hydrolyzing enzymes were first identified by Mazur in a 1946 report.[1] In the 1950s Mounter and colleagues[2] reported similar types of activities found in various types of bacteria. In a comprehensive 1963 review,[3] Mounter summarized the extent of the knowledge of these peculiar xenobiotic degrading enzymes, which were common to both bacterial and mammalian sources. In 1965, Hoskin and co-workers[4] accidentally discovered a diisopropyl fluorophosphate (DFP) hydrolyzing enzyme in the giant nerve axon of the squid. DFP is one of the most commonly used organophosphate compounds that are potent acetylcholinesterase inhibitors. During the next several years, Hoskin and colleagues published numerous reports on the characterization of the squid-type DFPase, the DFPases found in mammalian tissues, and a similar enzyme in *Escherichia coli*.[5-10] In 1975, Storkebaum and Witzel[11] isolated, purified, and elucidated the dimeric nature of the hog kidney DFPase. In the same year, Zech and Wigand,[12] using electrofocusing, separated two enzymes from *Escherichia coli*, one able to hydrolyze DFP, the other paraoxon (diethyl 4-nitrophenyl phosphate).

There was considerable renewed interest in this class of enzymes in the early 1980s with the report by Hoskin and Roush[13] of the immobilization of the squid DFPase on agarose resin. The interest was generated by the possible practical application of these enzymes for the detoxification of organophosphate materials. Landis and coworkers[14-17] initiated a study of the DFPases of the ciliate protozoan, *Tetrahymena thermophila*, and the clam, *Rangia cuneata*, that led to the realization that many different forms of DFP hydrolyzing enzymes may exist within the same organism.

Nomenclature

The early literature in this field contains an almost bewildering number of names for enzymes with the same basic activity. In the past, the enzymes were called DFPases, somanases, sarinases, paraoxonases, and parathion hydrolases, among others, depending primarily on the substrate the investigator was using to screen for activity. These have been conventionally classified as either DFPase (EC 3.8.2.1) or paraoxonase (arylesterase, EC 3.1.1.2). In order to consolidate these enzymes under one descriptive name, the participants of the First DFPase Workshop (Marine Biological Laboratory, Woods Hole, MA, June 1987) selected the designation of organophosphorus acid (OPA) anhydrase. This name is now used for any enzyme able to catalytically hydrolyze an organophosphate that has an acidic leaving group. The convention used in this review is to call everything an OPA anhydrase, with a specific identifier. For example, squid DFPase becomes squid OPA anhydrase.

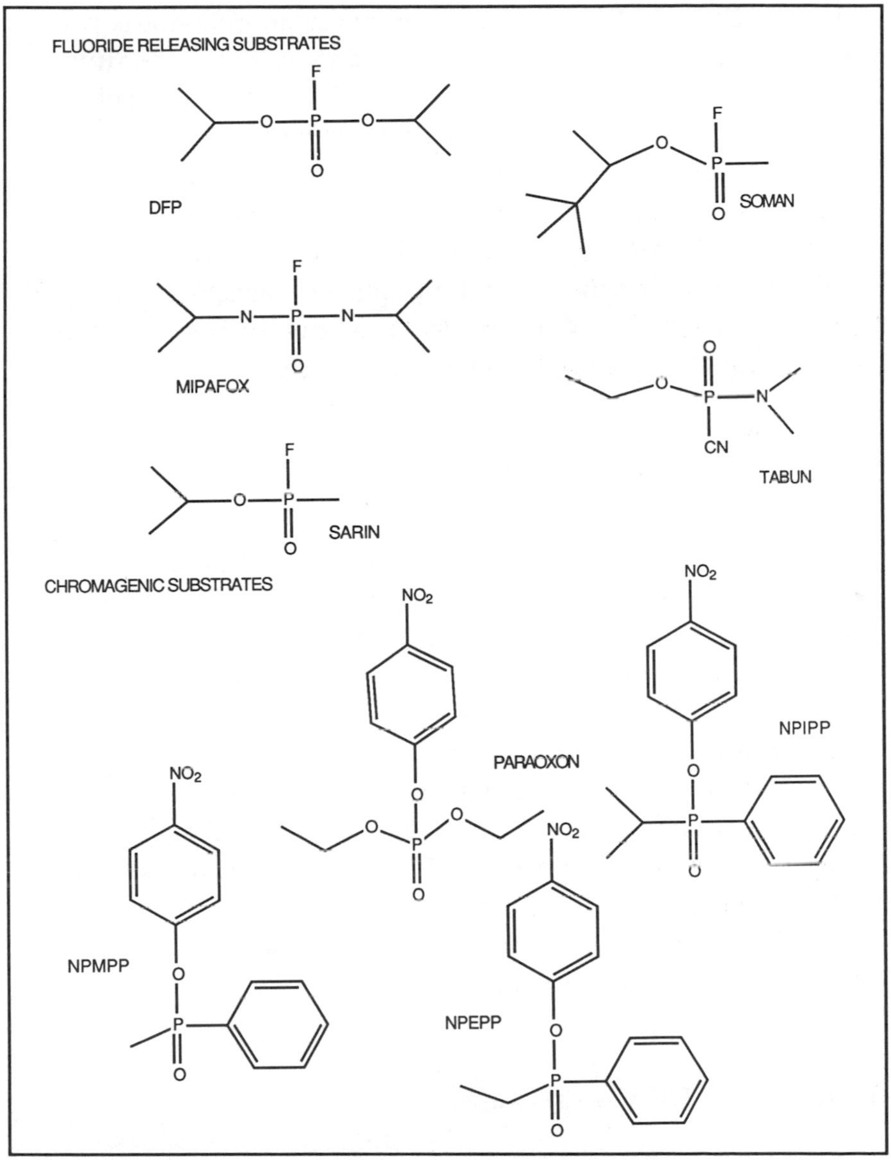

Figure 1. Structures of several common substrates and inhibitors used in the study of OPA anhydrases.

The OPA anhydrases described in this report are able to hydrolyze a surprising variety of substrates. The structures of some substrates are depicted in Figure 1. In addition to the already mentioned DFP, these include soman (1,2,2-tri-methylpropyl methylphosphonofluoridate); sarin (isopropyl methylphosphonofluoridate); tabun (N,N-dimethyl ethyl phosphororamidocyanidate); and mipafox (diisopropyl phosphorodiamidofluoridate). Among the substrates that have been examined that have a nitrophenol leaving group (thus providing a chromogenic assay) are paraoxon; parathion (diethyl 4-nitrophenylphosphorothioate); 4-nitrophenylmethyl(phenyl) phosphinate (NPMPP); 4-nitrophenyl ethyl (phenyl) phosphinate (NPEPP); and 4-nitrophenyl isopropyl (phenyl) phosphinate (NPIPP). The yellow color of the 4-nitrophenol can be easily seen with the eye and measured by spectrophotometer at 402nm.

Assay Methods

Although the activity of the OPA anhydrases can be monitored by several methods, including pH stat and acetylcholinesterase inhibition assay, the technique that has been used for the bulk of these studies involves the use of a fluoride-specific electrode. The assay has been described previously.[13,15] In general, 5ml of a buffered solution (5 to 50mM bis-tris propane, 500mM NaCl or KCl, pH 7.2) is added to a reaction vessel equipped with a magnetic stirrer and a fluoride-specific electrode that has been calibrated with NaF standards. Although techniques vary somewhat, 50 to 100μl of enzyme sample and 1 to 3mM of the substrate are used in each assay. The spontaneous rate of hydrolysis for each substrate under the conditions of the reaction is subtracted from the experimental rate.

Review of the OPA Anhydrases

Until approximately five years ago, it appeared that the OPA anhydrases could be divided into two classes, the "squid-type" and all the rest, which were referred to as "Mazur type."[18] Typically, the squid-type OPA anhydrase hydrolyzes DFP faster than soman, is stable, can be purified using ammonium sulfate, has a molecular weight of ~26,000 daltons, is usually unaffected or slightly inhibited by Mn^{2+}, experiences no inhibition of DFP hydrolysis by mipafox,[19] and does not demonstrate stereospecificity in the hydrolysis of soman. The Mazur type OPA anhydrase, as typified by the hog kidney enzyme, is characterized by hydrolyzing soman faster than DFP, is non-tolerant of ammonium sulfate precipitation, is stimulated by Mn^{2+}, is usually a dimer of ~62,000 daltons, and is competitively or reversibly inhibited by mipafox. The Mazur type enzyme also demonstrates a stereospecificity in the hydrolysis of tabun and soman.

The results of the past five years have shown that the OPA anhydrases can no longer be separated into only two distinct classes but probably belong to many diverse classes of enzymes that have similar catalytic mechanisms and overlapping substrate specificities. As will be seen in the following sections, there are often several distinguishable enzymes within the same organism. Substrate ranges vary tremendously, as do the effects of possible inhibitors and metal ions. The enzymatic mechanism has been described for the *opd* gene product (parathion hydrolase) but is still unknown for the remaining OPA anhydrases. Currently, the natural role of these enzymes is unknown, although suggestions have recently been made that the OPA anhydrases evolved for the degradation of naturally occurring organophosphates and halogenated organics. Table 1 summarizes the characteristics of many of the best studied OPA anhydrases.

Squid OPA anhydrases. Of all the conventionally recognized OPA anhydrases, the squid-type is the best studied. The OPA anhydrases of the squid have recently been reviewed by Hoskin,[20] the principal contributor to the body of knowledge on this enzymatic system. Our report will summarize some of the major findings covered in the review.

The distribution of the squid-type OPA anhydrase is relatively narrow, being found in only the nervous tissue, saliva, and hepatopancreas of cephalopods. The molecular weight of the squid-type OPA anhydrase is approximately 23 to 30,000 daltons. The term squid-type is specific to the activities found in these tissues. At times, more than one peak is apparent on molecular sizing chromatography at this

Table 1
Characteristics of OPA Anhydrase Activities

Enzyme	Substrate Hydrolysis MW*	Soman/DFP ratio	Mn2+ stimulation	Mipafox inhibition
T. thermophila				
Tt DFPase-1	80,000	1.12	2.5-4.0	+
Tt DFPase-2	75,000	1.26	2.0	+
Tt DFPase-3	72,000	0.71	1.7-2.5	+
Tt DFPase-4	96,000	1.95	17-30	nt
Tt DFPase-5	67,000	0.34	8.0	nt
R. cuneata				
Rc opa-1	19-35,000	nt[§]	1.0	−
Rc opa-2[†]	73-82,000		1.0	−
Rc opa-3	82-138,000	nt	nt	
Thermophile isolate OT				
(JD100)	84,000	−	+	−
Halophile isolate JD6.5				
OPAA-1A	145,000[‡]	nt	+	nt
OPAA-1B	124,000[‡]	nt	+	nt
OPAA-2	62,000[‡]	0.5	3-5	nt
Halophile isolate JD30.3				
OPAA-1	76,000		+	nt
opd gene product				
(parathion hydrolase)	60-65,000		nt	+
	(35,418 x 2)			
Squid-type OPA anhydrase (*Loligo peali*)	23-30,000	0.25	1.0	−
Mazur-type OPA anhydrase (hog kidney)	62-66,000	6.54	3.0	+

*Molecular weight as determined by column chromatography unless otherwise stated.
[§]nt=not tested.
[†]tentative designation, may be artifactual.
[‡]molecular weight by SDS and non-SDS PAGE.

molecular weight range.[21] It has been estimated that the squid-type OPA anhydrase constitutes approximately 0.002 percent of the intracellular tissue.[20]

Squid-type OPA anhydrase hydrolyzes soman at a rate that is only approximately 0.25 that of DFP. It apparently hydrolyzes all of the four stereoisomers of soman, but with some selectivity in rates.

Hoskin and Brande[7] examined a variety of materials as potential inhibitors and substrates of the squid-type OPA anhydrase. The compounds methanesulfonyl fluoride, phenyl-methanesulfonyl-fluoride (PMSF), monofluorophosphate, *p*-nitro-phenyl phosphate, octamethyl pyrophosphoramide (OMPA), tetra-monoisopropylphosphoramide (isoOMPA), sulfanilamide, and isethionate showed little or no inhibition of DFP hydrolysis. Methanesulfonyl fluoride, PMSF, monofluorophosphate, *p*-nitrophenyl phosphate, OMPA, isoOMPA, and aderosine triphosphate were not substrates. Paraoxon was also found to be resistant to hydrolysis in a later study.[8]

Among the most exciting results of recent research on the squid-type activity has been the elucidation of the role of various metal ions. It has long been known that Mn^{2+} either has no effect on or is inhibitory to the squid-type OPA anhydrase. In order to further characterize the effects of metal ions, Hoskin[20] used the chelators ethylenedinitrilo tetra-acetic acid (EDTA), ethylene glycol tetra-acetic, 1,10-phenanthroline; and 8-hydroxyquinoline-5-sulfonate. As a result of these experiments, it was surmised that the squid-type OPA anhydrase is Ca^{++} requiring but is not stimulated by other divalent cations. After chelation of the Ca^{++} by EGTA, it was demonstrated that the activity of the enzyme could be restored by the addition of Ca^{++}. Although the squid-type OPA anhydrase is apparently a Ca^{++} requiring enzyme, it is not stimulated by the addition of excess Ca^{++}.

Unlike many of the OPA anhydrases, mipafox is not inhibitory to this enzyme. The squid-type OPA anhydrase also has little, if any, activity with the chromogenic substrate NPEPP. It has been reported that the enzyme prefers an isopropyl side chain compared with an ethyl or methyl group.[10]

Although the primary investigations into the OPA anhydrases of squid tissue here been of the squid-type OPA anhydrase, squid also contains the more widespread "Mazur-type" enzyme. Gill, heart, mantle, and blood tissues all exhibit OPA anhydrase activities that are Mn^{2+} stimulated and hydrolyze soman faster than DFP.[20] The differential expression of these enzymes in such a variety of tissues is an extremely interesting area for speculation.

Tetrahymena OPA anhydrase. The ability of crude extracts of the protozoan *Tetrahymena thermophila* to hydrolyze DFP was discovered by Landis.[14] In the crude extracts, Mn^{2+} stimulated the DFP hydrolysis by a factor of 2.3. Addition of 0.01 percent EDTA halted the hydrolysis of the substrate, indicating a divalent cation requirement. Triton X-100 detergent at less than 0.5 percent had no effect on the reaction. Initial purification efforts using a Sephacryl S-200 (Pharmacia) molecular sizing column resulted in a somewhat broad peak in which the DFP hydrolyzing activity increased nine- to 12-fold. Interestingly, the rate of soman hydrolysis increased only two- to three-fold, indicating the possible presence of more that one OPA anhydrase. DFP was the substrate used in the screening of the column fractions.

Using material that had been fractionated with ammonium sulfate, chromatographed on Sephadex G-100, and lyophilized, we conducted a number of studies to characterize the DFP hydrolyzing activity.[15] Salt concentrations ranging from 0 to 500mM NaCl had little effect on activity. Three regions of activity were apparent in the pH-versus-activity curve: pH 4 to 6, 6 to 7.5, and greater than 7.5. Accurate activity measurements below pH 3 or above pH 10 are quite difficult due to the limitations of the fluoride-selective electrode. The temperature range was also fairly broad, from 20 to 55°C, with a plateau from 35 to 50°C.

Further purification of the *T. thermophila* OPA anhydrase activity by chromatography on DEAE-Sepharose and Sephacryl S-300 resulted in the identification of three peaks of activity with DFP. On addition of Mn^{2+}, a fourth peak was observed (Figure 2). These activities, designated as *Tt* DFPases, and their characteristics can be found in Table 1. Although there is a considerable variation in

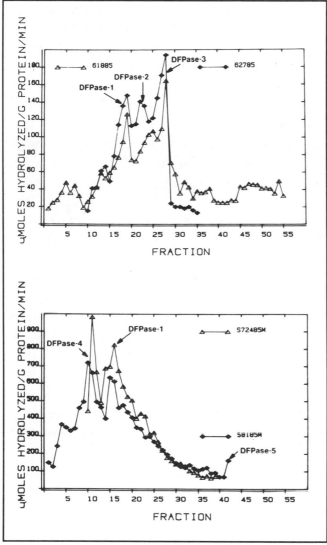

Figure 2. Initial elucidation of the *Tetrahymena thermophila* OPA anhydrases by Sephacryl S-300 chromatography. Top assays with DFP; bottom, assays with soman and manganese.

molecular weights (67 to 96,000 daltons) and stimulation by Mn^{2+} (two- to 30-fold), all the enzymes have a soman-to-DFP ratio of approximately 1:1. The existence of multiple OPA anhydrase activities was confirmed by isoelectric focusing, which gave three bands with isoelectric points of 5.2, 4.7, and 4.2.

Mipafox, which is a competitive inhibitor of the classical Mazur-type OPA anhydrases of hog kidney and *E. coli*, competitively inhibits *Tt* DFPases 1, 2, and 3.[17] Studies with partially purified extracts gave a $K_i \approx 1.3mM$ and a pattern that qualitatively resembled that of the inhibition of the hog kidney OPA anhydrase.

Several substrates were used in the search for a chromogenic assay for OPA anhydrase activity. These included paraoxon, NPEPP, NPIPP, NPMPP, and 4-nitrophenyl dimethylphosphinate. Only NPEPP was found to provide a reaction that corresponded to the hydrolysis by an OPA anhydrase, *Tt* DFPase 2.[17] In a comparative study, NPEPP was hydrolyzed by hog kidney OPA anhydrase but not by the squid-type enzyme.

Clam OPA anhydrases. The estuarine clam *Rangia cuneata* was discovered to possess OPA anhydrase activity by Anderson and co-workers[22] Clams collected from sediment samples from Chesapeake Bay were dissected at 1°C, and tissue weights were determined. Tissue homogenates (33 percent by weight) were prepared with Hank's balanced salt solution.

Of the tissues examined, levels of OPA anhydrase were highest in the digestive gland and lowest in the foot muscle.[22] Soman was hydrolyzed faster than DFP. Exogenous Mn^{2+} did not increase the rate of DFP hydrolysis, although soman hydrolysis was increased by 40 percent in the presence of 1mM Mn^{2+}. As with *Tetrahymena*, the temperature range of the activity in crude extracts was fairly broad, from 15 to 50°C. The pH optimum could not be accurately determined but was at least pH 9 or higher. An initial estimate of molecular weight at 22,000 daltons was determined by gel permeation chromatography. Interestingly, the molecular weight of the OPA anhydrase from the visceral mass was higher, implying a different enzyme and some tissue specificity. Except for molecular weight, the clam activity appeared to more closely resemble Mazur-type OPA anhydrase.

Because mipafox is a potent inhibitor of the Mazur-type OPA anhydrases, it was tested with the crude extract from *R. cuneata*. Surprisingly, the rate of fluoride release was even higher when 3mM mipafox was added to a solution of 3mM DFP.[22] The effect appeared to be the additive result of DFP and mipafox hydrolysis, as shown in Figure 3.

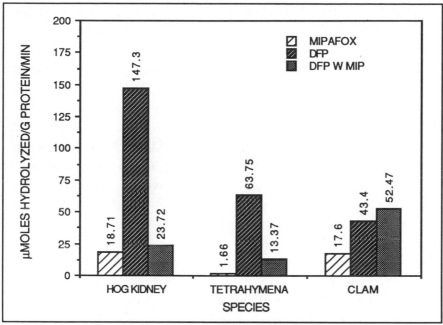

Figure 3. DFP and mipafox hydrolysis by *Rangia cuneata* extracts.

On separation using gel permeation chromatography, a distinct mipafox hydrolyzing activity was detected at a higher molecular weight than the DFP hydrolyzing OPA anhydrase. Currently, the mipafox hydrolyzing activity, which does not hydrolyze DFP, is being referred to as an OPA anhydrase until further studies can be conducted to ascertain its substrate specificity.

Mammalian OPA anhydrases. The best characterized mammalian OPA anhydrase is that of the hog kidney. A series of purification and characterization studies[11] resulted in a molecular weight determination of 62,000 daltons by sodium dodecylsulfate–polyacrylamide gel electrophoresis. Above pH 9.0 and below pH 3.5, two bands appeared with molecular weights of ~30,000. After this dissociation, the activity was reported to be lost. Mn^{2+} was important for the stability of the enzyme during the purification procedure. EDTA rapidly destroys enzymatic activity. According to the authors,[11] the active enzyme is a manganese-protein complex in a 1:1 ratio.

The substrate specificity of the hog kidney OPA anhydrase was extensively examined. Intact nucleic acid esters, phosphoric mono- and diesters, and phosphoric acid triesters with a nitrophenyl leaving group were not hydrolyzed by this enzyme. In addition to soman, sarin, and DFP, the hog kidney OPA anhydrase hydrolyzed a variety of substituted (2,2-dichlorovinyl)-phosphoric (DVP) acid esters. These included O,O-dimethyl-O"-DVP (DDVP); O-methyl-O'-2-methoxyethyl-O"-DVP (Sir 6091); O-methyl-O' cyclohexyl-O"-DVP (Sir 6089); O- methyl-O'-benzyl-O"-DVP (Sir 6115); and O-methyl-O'-butyl-O"-DVP. In a series of inhibition studies using Mevinphos and trimethylphosphate, both compounds were competitive inhibitors, with K_is of 1.5 and 5mM, respectively. Mipafox has also been demonstrated to be a powerful inhibitor of hog kidney OPA anhydrase activity.

Numerous other eukaryotic organisms have been screened for OPA anhydrase activity. For the purpose of this paper, it is sufficient to state that a variety of both squid- and Mazur-type enzymes have been detected that show differences in substrate specificity and Mn2+ stimulation. A great deal more research, including DNA and protein sequence homologies, will be required to work out the properties and possible relationships of these diverse enzymes.

Bacterial OPA anhydrases. In his extensive review, Mounter[2] showed that many bacteria exhibit OPA anhydrase activity. Several bacterial isolates have been recently examined in greater depth for OPA anhydrase activity and will be compared in this section to the *opd* gene product enzyme (parathion hydrolase). Chettur *et al.,*[23] published findings on the OPA anhydrase from an obligate thermophile (OT), also known as JD100 (from the DeFrank collection). This organism, which has been tentatively identified as a strain of *Bacillus stearothermophilus,* was isolated from soil samples from the Edgewood Area of the Aberdeen Proving Ground, Maryland. The enzyme was partially purified by gel permeation chromatography on Sephadex G-100, followed by DEAE-cellulose ion exchange chromatography. The estimated molecular weight of the enzyme is 84,000 daltons. The OT enzyme hydrolyzes soman, sarin, and dimebu (3,3-dimethylbutylmethyl-phosphonofluoridate) but not DFP. The catalysis is markedly stimulated by Mn^{2+} and is not inhibited by mipafox. DFP is a slight (~7 percent) noncompetitive inhibitor of soman hydrolysis. Because hydrolysis and the reduction of acetylcholinesterase inhibition coincide, the OT enzyme may hydrolyze all four isomers of soman simultaneously, similar to the squid-type enzyme.

Several halophilic bacterial isolates that have exhibited high levels of OPA anhydrase activity were obtained by DeFrank from salt springs in Utah. One isolate, designated JD6.5, has been the subject of considerable study.[24] This organism, which, based on fatty acid analysis (Microbial ID, Inc., Newark, DE), appears to be a strain of *Alteromonas*, was obtained from Grantsville Warm Springs near Salt Lake City, Utah.

As with many organisms, at least two or three different DFP hydrolyzing OPA anhydrases are found in JD6.5; however, ~90 percent of the activity is contributed by one enzyme, OPAA-2 (Figure 4). The enzyme has been purified 300-fold to near homogeneity by ammonium sulfate fractionation and chromatography on DEAE-Sephacel, HA Ultrogel (hydroxyapatite), and gel permeation high-pressure liquid chromatography. OPAA-2 appears to be a single polypeptide of 62,000 daltons molecular weight based on gel permeation and SDS- and nondenaturing PAGE. It is stimulated approximately fourfold by Mn^{2+} and twofold by Ca^{++}. In addition to DFP, the enzyme hydrolyzes soman and NPEPP and has a pH optimum of ~7.5.

Parathion hydrolase (opd OPA anhydrase). Parathion hydrolase, the product of the *opd* gene of *Pseudomonas diminuta*, is the best studied of the bacterial OPA anhydrases. This enzyme has the capability to hydrolyze DFP and other organofluorophosphates[25] in addition to its more commonly associated substrates of parathion and paraoxon. This OPA anhydrase, which until recently was labeled as a phosphotriesterase, is apparently widely distributed among bacteria. The genetic code has been sequenced, and the mechanism of hydrolysis has been elucidated. The pertinent facts are included for comparison to the OPA anhydrases just discussed.

The *opd* OPA anhydrase is coded for by a plasmid-borne gene of 1079 base pairs.[26] The gene sequence is identical in both *Flavobacterium* and *P. diminuta* , although the plasmids bearing this gene are not. Crude preparations of bacteria containing the *opd* gene

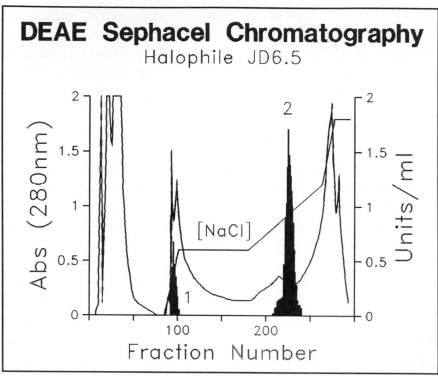

Figure 4. Separation of halophile JD6.5 OPA anhydrases by DEAE-Sephacel chromatography.

have been demonstrated to have the ability to hydrolyze a variety of phosphotriesters such as paraoxon; parathion; fensulfothion; O-ethyl O-p-nitrophenyl phenylphosphothioate (EPN); and chlorofenvinophos.[27,28] However, in at least the case of malathion hydrolysis, the active agent is not the *opd* OPA anhydrase. Activity that can degrade malathion even exists in *P. diminuta* cured of the plasmid containing the *opd* gene (J.R. Wild and F.M. Raushel, personal communication), indicating the possible existence of other OPA anhydrases in this organism. Eighty to ninety percent of the OPA anhydrase activity is associated with the pseudomonad membrane. The *opd* OPA anhydrase has a molecular weight of 35,418 daltons,[26] as determined by analysis of the gene sequence. However, the apparent molecular weight of the enzyme removed from the membrane is estimated to be in the 60 to 65,000 range, indicating that the active enzyme is dimeric.

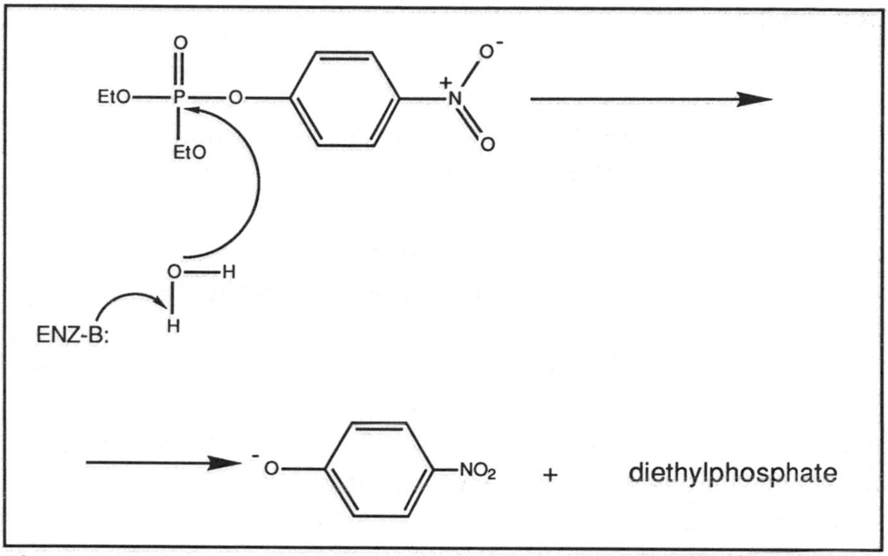

Figure 5. Mechanism of hydrolysis of paraoxon by the *opd* OPA anhydrase.

Recently, Dumas and co-workers[25] examined the hydrolysis of DFP by purified *opd* OPA anhydrase derived from an *E. coli* strain containing the *opd* gene and no other OPA anhydrase activity. DFP was hydrolyzed but at a rate of only 3.6 percent that of paraoxon. The K_m for DFP was 0.12mM versus 0.012mM for paraoxon. Diisopropyl-*p*-nitrophenylphosphate(DINPP), a nitrophenyl containing analoguc of DFP, was also hydrolyzed but at a rate of 9 percent that of paraoxon. The K_m for DINPP was similar to paraoxon at 0.013mM. DFP is a competitive inhibitor of paraoxon hydrolysis, suggesting that the active site is the same for both reactions. Mipafox also has been demonstrated to act as a competive inhibitor of DFP hydrolysis by this enzyme.

In an elegant series of experiments, the mechanism of the *opd* OPA anhydrase has been derived.[29] Using[18] containing water and the (+) and (–) enantiomers of O-ethyl phenylphosphonothioic acid, it was determined that the reaction was a single in-line displacement by an activated water molecule at the phosphorus center of the substrate (Figure 5). It is significant that this same active site was able to hydrolyze DFP and some other related organofluorophosphates.

Conclusions

Dramatically different organisms—bacteria, protozoans, clams, squid, and mammals—contain similar activities against compounds that are artificially synthesized and relatively rare in the environment. The production of organofluorophosphates only began in World War II, so the widespread phylogenetic distribution of these enzymes is more likely due to natural selection for the metabolism of some natural substances.

It is natural to wish to impose some sort of classification scheme on the OPA anhydrases that implies a set of phylogenetic relationships. The classification scheme of squid-type and Mazur-type OPA anhydrases has proved useful in that it was quickly possible to differentiate the squid-type enzyme from the other forms. However, as discussed previously, many of the more recently described OPA anhydrase activities appear to fall somewhere in between the classical types.

Even though they are a diverse set of enzymes, some generalization on the OPA anhydrases can be reached. The substrate range of the OPA anhydrases is quite broad. With a few exceptions, most of the enzymes are not sensitive to ammonium sulfate. A variety of OPA anhydrases are routinely found within an organism, be it squid, protozoan, bacteria, or clam. In addition, differentiation among OPA anhydrase of various tissues has been demonstrated.

To date, the active site of any of the OPA anhydrases has not been mapped by x-ray crystallography, yet some indications of the topography can be made. The size of the leaving group does not seem to be important. Enzymes from a variety of sources can hydrolyze compounds with both fluoride and nitrophenol leaving groups. It appears as if the leaving group is either perpendicular to the surface of the enzyme, with the rest of the molecule inserted into the active site, or lies in a large cavity on the enzyme surface. The latter case would indicate that the natural substrate of the enzyme is quite bulky. If the mechanism for the *opd* OPA anhydrase can be generalized as an attack at the phosphorus by an activated water, the configuration may be very important to catalytic activity. Indeed, small changes in side chains apparently make a tremendous difference for at least some of the OPA anhydrases. The *Tetrahymena* enzymes readily hydrolyze NPEPP but not its close analogue NPIPP. The squid-type OPA anhydrase does not hydrolyze either NPEPP or NPIPP.

An enzymatic activity that phylogenetically is as widespread as that of the OPA anhydrases must be important to the cellular metabolism and survival of the organism. The strength of the selective pressure for the *opd* OPA anhydrase is evident; divergent plasmids in *Pseudomonas* and *Flavobacterium* share identical *opd* sequences. The widespread nature of the OPA anhydrases also argues for a strong selective pressure over a much longer period than the last 45 years. However, the natural substrate and role(s) of the OPA anhydrase remain unknown. There are numerous candidate organophosphorus compounds that may be the natural substrate such as glycerophosphon-olipids, sphingophosphonolipids, phosphonoproteins, and nucleic acids and their many derivatives. It is possible, because these enzymes are generally found at relatively low concentrations within the cell or organism, that the natural substrate may be a substance that has not yet been described.

The diversity of the OPA anhydrases could be accounted for by at least two different evolutionary mechanisms. The enzymes may be all derived from a common ancestral protein and may have diverged significantly. Alternatively, over the last 3.5 billion years, numerous enzymes may have converged in activity due to the selection of a particularly narrow set of enzymatic mechanisms. Antigenic relationships, DNA and protein sequencing, and determination of the three-dimensional structures will help refine the classification of the OPA anhydrases and facilitate their use in biodegradation.

References

1. A. Mazur, *J. Biol. Chem.* **164**, 271 (1946).
2. L.A. Mounter, R.F. Baxter, and A. Chautin, *J. Biol. Chem.* **215**, 699 (1955).
3. L.A. Mounter, in *Hanbuch de Experimentellen Pharmakologie: Cholinesterases and Anticholinesterase Agents.* G.B. Kolle, Ed. (Springer-Verlag, Berlin, 1963) pp. 486-504.

4. F.C.G. Hoskin, P. Rosenberg, and M. Brzin, *Proc. Natl. Acad. Sci. USA* **55**,1231 (1966).
5. F.C.G. Hoskin, *Science* **172**, 1243 (1971).
6. F.C.G. Hoskin and R.J. Long, *Arch. Biochem. Biophys.* **150**, 548 (1972).
7. F.C.G. Hoskin and M. Brande, *J. Neurochem.* **20**, 1317 (1973).
8. J.M. Garden *et al., Comp. Biochem. Physiol.* **52C**, 95 (1975).
9. F.C.G. Hoskin, *J. Neurochem.* **26**, 1043 (1976).
10. D.D. Gay and F.C.G. Hoskin, *Biochem. Pharmacol.* **128**, 1259 (1979).
11. W. Storkebaum and H. Witzel, *Study on the Enzyme Catalyzed Splitting of Triphosphates* (Forschungsber. Landes Nordrhein-Westfalen, Federal Republic of Germany) **2523**, 1 (1975).
12. R. Zech and K.D. Wigand, *Experientia* **37**, 157 (1975).
13. F.C.G. Hoskin and A.H. Roush, *Science* **215**, 1255 (1982).
14. W.G. Landis, R.E. Savage, Jr., and F.C.G. Hoskin, *J. Protozool.* **32**, 517 (1985).
15. W.G. Landis, M.V. Haley, and D.W. Johnson, *J. Protozool.* **33**, 216 (1986).
16. W.G. Landis *et al.*, *J. Appl. Tox.* **7**, 35 (1987).
17. W.G. Landis *et al., Comp. Biochem. Phys.*, in press.
18. F.C.G. Hoskin, M.A. Kirkish, and K.E. Steinman, *Fund. Appl. Tox.* **4**, 5165 (1984).
19. F.C.G. Hoskin, *Biochem. Pharmacol.* **34**, 2069 (1985).
20. F.C.G. Hoskin, *in Squid as Experimental Animals*, D.L. Gilbert, W.J. Adelman, Jr., and J.M. Arnold, Eds. (Plenum Press, New York, 1989), in press.
21. K.E. Steinmann, personal communication, 1988.
22. R.S. Anderson, H.D. Durst, and W.G. Landis, *Comp. Biochem. Physiol.* **91C**, 575 (1988).
23. G. Chettur *et al., Fund. Appl. Tox.* **11**, 373 (1988).
24. J.J. DeFrank and T.-C. Cheng, *Abstr. Annu. Meet. Am. Soc. Microbiol.* **K186**, 276 (1989).
25. D.P. Dumas, J.R. Wild, and F.M. Raushel, *J. Appl. Biotech.*, in press.
26. C.S. McDaniel, L.L. Harper, and J.R.Wild, *J. Bacteriol.* **170**, 2306 (1988).
27. K.A. Brown, *Soil Biol. Biochem.* **12**, 105 (1980).
28. T. Chiang, M.C. Dean, and C.S. McDaniel, *Bull. Environ. Contam. Toxicol.* **34**, 809 (1985).
29. V.E. Lewis *et al., Biochem.* **27**, 1591 (1988).

Discussion

Buswell: Does the OPA anhydrase from your *Bacillus stearothermophilus* show any enhanced stability; have you looked at any of the more extreme thermophiles?

DeFrank: I have looked at *Thermus thermophilus* and *Thermus aquaticus*. They do not have activity that I could detect with diisopropyl fluorophosphate (DFP). I have not been working with *Bacillus stearothermophilus* myself. I know it has been immobilized on cotton and some other materials and has shown fairly good stability. I do not think that Frank Hoskin has done any long-term stability tests with it at different temperatures. Many experiments still need to be done, but from initial indications the enzyme appears to be quite stable. By contrast, an *Escherichia coli* enzyme that is somewhat similar is quite unstable.

Manuel Mota (Oporto University, Portugal): Are you using the DFP activity with these kinds of microorganisms in direct contact?

DeFrank: No. DFP, soman, and the other compounds will degrade spontaneously in soil. We are interested in using enzyme systems that can rapidly degrade compounds of this type either in a bioreactor or on contaminated surfaces. I do not think there has ever been an attempt to find organisms that would grow on these compounds.

Mota: I do not mean growing but the screening.

DeFrank: All the screening has been done with cell extracts, not with intact cells. Bacteria have been broken open, and squid have been homogenized before assays have been done. I am not sure how well the compounds would get into the cell.

Gunsalus: I have often said that there are not very many unstable enzymes, but there are many unstable investigators. It is a question of working out under what conditions these enzymes will withstand whatever kind of treatment. They did not stand ammonium sulfate until you learned how to handle it. Also bothersome in this exploratory work is the fact that when you have very low binding constants and low affinities, you often have "very broad substrate activity." As is known with oxygenases and microsomal enzymes, inducers and substrates may not be the same compounds.

DeFrank: For the few enzymes that have been characterized, their K_m has been usually in the range of 1 to 5mM.

Gunsalus: Enzymes that are selective typically have micromolar affinity constants.

12

Microorganism Stabilization for *In Situ* Degradation of Toxic Chemicals

Ronald L. Crawford
Kirk T. O'Reilly
Hong-Lei Tao
Department of Bacteriology
University of Idaho
Moscow, ID 83843

When pure cultures of bacteria are introduced into natural environments such as soil or subsurface waters, they often do not persist because they are not competitive with natural microbial populations, or these environments are too toxic or oligotrophic to support growth or maintenance requirements of the added cells. To improve prospects for successful *in situ* bioremediation of aquifers contaminated by toxic chemicals, methods are needed to stabilize microbial cells so that they persist following introduction into hostile natural environments. We have found that immobilization of pollutant-degrading bacteria in polymeric matrices such as alginate or polyurethane stabilizes them for introduction into surface soils or waters. This stabilization is at least partly a result of protection of the immobilized microbial cells from pollutant toxicity.

Introduction

In recent years, researchers in our laboratory have investigated the use of a pentachlorophenol-degrading *Flavobacterium* and other bacteria as bioremediation tools in soil,[1] groundwater,[2] and free-cell bioreactors.[3] We have observed repeatedly that when free cells of pure cultures are added to nonsterile soil or water, they usually persist for relatively short periods of time. These periods of time often have been insufficient to accomplish complete mineralization of the pollutants targeted for decontamination.[1,4]

Stotzky and Babich[5] reviewed the literature concerning survival of genetically engineered bacteria in natural environments. This work is relevant to the use of bacteria to treat polluted waters and soils, although one should recognize that the presence of foreign DNA in a bacterium may be detrimental to its competitive abilities in nature.[6,7] Representative examples of research in this area show that survivability of introduced strains in nonsterile soils and waters is highly strain-specific and greatly influenced by the presence and absence of selective pressures associated with cloned genes (for example, antibiotic resistance). However, under most competitive situations, introduced strains die back very quickly.

Sagik and colleagues[8,9] studied the survival of various *E. coli* host-vector systems in an activated sludge domestic sewage plant microcosm. These authors reported rapid diebacks of the added strains over periods of 20 to 30 hours. Schilf and Klingmüller[10] added various plasmid-bearing *E. coli* and *Pseudomonas* strains to natural soils and waters. In both environments, the authors observed diebacks of the introduced strains, but titers of indigenous bacteria remained constant during the experiments.

Pertsova and co-workers[11] inoculated soil columns with various *Pseudomonas putida* and *P. aeruginosa* isolates capable of degrading 3-chlorobenzoate. Uninoculated soils did not degrade 3-chlorobenzoate, but inoculated soils did. However, chlorobenzoate-degraders isolated from inoculated soils appeared not to be like the originally added *P. putida* and *P. aeruginosa* strains. This suggested that there had been death of the added cells, but exchange of genetic information from added cells to the indigenous microbial population had occurred.

Devanas and colleagues[12] added plasmid-bearing *E. coli* strains to soil at levels of 10^4 to 10^5 cells/gram soil. The added strains either maintained populations of about 10^4 cells/gram soil or died back to nondetectable levels during a 28-day incubation period. In similar experiments[13] this research group observed that populations of *E. coli* host-plasmid systems such as strains HB101, HB101 (C357), and HB101 (pBR322) declined after inoculation into soils, often to nondetectable levels after 28 days (the level of detection was 1 to 20 CFU/gram soil). However, survival was sufficiently long to allow transfer of genes within the microbiota and the added strains.

Liang and co-workers[14] found that *R. meliloti, A. tumefaciens, K. pneumoniae*, and *S. typhimurium* did not survive for extended periods when added to nonsterile sewage. In natural lake water, *R. meliloti* and *A. tumefaciens* declined to stable populations; *K. pneumoniae* and *S. typhimurium* populations declined rapidly.

In our initial work with alginate-immobilized *Flavobacterium* cells,[15] we found that pentachlorophenol (PCP) was degraded at initial concentrations as high as 150mg/l in batch reactors. Such concentrations are considerably higher than those tolerated by free cells. Even higher PCP concentrations could be degraded in continuous reactors if the flow rate was slow enough to maintain a low steady-state PCP concentration within a reactor. Other investigators have also shown that catalytic stability can be greater for immobilized cells compared with free cells and that some immobilized microorganisms tolerate higher concentrations of toxic compounds than their nonimmobilized counterparts.[16-18] These observations led us to examine the possible uses of polymeric immobilization matrices to protect cells from the hostile environments of natural soils and waters.

Immobilization of Bacterial Cells

We have employed immobilization matrices of alginate and polyurethane for our investigations. Alginate is a polysaccharide that when cross-linked by cations such as Ca^{++} forms a gel that is highly effective as a cell-entrapping matrix. Alginate, however, has somewhat low mechanical strength and is incompatible with anions such as phosphate, which promote disintegration of alginate beads. Alginate also is susceptible to biodegradation. These characteristics make alginate the preferred matrix for environments where persistence of the added matrix is not desirable, but alginate is less desirable for applications where long life and/or mehanical strength are needed.

Polyurethanes are a class of nonbiodegradable polymers synthesized as a result of the reactions between compounds containing an isocyanate group (R–N=C=0) and compounds containing a hydroxyl group. They have been investigated as immobilization matrices for microbial cells,[17] enzymes,[19] and organelles.[20] The use of polyurethane-immobilized microorganisms for the degradation of aromatic compounds was patented in U.S. patent No. 4,634,672.[21] The method included the addition of absorbents such as activated carbon or coal dust. All losses of compounds using the system were attributed to biodegradation, although the matrix was exposed to nonsterile wastewater for times as long as a few weeks before use. Although not discussed by the authors, the foam also might have served as a surface for chemical adsorption and/or biofilm formation.

We have isolated a group of PCP-degrading bacteria from a variety of environments contaminated with PCP.[22,23] All strains have been assigned to the genus *Flavobacterium*. A pure culture of one of the strains (ATCC 39723) was in the experiments reported here. Prior to immobilization, the *Flavobacterium* was grown in a minimal salts medium (3.6mM K_2HPO_4, 1.4mM KH_2PO_4, 5.9mM $NaNO_3$, 0.4mM $MgSO_4$, 50µM $FeSO_4$; pH 7.3). Sodium glutamate (4g/l) was supplied as the only carbon source. To induce the catabolic enzymes,[24] PCP (50mg /1) was added when the cultures reached mid-logarithmic phase. The disappearance of PCP was monitored spectrophotometrically at 320nm. When five percent of the PCP had been degraded, the cells were collected into a paste by centrifugation.[25]

The cells were mixed 1:1 (weight:weight) with cold (5°C), sterile four percent sodium alginate (Sigma type VII). Cold two percent sodium alginate was added to bring the mixture to the final desired volume. Five grams (wet weight) of cells were used for each 100ml (final volume) of alginate solution. The alginate-cell mixture was added dropwise to cold 50mM $CaCl_2$ for 30 minutes, and the beads that formed were collected by filtration. They were stored at

5°C in HEPES immobilization buffer (HIB: 50mM HEPES, 1mM CaCl$_2$, 1mM MgSO$_4$, 20μM FeSO$_4$, 0.5g/l sodium glutamate; pH 7.3) until used.

For immobilization in polyurethane,[26] a cell suspension was prepared by mixing 10g of the cell paste with 20ml of buffer (carbon-free growth medium). One part of polyurethane prepolymer (Hypol FHP2000®, W.R. Grace Co., Lexington, MA) was cooled on ice. One part (weight:weight) of buffer was added, and the mixture was stirred well for one minute. One part of the cell suspension was added, and mixing was continued for an additional one minute. An additional part of cell suspension was then added, and mixing was continued for another one minute. Cell-free foam was made for use as a control by substituting buffer for the cell suspensions. The reaction vessel was kept on ice for two hours while the polyurethane foam hardened. The foam was removed from the reaction vessel, rinsed with buffer to remove free cells, and stored at 4°C. At the beginning of each experiment, the foam was cut into 1cm³ pieces and rinsed three times with buffer to remove any free cells released during cutting of the foam.

Measurements of Pentachlorophenol (PCP) Degradation

Concentrations of PCP in liquid media were determined by measuring the absorbance of solutions at 320nm,[25] whenever possible. However, because of interferences by soil particles and because PCP adsorbs to polyurethane, PCP degradation was monitored by measuring the production of ^{14}C-CO$_2$ from ^{14}C-PCP in 250ml flask reactors.[26] Each flask was fitted with a CO$_2$ trap consisting of a small glass cup connected to the top of the flask. The cup contained 0.75ml of 1N NaOH. A rubber stopper was placed in the flask to prevent the loss of CO$_2$. At each sampling time, the NaOH was transferred to a liquid scintillation vial, the cup was rinsed twice with one milliliter of water, and the rinse water was also placed in the vial. Twenty milliliters of ReadySafe® scintillation cocktail were added, and the vial counted in a liquid scintillation counter. Concentrations of free PCP in media were determined by measuring the disintegration per minute in one milliliter of liquid.

Adsorption and Desorption of PCP to Polyurethane

Hypol FHP2000® was prepared using our usual method except that cells were omitted. Six flasks were prepared, each containing 50ml of water. Two flasks each received 10, 50, and 100ppm of PCP (concentrations used in typical biodegradation experiments).

At time 0, one gram of foam was added to each flask. At 15, 30, and 70 minutes, and then every hour for three hours, PCP concentration was measured spectrophotometrically. The blank employed was 50ml water plus one gram foam, without PCP. At 3.5 hours, additional PCP was added to one flask of each concentration. Measurements of PCP in solution over time, including the next morning, were used to calculate partition coefficients (Q).[27]

To measure desorption rates of PCP from polyurethane foam, we added one gram foam to 200ppm PCP in 50ml of water and let this mixture sit overnight. The foam then was placed in distilled water, and the release of PCP was monitored. We observed quick desorption (similar to adsorption).

To look at the effect of surface area on PCP adsorption-desorption rates, three flasks were prepared using media with 500ppm PCP. One gram of foam was added to each flask as either one piece, seven pieces, or 40+ pieces. No differences were observed in amounts of PCP bound or the calculated Q.

On day one (foam made on day 0), the calculated Q averaged approximately 25 and was consistent over the range of PCP concentrations tested (up to 200ppm), indicating that the foam had not been saturated with PCP. With three-day-old foam, the Q was 10. The Q still was approximately 10 using nine-day-old foam. The surface area or number of pieces of foam per gram did not influence the Q. There was no obvious difference in rates of adsorption and desorption. The graphs of PCP bound or released over time could be superimposed for the two events. Near steady state was obtained in about 10 minutes.

Biodegradation of PCP by Immobilized *Flavobacterium* Cells

Flavobacterium cells were immobilized in calcium alginate and used to degrade PCP in soil environments. Immobilized cells were compared with free cells. Ten ppm of ^{14}C-PCP were added to sand slurries in which either immobilized cells or free cells were present at approximately 2×10^6 cells/ml·CO$_2$ traps were used to trap the evolved ^{14}C-CO$_2$, and the flasks were incubated on a shaker at 27°C. The production of ^{14}C-CO$_2$ was checked weekly. After 42 days, the immobilized cells degraded 71 percent of the radiolabeled PCP. Most of the degradation occurred within the first 16 days. When incorporation of ^{14}C into cell mass is considered, this level of ^{14}C-CO$_2$ production represents total degradation of PCP. Similar inoculation with nonimmobilized cells showed that the free cells degraded less than 0.1 percent of the PCP over the 42 days.

We examined the ability of polyurethane-immobilized *Flavobacterium* cells to degrade 100 to 300ppm of PCP.[26] These are concentrations known to severely inhibit free cells. At 100ppm, half the degradation occurred over the first 24 hours. The degradation was complete by 48 hours. At 200ppm, degradation was fairly steady over the first three days. Half the PCP was degraded over this time, whereas the remaining PCP was degraded on the fourth day. At 300ppm, slight degradation occurred over the first few days, then on either the fourth or fifth day degradation was complete. Thus, polyurethane appears to protect the cells from inactivation by high concentrations of PCP.

The adsorption of PCP to the polyurethane appeared to protect the cells from PCP inhibition. Although the total PCP concentration, for example, was 200mg/l., the soluble concentration in the presence of the foam was about 120mg/l. The reversible binding of PCP to the polyurethane maintained the soluble PCP concentration below the toxic level while keeping the PCP available for degradation. The results were similar to those of Apajalahti and Salkinoja-Salonen[28] who found that the reversible binding of PCP to bark chips allowed a mixed culture to degrade PCP at higher initial concentrations.

Acknowledgments

This work was supported by U.S. Geological Survey Grant No. 14-O8OOO1-G1417 in collaboration with BioTrol, Inc., Chaska, MN.

References

1. R.L. Crawford and W. Mohn, *Enz. Microbiol. Technol.* **7**, 617 (1985).
2. M. Martinson *et al.*, in *Biodeterioration 6*, G. Llewellyn and O'Rear, Eds. (Commonwealth Agricultural Bureau, Slough, United Kingdom, 1986), pp. 529-534.
3. E. Brown *et al.*, *Appl. Environ. Microbiol.* **52**, 92 (1986).
4. E. Topp, R. Crawford, and R. Hanson, *Appl. Environ. Microbiol.* **54**, 2452 (1988).
5. G. Stotzy and H. Babich, *Adv. Appl. Microbiol.* **31**, 93 (1986).
6. R. Curtiss, *Ann. Rev. Microbiol.* **30**, 507 (1976).
7. R.B. Helling, T. Kinney, and J. Adams, *J. Gen. Microbiol.* **123**, 129 (1981).
8. B.P. Sagik and C.A Sorber, *Recomb. DNA Tech. Bull.* **2**, 55 (1979).
9. B.P. Sagik, C.A Sorber, and B.E. Morse, in *Molecular Biology, Pathogenicity, and Ecology of Bacterial Plasmids*, S.B.Levy, R.C. Clowes, and E.L. Koenig, Eds. (Plenum Press, New York, 1981), pp. 449-460.
10. W. Schilf and W. Klingmüller, *Recomb. DNA Tech. Bull.* **6**, 101 (1983).
11. R.N. Pertsova, F. Kunc, and L.A. Golovleva, *Folia Microbiol.* **29**, 242 (1984).
12. M.A. Devanas, D. Rafaelli-Eshkol, and G. Stotzky, *Curr. Microbiol.* **13**, 269 (1986).
13. M.A Devanas and G. Stotzky, *Curr. Microbiol.* **13**, 279 (1986).
14. L.N. Liang *et al.*, *Appl. Environ. Microbiol.* **44**, 708 (1982).
15. K. O'Reilly *et al.*, in *Chemical and Biochemical Detoxification of Hazardous Waste*, J. Glasser, Ed. (American Chemical Society, New Orleans, LA, 1988), in press.
16. D.F. Dwyer et al., *Appl. Environ. Microbiol.* **52**, 345 (1986).
17. J. Klein and M. Kluge, *Biotechnol. Letters* **3**, 65 (1981).
18. F. Westmeier and H. Rehm, *Appl. Microbiol. Biotechnol.* **22**, 301 (1985).
19. S. Fukushima *et al.*, *Biotech. Bioeng.* **20**, 1465 (1978).
20. A Tanaka *et al.*, *Eur. J. Appl. Microb. Biotechnol.* **7**, 351 (1979).
21. W. Baumgarten *et al.*, (*U.S. Patent No. 4, 634, 672*, 1987).
22. J.J. Pignatello *et al.*, *Appl. Environ. Microbiol.* **46**, 1024 (1983).
23. D.L Saber and R.L Crawford, *Appl. Environ. Microbiol.* **50**, 1512 (1985).
24. K. Sonomoto *et al.*, *J. Fenn. Tech.* **59**, 465 (1981).
25. J.C. Steiert, J.J. Pignatello, and R.L. Crawford, *Appl. Environ. Microbiol.* **53**, 907 (1987).

26. K.T. O'Reilly and R.L Crawford, *Appl. Environ. Microbiol.* **55**, 866 (1989).
27. K. Sonomoto *et al.*, *Ag. Biol. Chem.* **44**, 1119 (1980).
28. J.H. Apajalahti and M.S. Salkinoja-Salonen, *Microb. Ecol.* **10**, 359 (1984).

13

Biodegradations Yield Novel Intermediates for Chemical Synthesis

correspondence

Douglas W. Ribbons
Stephen J.C. Taylor
Centre for Biotechnology
Imperial College of Science,
Technology, and Medicine
London, United Kingdom
and Enzymatix Ltd.
Cambridge Science Park
Milton Road
Cambridge, CB4 4WE
United Kingdom

Chris T. Evans
Steven D. Thomas
Enzymatix Ltd.

John T. Rossiter
Department of Biochemistry
Wye College,
University of London

David A. Widdowson
David J. Williams
Department of Chemistry
Imperial College of Science,
Technology, and Medicine
London , United Kingdom

It is rare for biotransformation processes to compete economically with chemical routes to provide compounds. The exceptions relate usually to the provision of chiral intermediates in high enantiomeric excess by: (1) kinetic resolution, (2) stereoselective synthesis, (3) specific discrimination of similar groups by regioselective modifications, and (4) processing of fragile products or precursors. The authors review here some relatively new microbial processes that yield frequently novel chemical intermediates that are interesting substances in themselves, but are also precursors to simple and complex products of biological, chemical, and physical interest by further chemical or biochemical modifications. The biotransformations described here are based on regio- and stereoselective oxygenations of arenes. Two groups of numerous families of novel products are highlighted as examples suitable for exploitation, namely chiral products and fluorinated compounds. It is conceivable that detoxification strategies in the future will include biotransformations to synthesize commercially and pharmacologically useful derivatives such as those described here.

Introduction

Some significant changes in perceptions of the chemical and pharmaceutical industries have occurred during the last two decades. One involves a move towards more high value–added materials rather than commodities. Biotechnological processes, particularly biotrans-formations, are being recognized as valuable auxiliary or essential procedures to achieve certain highly specific reactions to yield, for example, chiral products in high enantiomeric excess. These reactions occur under mild conditions, so they are also suitable for the synthesis of fragile precursors or products. Here we illustrate some reactions that proceed smoothly to novel chiral and sensitive products in high yields, some from inexpensive precursors. There is no single chemical process to date that permits the direct oxidation of benzene or other very simple arenes to synthetically useful substances. The philosophy of our approach is the development of biotransformation processes using enzyme-catalyzed reactions unique to bacteria, which chemists have not yet learned to emulate. We concentrate on reactions that are initiated by dioxygenations of arenes to give *cis*-1,2-diols of cyclo-hexadienes (of known and unknown absolute stereochemistry), which have not been described by synthetic routes. This approach to bio-transformations of arenes is significantly different from early work in the 1950s and 1960s that attempted to produce known high-volume chemicals of established commercial value by bacterial oxidations, for example, salicylic acid and 1-naphthol from naphthalene, or adipic acid from several monocyclic arenes. It is very difficult to imagine how these biological processes could ever compete with well-estab-lished chemistry; additionally, it would need retraining of personnel and new, expensive capital investment.

The second area of interest we discuss here is the biotransforma-tion of fluoroarenes to a variety of oxidized fluorochemicals. Al-though fluorine was isolated just over 100 years ago, and an ever-increasing interest in the synthesis of fluoro-organic chemicals has been sustained, the introduction of fluorine to provide several types or substitution patterns of fluorinated compounds has been either unattainable or not facile. Fluorine introduction often involves harsh chemistry; many desired precursors or products are too sensitive to survive these procedures. In 1982, approximately 600 fluoro-organic chemicals were readily available for purchase, but by 1985 this number had increased to 1,600 (in the catalogues of Aldrich, Fluoro-chem, Koch-Light [Genzyme], and Yarsley [now Shell]). Of these, few were hydroxylated arenes, and less than a handful were chiral molecules (if so, they were racemates). Biotransformations, with their mild reaction conditions and usually exquisite specificity, offer alternative and unique routes to new, interesting fluorochemicals.[1]

Various recent syntheses starting from the bacterial oxidation products of arenes are described to demonstrate the growing awareness that these compounds are suitable starting materials for further chemical (or enzymic) modifications to desired synthetic targets. Knowledge of their availability should stimulate more chemists to design alternative strategies for their synthetic programs. Furthermore, environmental biotechnologists may be stimulated to perceive valuable products from biotransformation of aromatic compounds that otherwise are a nuisance.

Chiral Synthons in Organic Synthesis

Frequently, the ability of a chemical, be it a drug or a pesticide to perform the task for which it was synthesized depends on its interaction with a specific enzyme or receptor within a target cell. The substrates for such enzymes and receptors are often complex chiral molecules of a highly specific three-dimensional array.

Currently, much synthetic chemistry is geared toward the production of a particular enantiomer of a chiral substrate, and it is desirable and/or necessary to avoid the presence of the alternative enantiomer in the final product. One enantiomer of a substrate may simply be inactive towards its target enzyme; hence the synthesis of a racemic substrate represents a waste of starting material. In other instances, one enantiomer may be antagonistic towards the other, may be toxic, or may cause some unwanted effect. In the tragic case of thalidomide, only the S-isomer was found to be teratogenic. With the drug propranolol, the R-isomer is a contraceptive, but the S-isomer acts as a ß-blocker. Hence, there is a frequent need to synthesize a particular enantiomer of a bioactive compound. Current methods of producing optically active compounds can be broadly classified as involving either chiral resolution or chiral synthesis. A racemate may be resolved by fractional crystallization, whereby the enantiomers are complexed with a chiral auxiliary, forming a pair of diastereomers that can be separated by differences in their physical properties, by use of chiral high-pressure liquid chromatography (HPLC); or by stereoselective enzymatic transformation of one of an enantiomeric pair.

Chiral synthesis is the synthesis of one optical isomer of a product in preference to all other stereoisomers. The task can be greatly simplified if chiral starting materials or intermediates are available; hence, there is great interest in novel methods for producing enantiomerically pure synthons.

Biotransformations in Organic Synthesis

Much attention has been focused on the use of enzymes as chiral catalysts to produce optically active products.[2,3] Enzymes are often highly selective for their substrate from a mixture of reactants; are often regioselective within the substrate; operate under mild reaction conditions with respect to temperature, pH, and pressure; may functionalize specifically one of a number of nonactivated positions in substrates; and can catalyze reactions of substrates that may be unstable under the conditions required for the desired chemical reaction.

A biotransformation may be catalyzed by a purified enzyme or by a whole-cell system. Each has its merits. Whole-cell systems are inexpensive and have a naturally immobilized cofactor regeneration ability but may give rise to a difficult workup for product, and also to side reactions. Isolated enzymes catalyze cleaner, more specific reactions but may be expensive to use, be unstable, and require addition or regeneration of cofactors.

Biotransformation of Aromatic Compounds to Produce Chirons

Dioxygenation of the Aromatic Ring. Microorganisms are capable of an enormous range of biotransformations and degradations of aromatic compounds, some of which occur naturally in the environment, and some of which are xenobiotic.[4,5] Evolution has provided microorganisms with the capability for inserting molecular dioxygen into the relatively inert benzenoid ring as a general strategy for growth when aromatic compounds are the only source of carbon available. This process requires reducing equivalents in the form of nicotinamide-adenine dinucleotide (NADH). The resulting dihydroxylated nonaromatic intermediates (neutral or ionic dihydrodiols) are then dehydrogenated to catechols, further transformed to central metabolites, and used for growth and respiration. In all cases examined so far, bacteria catalyze the formation of *cis* diols. Eukaryotic organisms are known to transform aromatic compounds to diols having a *trans* configuration. The dioxygenation of the benzene nucleus may or may not be the primary step in the degradation of these compounds; in some instances, sidechain modifications occur before attack on the aromatic ring.

Microoganisms are able to dioxygenate the aromatic ring with a high degree of regio- and enantioselectivity. This gives rise to several families of neutral or ionic cyclohexadienes that contain two hydroxylated asymmetric carbon atoms (Figure 1).

Such families of compounds can be obtained in high yield using mutant bacteria that cannot rearomatize the dioxygenated products. These accumulate and are excreted into the medium. Microorganisms can also biotransform many substituted analogues of the natural aromatic substrate (although such compounds may only be partially metabolized), permitting access to molecules with unusual and crowded functionalities and substitution patterns in high enantiomeric

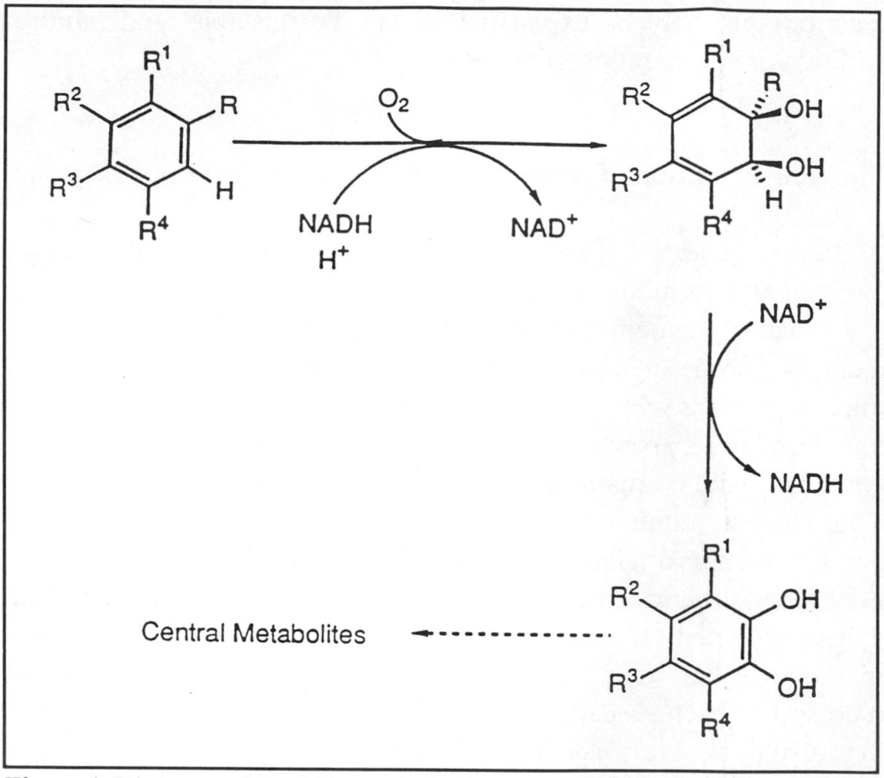

Figure 1. Dioxygenation of the aromatic ring.

excesses, many of which would be difficult if not impossible to synthesize using conventional chemistry. The starting materials for these biotransformations may be inexpensive and abundantly available from industrial sources, possibly even as byproducts of wastestreams.

Biotransformations of Fluoroaromatic Compounds

Although the fluorine atom is of a similar size to hydrogen and oxygen, it has a stronger electronegative character more akin to oxygen. The substitution of hydrogen or oxygen by fluorine in a molecule can greatly alter the biological and chemical properties of the compound. Hence, interest in the production of novel fluoro-chemicals, especially chiral fluorochemicals, is increasing. Synthetic fluorinated aromatic substrate analogues can have several conse-quences in microbes that degrade the nonfluorinated aromatics. The analogues may be inert. They may be degraded completely with excretion of the fluorine as fluoride ion. Toxic fluoroanalogues can provide a positive selection for new mutants defective in the catabolic pathway.[6] Finally, if an intermediate containing fluorine is not a substrate for a later enzyme in a reaction sequence, the fluorointerme-diate can accumulate and may be excreted from cells as a novel fluorochemical. Such compounds can also be obtained by provision of fluorinated substrates to mutant organisms, whereby the product accumulates due to a metabolic block. There are many new fluoro-chemicals potentially obtainable using microorganisms.

Dihydrodiols from Benzene and Toluenes

Initial reactions in the degradation of benzene and toluenes. The most studied and exploited systems that generate chirons from aro-matic compounds occur in bacteria able to metabolize benzenes or toluenes. Benzene oxidation by microorganisms has been recognized for many years, with catechol implicated as an intermediate.[7,8] The initial reactions in the metabolism of benzene and toluene are shown in Figure 2 for organisms that do not modify the sidechain of toluene.[9]

Studies by Gibson[10] provided a strain of *Pseudomonas putida* that could utilize benzene, toluene, and ethylbenzene as sole carbon sources. Nitrosoguanidine treatment yielded a mutant, *P. putida* 39/D, which was unable to grow on benzene but accumulated the dihydrodiol of benzene, benzene-*cis*-glycol.[11] The corresponding dihydrodiols from toluene, ethylbenzene, *p*-xylene, and halogenated benzenes and toluenes were all isolated and characterized using the same mutant *P. putida* 39/D.[12-15] Since then, other neutral dihydrodi-ols have been produced using mutants of *P. putida* [16-18] (Figure 3).

The absolute structure of the toluene-*cis*-glycol formed by *P.*

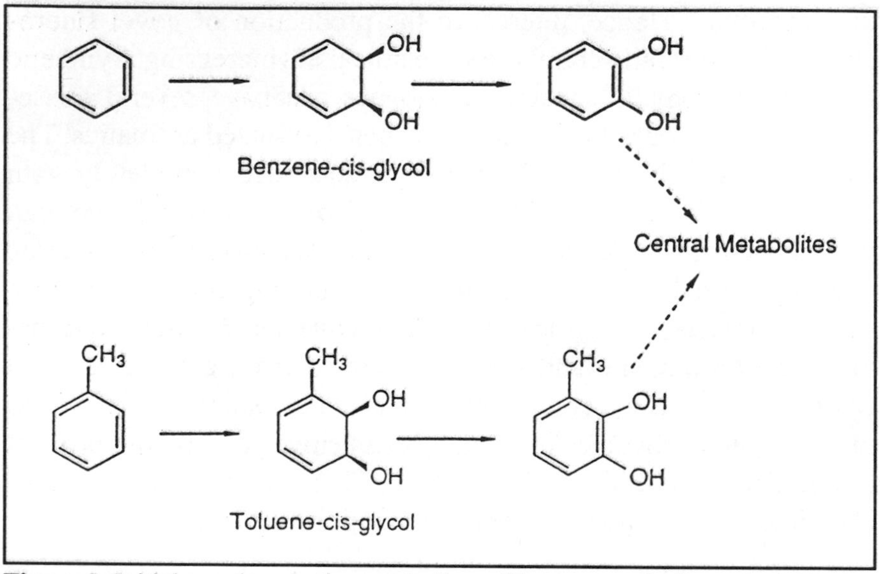

Figure 2. Initial reactions in the metabolism of benzene and toluene by bacteria.

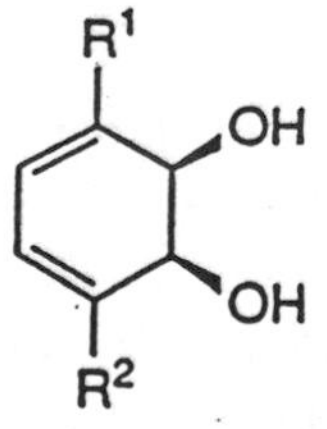

$R^1 = R^2 = H$ $R^1 = Ph, R^2 = H$ $R^1 = C{\equiv}CH, R^2 = H$

$R^1 = Cl, R^2 = H$ $R^1 = CF_3, R^2 = H$ $R^1 = CH_3, R^2 = F$

$R^1 = F, R^2 = H$ $R^1 = C_2H_5, R^2 = H$ $R^1 = CH_3, R^2 = Cl$

$R^1 = CH_3, R^2 = H$ $R^1 = HC{=}CH_2, R^2 = H$ $R^1 = CH_3, R^2 = Br$

Figure 3. Neutral dihydrodiols from mutants of *P. putida*.

putida 39/D was determined unambiguously in 1973 to be (+)-3-methyl-3,5-cyclohexadiene-1S, 2R-diol via x-ray studies of a diacetylated cycloaddition product of toluene-*cis*-glycol[19] (Figure 4).

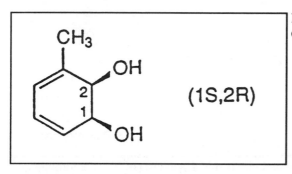

Figure 4. Absolute structure of toluene-*cis*-glycol.

(1S,2R)

Applications of Neutral Dihydrodiols

For several years, the interest in these neutral dihydrodiols remained purely academic. Only small quantities of these compounds were isolated using shaken-flask biotransformations (milligrams to a few grams), but using different mutants of *P. putida* containing lesions in dehydrogenase activity, accumulations of dihydrodiols to much higher concentrations have been achieved recently. For example, toluene-*cis*-glycol accumulated to 18 to 24 gm/l in fed-batch fermentation with *P. putida* strain NG1.[20]

Multinational companies such as ICI and Shell have recently issued patents claiming various neutral dihydrodiols, the fermentation processes for producing them, and the mutants used in the process.[21,22]

Phenols From Neutral Dihydrodiols

Rearomatization of these dihydrodiols yields phenols and catechols.[16] Dehydration under acidic or basic conditions will allow access to phenols that may be difficult to synthesize with the required substitution patterns. For example, dihydrodiol from 1,4-dichlorobenzene was synthesized and then dehydrated to yield 2,5-dichlorophenol (Figure 5). By contrast. the direct chemical chlorination of phenol results in 2,4- and 2,6-dichlorophenols.[16]

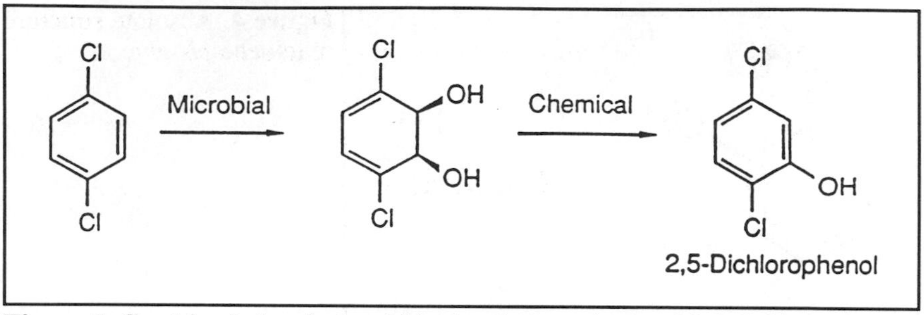

Figure 5. Combined chemical and biochemical synthesis of 2,5-dichlorophenol.

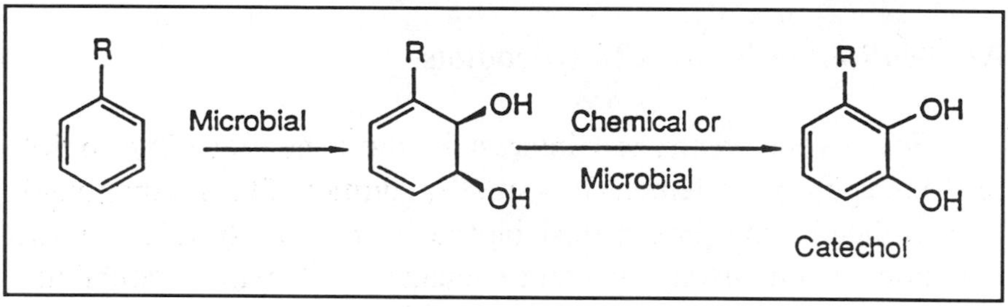

Figure 6. Biochemical and chemical synthesis of catechols.

Catechols From Neutral Dihydrodiols

Catechols can be synthesized by dehydrogenation of the dihydrodiol over a transition metal catalyst at low temperatures, providing high selectivity over the competing dehydration reaction[16] (Figure 6).

They have also been synthesized microbially by direct accumulation using a mutant organism with a lesion at the ring-cleavage stage. Such compounds and their production methods have been patented as have fluorophenol production processes (see Table 1).

The catechol moiety is found in many pharmacologically active compounds, especially anti-hypertensive agents. 3-Fluorocatechol is a valuable starting point because it can be readily methylated to 3-fluoroveratrole (Figure 7).

3-Fluoroveratrole is an intermediate used in the synthesis of neuroactive drugs related to fluorodimethoxyphenylethylamines.[23] The biological step represents a cost and labor-saving shortcut. 3-Fluoro-

Table 1
Substituted Aromatic Compounds Claimed in Patents by Multinational Companies

Compound	Description of Process	Patent
R=H,F	Accumulation of a catechol using a mutant of *P. putida* NCIB 12190.	0 253 438 (Shell, 1986)
R^1,R^2 selected from H, halogen, nitrile, carboxyl, alkyl, aryl, cycloalkyl	Accumulation of a catechol using a mutant benzene degrading organism.	0 268 331 (Shell, 1988)
Catechol (unspecified)	Accumulation of a catechol, using a mutant microbe, and molasses as carbon source.	0 252 567 (Shell, 1988)
Catechol or dihydrodiol	Accumulation of a cyclic dihydroxy compound using a mutant of *P. putida* NCIB 11680 or 11767; specifying method of growth and induction using pyridines.	0 250 122 (ICI, 2987)
R^1,R^2=H, halogen, nitrile, alkoxy, aryl, alkyl.	Catechols produced chemically by dehydrogenation of the dihydrodiol over Pd or Pt catalysts in the presence of O.	2 199 324 (GB) (Shell, 1986)
R^1=H, R^2=F R^1=F, R^2=H	Fluorophenols prepared Chemically by basic dehydration of the 3-fluorodihydrodiol	2 203 150 (GB) (Shell, 1988)

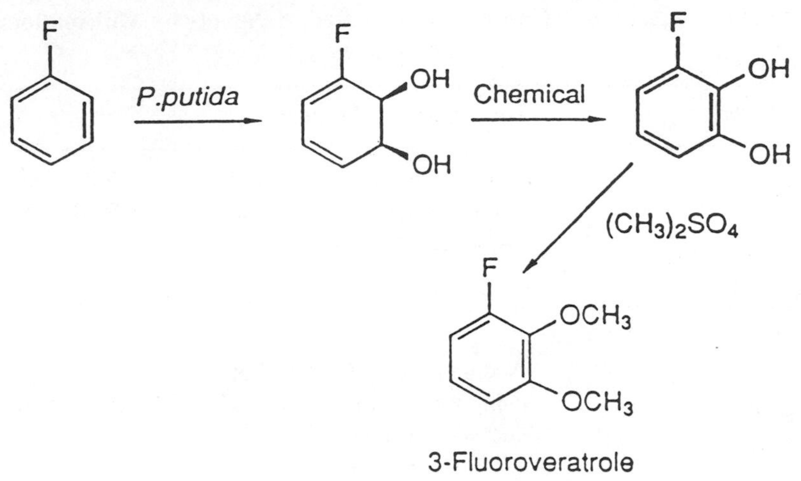

Figure 7. Combined biochemical chemical and synthesis of 3-fluoroveratrole.

catechol can be directly accumulated by mutant microorganisms blocked at the ring-cleavage stage, but accumulations of catechols are limited by their toxicity to the cells.[23]

Synthesis of Polyphenylene From Benzene-*cis*-Glycol

Benzene-*cis*-glycol has been used as a precursor for monomers in the production of polyphenylenes (Figure 8), which have electrical and electronic applications.[24] The polymer is of interest to scientists concerned with relationships between molecular structure and modulus, thermal stability, conductivity (when doped with metals such as ferric chloride), or insulation (when doped with electron donors).[25] Production of polyphenylene using conventional chemistry gave an inferior product of low molecular weight because of the poor solubility of intermediates in the reaction and fracture of the main chain under the severe conditions required for polymerization. The polymer derived from benzene-*cis*-glycol has a higher average molecular weight (from 600 to 1000 monomer units) and was readily cast into fibers and films.

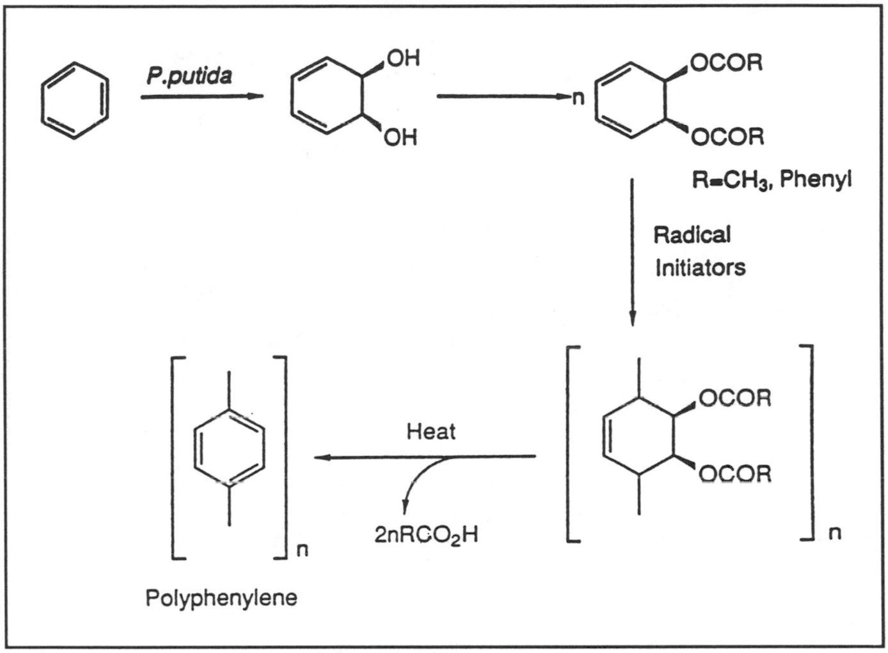

Figure 8. Polyphenylene synthesis from microbially derived precursors.

The production of phenols, catechols, and polymers from neutral dihydrodiols involves loss of any chirality that existed, with rearomatization of the diol. Other applications retain the chirality.

Synthesis of (±)–Pinitol from Benzene-*cis*-Glycol

Benzene-*cis*-glycol was used as a synthon in the synthesis of (±)–pinitol, a feeding stimulant in some larvae.[26] The synthesis was achieved in good yield in five steps from the dihydrodiol (Figure 9).

Synthesis of Inositol-1,4,5-Triphosphate from Benzene-*cis*-Glycol

The same *cis*-diol was used by our colleagues in the synthesis of inositol-1,4,5-triphosphate, an important cellular secondary messenger involved in many cellular processes[26,27] (Figure 10).

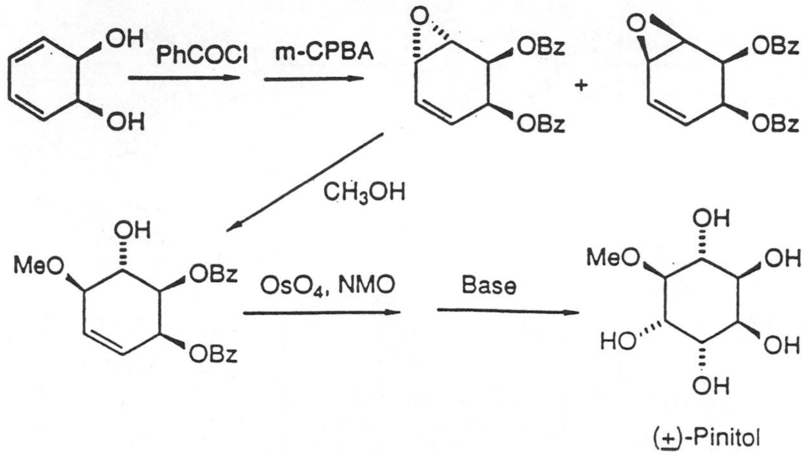

Figure 9. Synthesis of (+/-)-pinitol from benzene-*cis*-glycol.

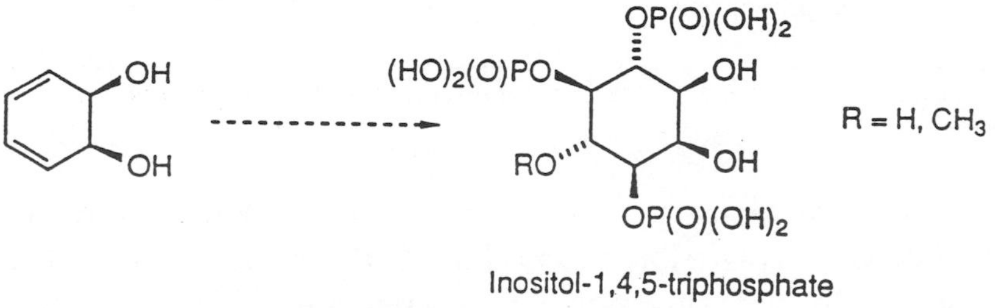

Figure 10. Inositol-1,4,5-triphosphate from benzene-*cis*-glycol.

Terpene and Prostaglandin Synthons From Toluene-*cis*-Glycol

Toluene-*cis*-glycol has been transformed to chirons of interest in the synthesis of terpenoids, prostaglandins, and cyclohexane oxides.[17] Terpene synthons were synthesized (Figure 11) in three operations from toluene-*cis*-glycol. The prostaglandin synthon PGE_{2a} was synthesized in three steps from toluene-*cis*-glycol in 45 percent overall yield (Figure 12). Epoxidation of the dihydrodiol acetonide (Figure 13) was achieved here in a regio- and enantio selective manner using 3-chloroperoxybenzoic acid. (This reaction is similar to the one that was performed in the synthesis of pinitol

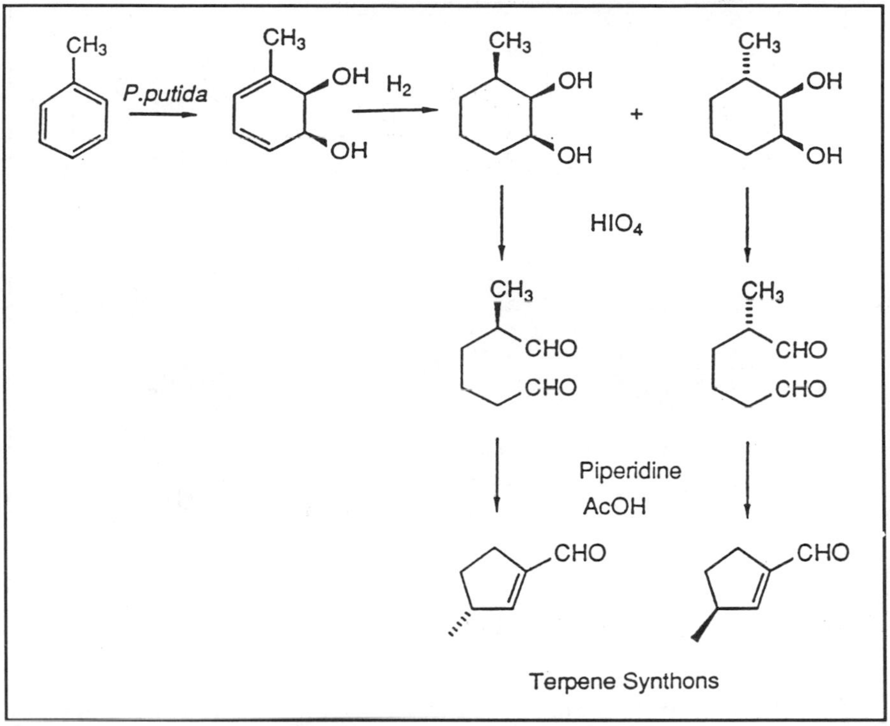

Figure 11. Terpene synthons from toluene-*cis*-glycol.

(Figure 9). Cyclohexane oxides may possibly have significant anti-tumor properties.[17]

Enzymic Transformation of a Benzene-*cis*-Glycol Derivative

In a combination of biological, chemical, then biological trans-formations, benzene-*cis*-glycol was derivatized in two stages to a pro-chiral diester (Figure 14). The diester was hydrolyzed by pig-liver esterase to produce an optically active mono-ester in 88 percent yield.[28]

Organometallic Complexes of Toluene-*cis*-Glycol

Toluene-*cis*-glycol has recently been used in the synthesis of homochiral organometallic complexes of the type seen in Figure

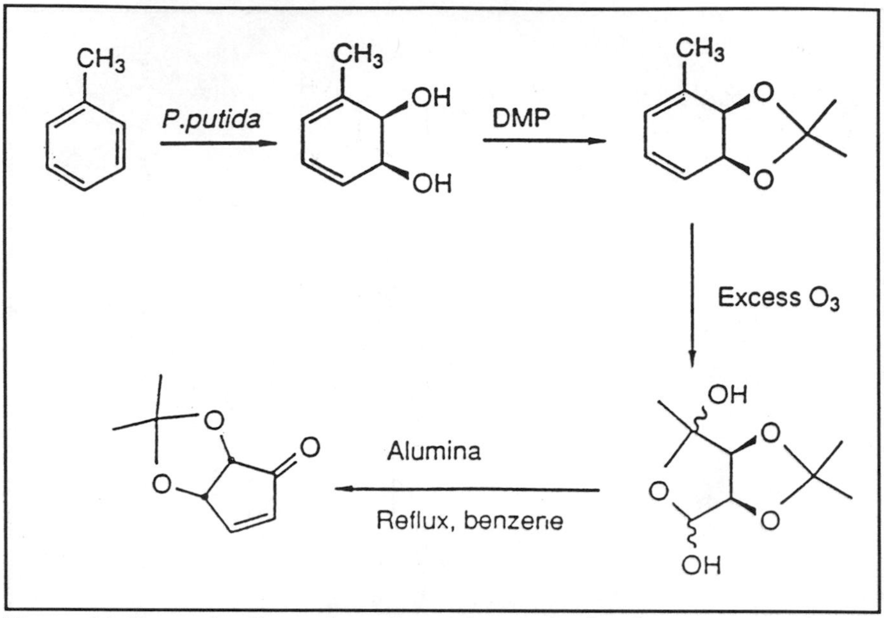

Figure 12. Prostaglandin synthons from toluene-*cis*-glycol.

15.[29,30] These complexes can react readily with nucleophiles in a fully stereocontrolled manner, a process of great value in organic stereospecific synthesis. The family of neutral *cis*-diols provides a valuable extension of the available dienes for such reactions.

Metabolism and Biotransformations of *p*-Cymene

Metabolism of p-cymene by pseudomonads. Whereas the degradation of some aromatic compounds involves the direct dioxygenation of the benzene ring, metabolism of other alkyl benzenes primarily involves oxidative attack of the alkyl sidechain. Commonly, the reaction sequence is the oxidation of a methyl group to the carboxylic acid via the alcohol and aldehyde, such as *p*- and *m*-xylenes to the toluates [31-33] and *p*-cymene (4-isopropyltoluene) to *p*-cumate.[31,34,35]

Figure 16 shows the degradation of *p*-cymene via a dihydrodiol.[36] A mutant of *P. putida* PL (JT107) that was unable to utilize *p*-cymene or *p*-cumate as carbon source for growth, accumulated a

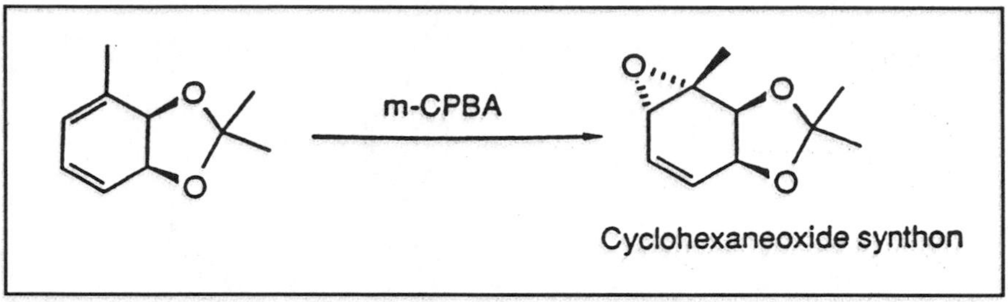

Figure 13. Epoxidation of a benzone-*cis*-glycol derivative.

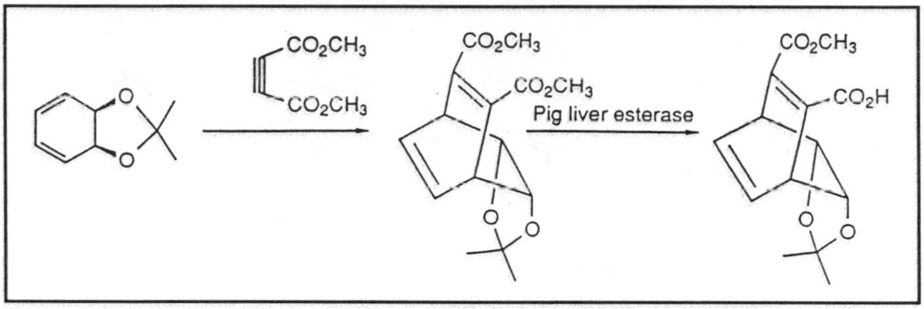

Figure 14. Enzymic transformation of a benzene-*cis*-glycol derivative.

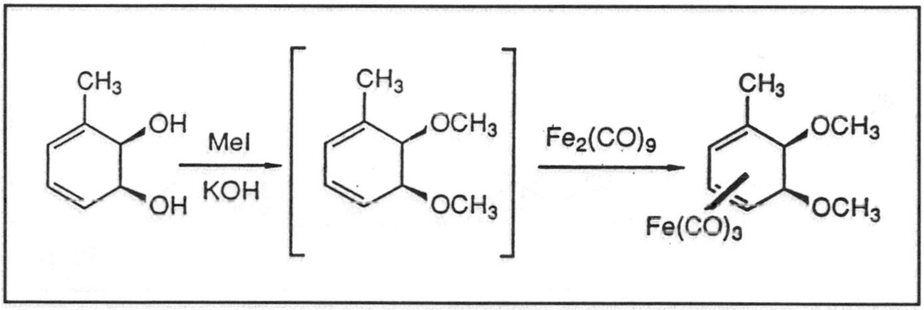

Figure 15. Tricarbonyliron complexes from toluene-*cis*-glycol.

compound that was identified as 4-isopropyl-*cis*-2,3-dihydroxy-2,3-dihydrocyclohexa-4,6- diene-1-carboxylic acid. This dihydrodiol was enzymically oxidized by an NAD-dependent dehydrogenase present in wild-type cells but absent in the mutant JT107. The monohydroxylated 3-hydroxy-*p*-cumate failed to support growth of *P. putida* PL and was not oxidized by cells or cell extracts. In contrast, 2,3-dihydroxy-*p*-cumate underwent ring cleavage and oxidation by cell extracts to yield pyruvate, acetaldehyde, isobutyrate, and carbon dioxide (see Figure 16).[37] Both atoms of oxygen in the

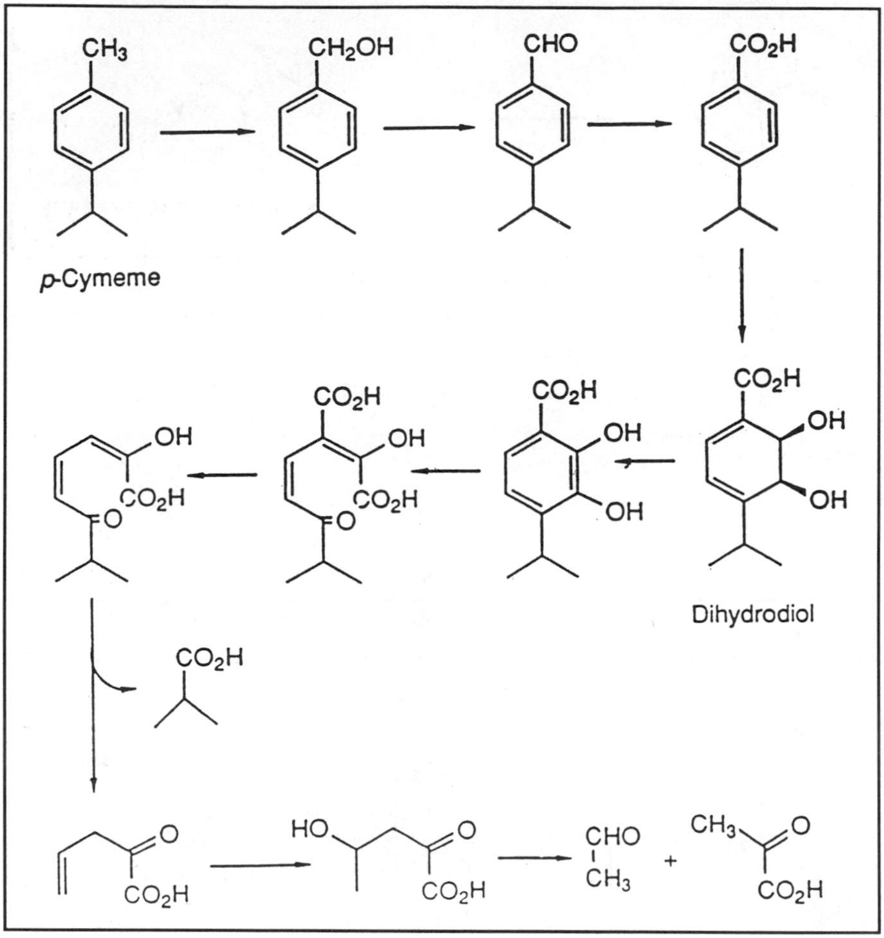

Figure 16. Metabolism of *p*-cymene by pseudomonads.

dihydrodiol were derived from molecular oxygen as shown by mass spectral analysis of the dihydrodiol produced in an $^{18}O_2$–enriched environment.

Production of Dihydrodiols by *Pseudomonad putida* JT107

Formation of a stable dihydrodiol from 4-trifluoromethylbenzo-ate (Figure 17),was the initial evidence for the involvement of a dihydrodiol in *p*-cymene metabolism.[38]

A *cis* configuration of the hydroxyl groups was inferred by the ease of formation of the acetonide derivative and the formation of a

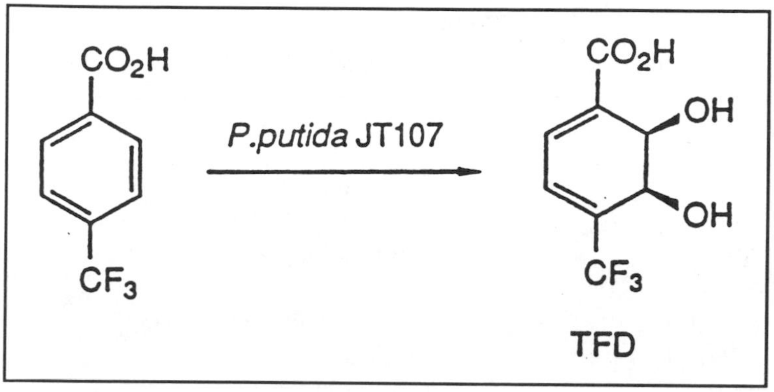

Figure 17. 4-Trifluoromethylbenzoate dihydrodiol (TFD) from *P. putida* JTIO7.

colored complex with triacetylosmate, which was stable to acetate ions. (The color of similar complexes of trans diols is discharged in the presence of acetate ions.) Acid dehydration of this dihydrodiol yielded 4-trifluoromethyl-3-hydroxybenzoate.

Many 4-substituted benzoates were tested as potential substrates for *P. putida* JT107; accumulation of dihydrodiols was inferred by ultraviolet spectroscopy of the diol and its dehydration product under acidic conditions.[36,39] A wide range of substrates are accepted (Table 2). The functionalities include primary, secondary, and tertiary alkyl groups; halogens; aryl, alkoxy and alkenyl groups; and 3,4-disubstituted benzoates. Some characteristics do emerge: a "bulky" group is needed at the 4-position as shown by the poor turnover with benzoate and 4-fluorobenzoate; groups in the 2-position are not tolerated nor are groups that are charged under physiological conditions; and 3-substituted benzoates appear to be poor substrates, which is in sharp contrast to the pathway encoded by the TOL plasmids that transform varied 3-substituted benzoates to dihydro-1,2-diols.[40]

Metabolism and Biotransformations of Benzoic Acids

Metabolism of benzoic acid and substituted benzoates. The metabolism of benzoic acid by bacteria has been known for many years to involve catechol.[41] In *P. putida, Alcaligenes eutrophus, Acinetobacter* sp., and *Azotobacter* sp., catechol is further oxidized via the ß-

Table 2
Substrate Specificity of *P. putida* JT107

Substrates	Non-substrates
p-Toluate	*o*-Toluate
3,4-Dimethylbenzoate	2,4-Dimethylbenzoate
4-Ethylbenzoate	2-Fluorobenzoate
4-Ethyl-*m*-xylene	Salicylate
4-Vinyltoluene	2,3-Dimethoxybenzoate
4-*n*—Propyltoluene	Anthranilate
p-Cumate	4-Methylaminobenzoate
4-Allyltoluene	4-Dimethylaminobenzoate
4-*t*—Butylbenzoate	4-Aminobenzoate
4-Phenylbenzoate	4-Methylsulphonylbenzoate
4-Benzylbenzoate	3-Chlorobenzoate
4-Benzoylbenzoate	*m*-Toluate
4-Ethoxybenzoate	3-Hydroxybenzoate
4-Propyloxybenzoate	*m*-Anisate
4-*n*-Butyloxybenzoate	3-Fluorobenzoate
4-Chlorobenzoate	
4-Bromobenzoate	
4-Iodobenzoate	
3-Fluoro-*p*-toluate	
3-Chloro-*p*-toluate	
4-Bromo-*m*-toluate	
4-Bromomethylbenzoate	
3,4-Dichlorobenzoate	
4-Trifluoromethylbenzoate	

ketoadipate pathway as shown in Figure 18. The involvement of a chiral intermediate containing two asymmetric carbon atoms was shown in mutant strain B9 of *A. eutrophus* that was blocked at the rearomatization stage.

The chiral intermediate was identified as *cis*-1,2-dihydroxy-cyclohexa-3,5-diene-l-carboxylic acid. Further investigations in the recalcitrance of halo-substituted aromatic compounds (using halo-substituted benzoates as models) revealed a range of novel chiral halogen and methyl substituted dihydrohydrodiol derivatives.

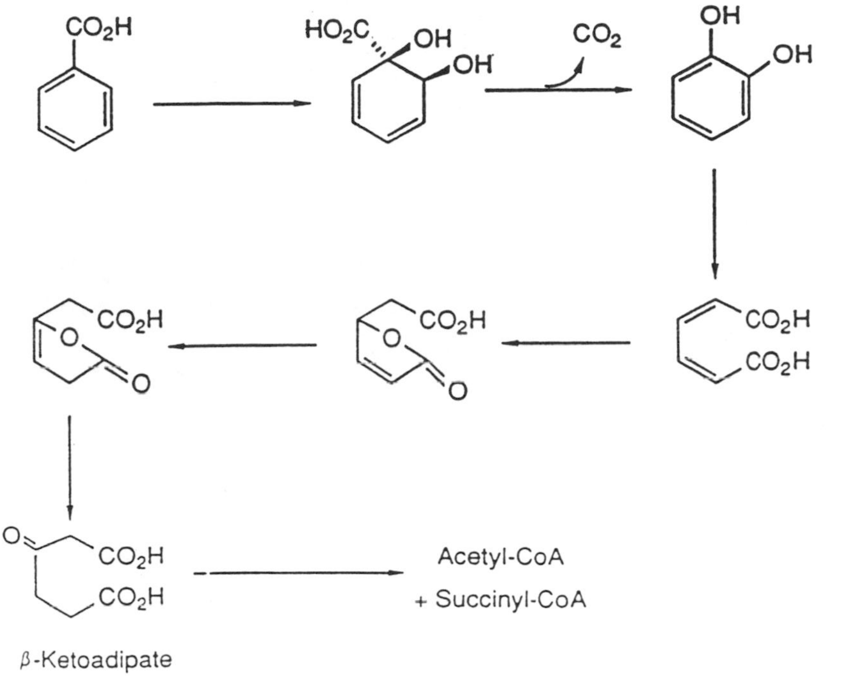

Figure 18. Metabolism of benzoic acid by the ß-ketoadipate path.

Biotransformations of Fluorinated Benzoates

All three isomers of fluorobenzoate are transformed by *A. eutrophus* B9, yielding a series of monofluorinated dihydrodiols[1,43] (Figure 19). 3-Fluorobenzoate is dioxygenated in the 1,2 and 1,6 positions, yielding two products. Only one product accumulated from 2-fluorobenzoate. The product arising from 1,2-dioxygenation overcomes the metabolic block by eliminating the fluorine as fluoride ion to yield catechol, which can then be further metabolized. Also all six isomers of difluorobenzoate were transformed by *P. putida* U103, a mutant that lacks diol dehydrogenase activity.[1,44,45] Three novel fluorinated dihydrodiols were isolated (as the methyl esters) from 3,4- and 3,5-difluorobenzoate as shown in Figure 20.

The transformations of 3.5- and 2,5-difluorobenzoate by *P. putida* U103 were investigated using ¹⁹F-NMR,[45] demonstrating the

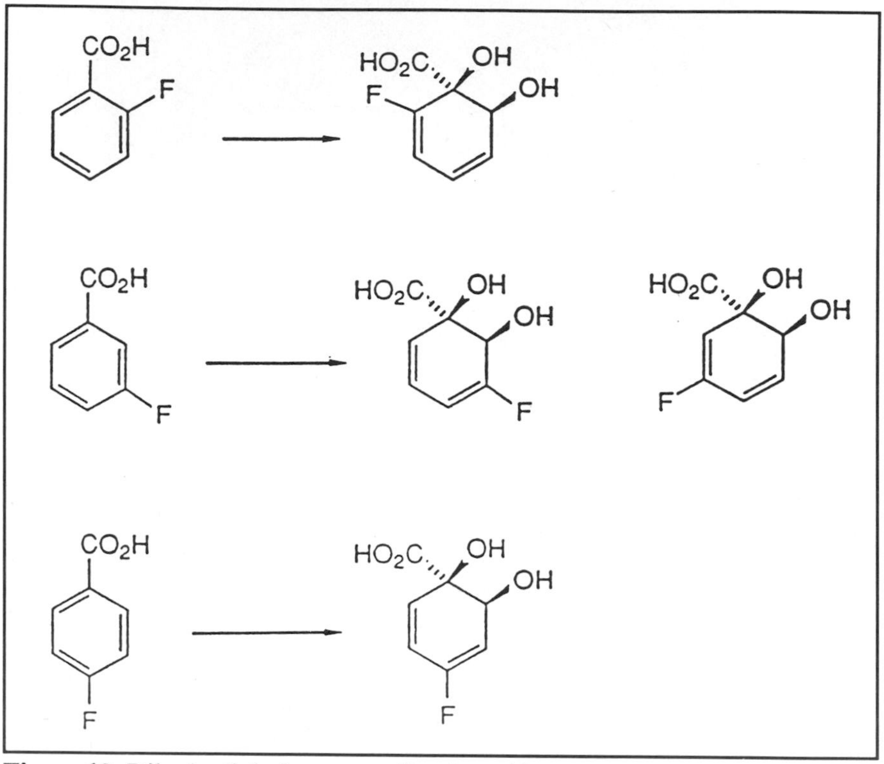

Figure 19. Dihydrodiols from monofluorinated benzoates.

spontaneous elimination of the fluoride ion when the 2,5-difluoroben-zoate substrate was putatively dihydroxylated in the 1,2 position.

Other Biotransformation Products of Benzoates

Pseudomonas sp. strain B13 and *Alcaligenes* sp. A7-2 accumu-lated up to 1.6gm/L 2-fluoro-*cis.cis*-muconate as a dead-end metabolite from 3-fluorobenzoate[46] (Figure 21) and 7.4gm/L of *cis,cis*-muconate from benzoate. No muconate cycloisomerase, the enzyme required for metabolism of *cis,cis*-muconate, was induced within the first 24 hours, whereas the three enzymes required for *cis,cis*-muconate production were induced to high level within 1 to 2 hours during exponential growth on succinate in the presence of benzoate. Mu-

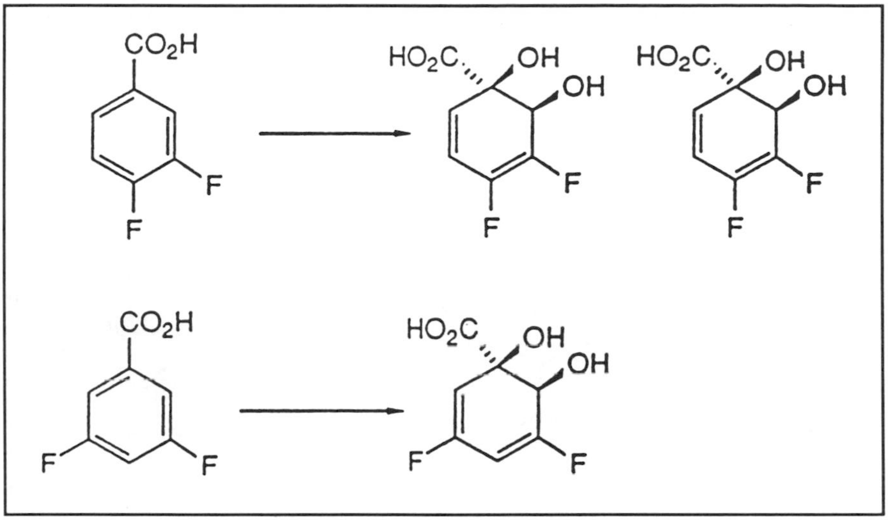

Figure 20. Dihydrodiols isolated from difluorinated benzoates.

conic acids are potentially useful for the synthesis of surfactants, antioxidants, and flame retardants (and may be the active metabolites in benzene toxicity).

Metabolism and Biotransformations of *o*-Phthalates

One degradative pathway of o-phthalate by pseudomonads involves oxidative attack about carbons 4 and 5 as shown in Figure 22.[47-49] Ring opening of protocatechuate occurs by *ortho* fission in fluorescent pseudomonads, but in strains of *P. testosteroni* occurs by a 4,5-*meta* fission.[49,50] 3-Fluorophthalate is a substrate for phthalate-utilizing strains of *P. testosteroni*. Novel fluorinated analogues of phthalate metabolic intermediates were isolated from catabolic mutants.[51]

Recent Results and Projections

Absolute stereochemistry of cis-diol carboxylates with 2,3-regioselectivity. We have crystallized the *cis*-diol analogues derived

Figure   21.
Degradation of
3 - f l u o r o -
benzoate by
Pseudomonas
sp. B13.

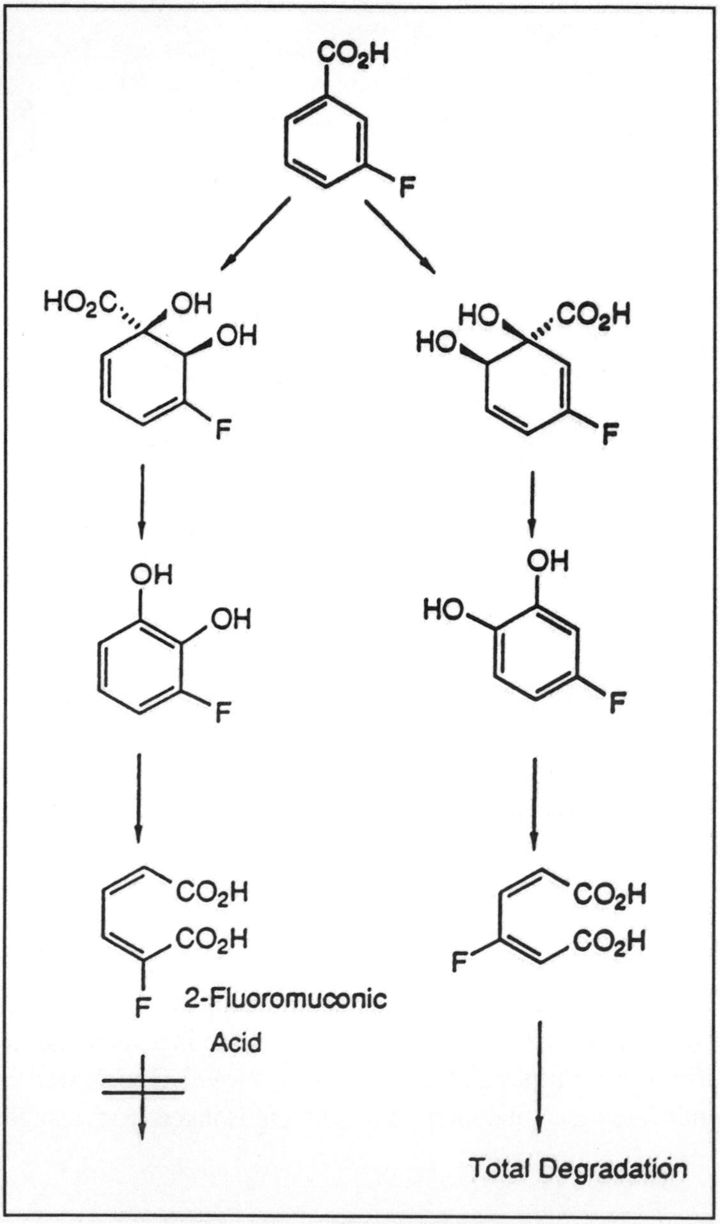

from 4-bromo- and 4-chlorobenzoate as the free acid, obtaining large prisms. In both cases, the absolute structure was determined by x-ray diffraction analysis (configurations 2R, 3R in Figure 23).

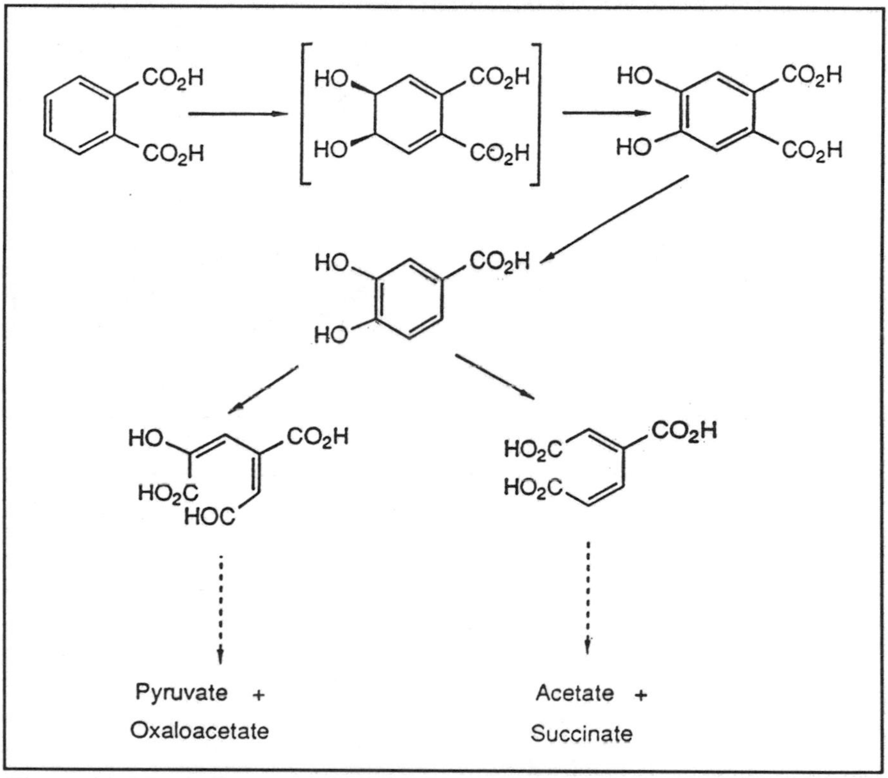

Figure 22. Metabolism of *o*-phthalate by pseudomonads.

To determine the enantiomeric excess of the 2R, 3R, -4-bromo-2,3-dihydroxycyclohexa-4,6-diene-1-carboxylic acid (BRD), the acid was derivatized to its 4-nitrobenzyl ester. The enantiomeric excess of the BRD ester was investigated by proton NMR with a chiral shift reagent. No enantiomer could be detected, suggesting an enantiomeric excess of the 2R, 3R isomer of at least 98 percent.

Formation of *cis*-Diol Carboxylates with 1,2-Regioselectivity

Benzoate is usually catabolized by aerobic bacteria to catechol via a chiral intermediate, the dihydroxylation occurring on carbon atoms 1 and 2. We have now determined the absolute stereochemistry of the methyl ester of the *cis*-diol produced from 3,5-difluorobenzoate

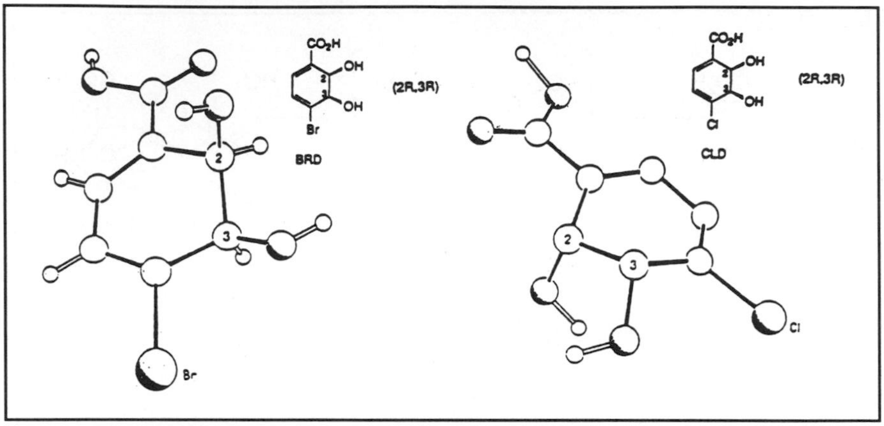

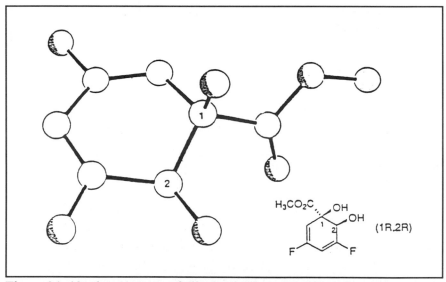

Figure 23. Absolute structure of BRD. Absolute structure of CLD.

Figure 24. Absolute structure of dihydrodiol from 3,5-difluorobenzoate.

by *P. putida* U103. X-ray diffraction patterns gave a structure with 95 percent certainty as 1R, 2R about carbons 1 and 2. Crystals of bromoester derivatives of the 1,2-diol from benzoate itself failed to provide the absolute stereochemistry, even though suitable x-ray diffractions were produced. The optical rotations given by the benzoate 1,2-diol obtained from culture filtrates of *P. putida* U103 and *A. eutrophus* B9 were shown to be of the same sign; therefore, they possess the same absolute stereochemistry (Figure 24).

New Fluorinated Chiral Products

All three isomers of monofluorobenzoate and all six isomers of difluorobenzoate were converted by *P. putida* U103 to *cis*-diols,as noted previously. The diols that were produced from the monofluorobenzoates and 3,4- and 3,5-difluorobenzoate have been well characterized. [40,42-44,52] It seems that *P. putida* U103 preferentially hydroxylates in the 1,2-positions when fluorine occupies the 2-position. This allows growth of *P. putida* U103 on 2-fluorobenzoate, as spontaneous elimination of fluoride occurs with decarboxylation to catechol, thus overcoming the lesion in the *cis*-diol dehydrogenase. Small amounts of 2-fluorobenzoate are metabolized via 1,6-dihydroxylation, producing a fluorodiol that accumulates in accord with the formation of two difluoro products from 3,4-difluorobenzoate. [44]

The isomers 2,3-, 2,4-, 2,5-, and 2,6-difluorobenzoate are all metabolized by benzoate induced *P. putida* U103. The 2,6-isomer is a very poor substrate and leads to the same monofluorodiol that accumulates from 2-fluorobenzoate (see Figure 19). We infer that the compounds accumulating from 2,3- and 2,4- difluorinated benzoates are mixtures of difluoro-*cis*-diols. 2,5-Difluorobenzoate catabolism by *P. putida* U103 has been studied by ^{19}F-NMR,[45] generating a vast amount of information, including the putative pathway (Figure 26), substrate specificities of the hydroxylation system, all of the enzymes of the *ortho*-cleavage pathway to 3-oxoadipate and the specificity of induction by fluorinated substrate analogues. [45]

Just as 4-trifluoromethylbenzoate is readily metabolized by *P. putida* JT101 and JT107,[38,53] 3-trifluoromethylbenzoate is metabolized to various products by pseudomonads harboring the TOL plasmid. But products beyond ring-fission products are not obtained.

Three New Families of *cis*-Diol Carboxylates From *o*-Phthalate and Its Analogues

We have shown that *o*-phthalate or its analogues are hydroxylated specifically with three different regioselectivities by different

Figure 25. Oxidation of 3,5- and 3,4-difluorobenzoate by a mutant of *P. putida* U-JT103 defective in the diol dehydrogenase.

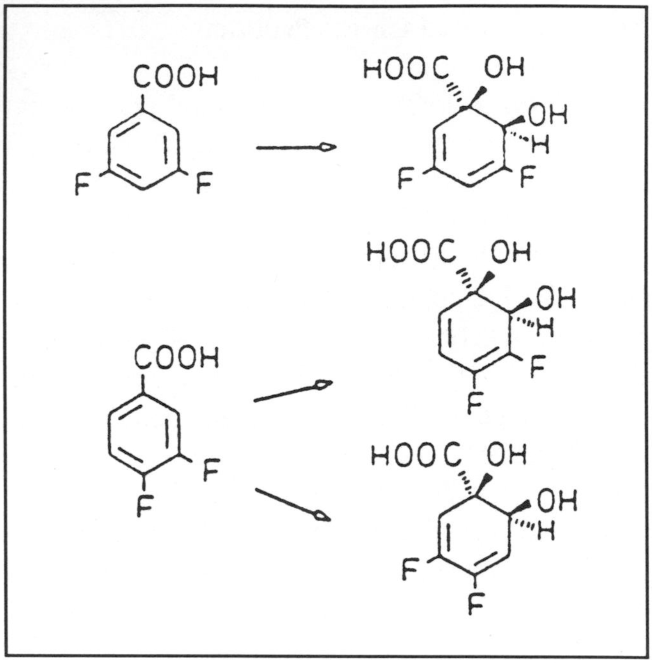

bacterial species. Thus, the regioselectivities of dihydroxylation by *P. cepacia* JT107, *Micrococcus* sp. strain 12B, and several fluorescent and nonfluorescent pseudomonads are 2,3-, 3,4- and 4,5-, respectively (Figure 27).[48,50,54-56] The 2,3- and 4,5-dihydrodiols have been isolated and characterized, but their absolute stereochemistry is still under investigation. The 3,4-*cis*-diol has not been isolated because appropriate mutants of *Micrococcus* sp. strain 12B are not yet available; however, the existence of the 3,4-diol can be inferred from $^{18}O_2$ experiments showing that both atoms of oxygen are incorporated into the substrate analogue phthalaldehydate (2-formylbenzoate).[54]

Discussion

We have described two groups of novel compounds that can be made by microbial oxidations, cyclohexadiene-*cis*-1,2-diols and fluorinated intermediates. Some of the products possess both features.

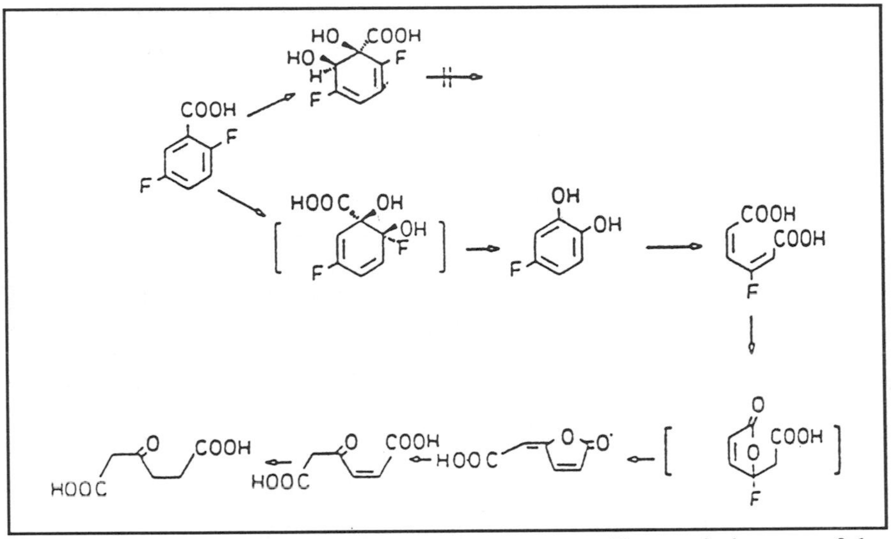

Figure 26. Bacterial oxidation of 2,5-difluorobenzoate. Two regio isomers of the first intermediate are formed; one eliminates F⁻ spontaneously, so it fortuitously bypasses the dehydrogenase lesion.

Provision of two chiral centers in a single hydroxylation reaction by bacterial oxidation of arenes is a valuable asset for synthesis. This expands the traditional pool of chiral molecules that can be used to initiate synthesis of compounds with asymmetric centers, namely, amino acids, hydroxy acids, terpenes, and carbohydrates. The first use of these bacterial oxidation products for synthesis started with pro-chiral benzene-*cis*-1,2-diol. The prochiral intermediate *cis*-4,5dihy-dro-4,5-dihydroxyphthalic acid is much more stable than the benzene diol and possesses added functionality with its two carboxyl groups. This is one of the rare dihydroxylation products of arenes with two *para* positions occupied by hydrogen, like the 1,2-diol carboxylate derived from benzoic acid. Other examples of this substitution pattern are the formation of: (1) 3,4-difluoro-*cis*-1,6-dihydroxy-cyclohexa-2,4-diene-1-carboxylate from 3,4-difluorobenzoate, (2) 4-fluoro-*cis*-1,2-dihydroxycyclo-hexa-3,5-diene-1-carboxylate from 4-fluoroben-zoate, and (3) 5-fluoro-*cis*-1,2-dihydroxycyclohexa-3,5-diene-1-car-boxylate from 3-fluorobenzoate. The three latter compounds also might be made available from the respective fluorinated toluenes with

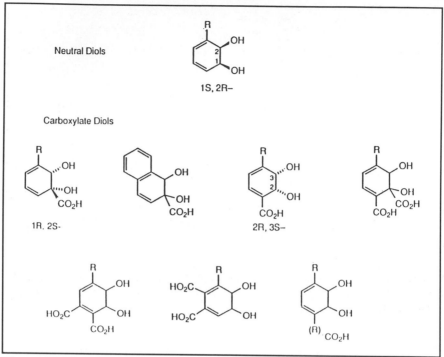

Figure 27. Eight families of *cis*-diols.

suitable microbial strains. These compounds can be used to form highly functionalized or fluorinated polyphenylenes or both. In such applications the chirality is lost, but regioselectivity of the dihydroxylation is utilized.

We now have access to eight families of *cis*-dihydrodiols by bacterial oxidations (Figure 27). Limitations of the size of each family are due to the availability of starting substrates for biotransformations. It is noteworthy that the absolute configurations of the carboxylate *cis*-diols of 1,2- and 2,3-regioselectivities are antipodal to the neutral R function (see Figure 27). The optical purity of the various *cis*-diol products has not usually been assessed. In the single neutral diol family, *para*-substituents of similar size are not always discriminated by the hydroxylation enzyme system. Biotransformation of 4-fluorotoluene by *P. putida* yields an optically active product, but 4-chlorotoluene is oxidized to a racemate. In contrast, the hydroxylation products of the seven carboxylate families (see Figure 27) are largely determined by regioselectivity, due to the anionic substituent. It is inferred but not proved that all of the *cis*-diols formed from various benzoates and phthalates are essentially optically pure substances, based on the absolute structure of the *cis*-diol derived from 4-bromo-, 4-chloro-, and 3,5-difluorobenzoic acids. We predict that the carboxylic (or carbonyl) functions are crucial for the substrate–enzyme binding and subsequent reaction.

It is now obvious that the specificities of oxygenases are much more relaxed than previously supposed, such that a multitude of substituents may be accommodated for transformations. Regioselective ring opening dioxygenations of catechols (and carboxycatechols) offer an additional range of chiral synthons, which include butenolides (see Figure 18) and 2-oxo-4-hydroxyal-kenoates (see Figure 16) in high enantiomeric excess, as well as access to both antipodes. Several aliphatic intermediates of the *ortho-* and *meta*-cleavage pathways will be useful for the provision of many heterocyclic compounds such as pyridines, pyrones, and butenolides.

References

1. D.W. Ribbons *et al.*, *J. Fluorine Chem.* **37**, 299 (1987).
2. J.B. Jones, *Tetrahedron* **43**, 3351 (1986).
3. S. Butt and S.M. Roberts, *Nat. Prod. Rep.* **28**, 489 (1986).
4. A.M. Chakrabarty, in *Biodegradation and Detoxification of Environmental Pollutants*, A.M. Chakrabarty, Ed. (C.R.C. Press, Boca Raton, FL (1982).
5. D.T. Gibson, in *Microbial Degradation of Organic Compounds*, D.T. Gibson, Ed. (Marcel Dekker, New York, 1984).
6. G.J. Wigmore and D.W. Ribbons, *J. Bacteriol.* **146**, 920 (1981).
7. T. Wieland, G. Griss, and B. Haccius, *Arch. Mikrobiol.* **28**, 383 (1958).
8. E.K. Marr and R.W. Stone, *J. Bacteriol.* **81**, 425 (1961).
9. S. Dagley, in *Biodegradation of Synthetic Organic Molecules in the Biosphere* (Proceedings of a conference, National Academy of Sciences, 1972).
10. D.T. Gibson, J.R. Koch, and R.E. Kallio, *Biochemistry* **7**, 2653 (1968a).
11. D.T. Gibson *et al.*, *Biochemistry* **9**, 1631 (1970a).
12. D.T. Gibson *et al.*, *Biochemistry* **9**, 1626 (1970b).
13. D.T. Gibson *et al.*, *Biochemistry* **12**, 1520 (1973).
14. D.T. Gibson *et al.*, *Biochemistry* **7**, 3795 (1968b).
15. D.T. Gibson., V. Mahadevon, and J.F. Davey, *J. Bacteriol.* **119**, 930 (1974).

16. S.C. Taylor and S. Brown, *Performance Chem.* **11**, 20 (1986).
17. T. Hudlicky *et al., J. Am. Chem. Soc.* **110**, 4735 (1988).
18. H. Ziffer *et al., Tetrahedron* **33**, 2491 (1977).
19. V.M. Kobal *et al., J. Am. Chem. Soc.* **95**, 4420 (1973).
20. R.O. Jenkins, G.M. Stephens, and H. Dalton, *Biotechnol. Bioeng.* **24**, 873 (1987).
21. J.A. Schofield, P.R. Betteridge, and G. Ryback, *European Patent Application 0 253 438* (1988).
22. S.C. Taylor and M.D. Turnbull, *European Patent Application 0 253 485* (1988).
23. J.B. Jonston, H. Winicov, V.L. Cunningham, *Biotechnol. Progress* **3**, 127 (1987).
24. D.G.H. Ballard *et al., Chem. Comms.* **17**, 954 (1983).
25. D.G.H. Ballard, European Patent Application 0 122 079 (1984).
26. S.V. Ley, F. Sternfeld, and S.C. Taylor, *Tetrahedron Lett.*, **28**, 225 (1987).
27. J.M. Berridge and R.F. Irvine, *Nature* **312**, 315 (1984).
28. I.C. Cotterill, S.M. Roberts, J.O. Williams, *Chem. Comms.* **24**, 1628 (1988).
29. P.W. Howard, G.R. Stephenson, and S.C. Taylor, *J. Organomet. Chem.* **339**, C5 (1988a).
30. P.W. Howard, G.R. Stephenson, and S.C. Taylor, *Chem. Comms.* **24**, 1603 (1988b).
31. J.B. Davis and R.L. Raymond, *Appl. Microbiol.* **9**, 383 (1961).
32. R.S. Davis, F.E. Hossler, and R.W. Stone, *Can J. Microbiol.* **14**, 1005 (1968).
33. J.F. Davey and D.T. Gibson, *J. Bacteriol.* **119**, 923 (1974).
34. K. Yamada, S. Horiguchi, and J. Takahashi, *Agric. Biol. Chem.* **29**, 943 (1965).
35. R.I. Leavitt, *J. Gen. Microbiol.* **49**, 411 (1967).
36. J.J. De Frank and D.W. Ribbons, *J. Bacteriol.* **129**, 1356 (1977a).
37. J.J. De Frank and D.W. Ribbons, *J. Bacteriol.* **129**, 1365 (1977b).
38. J.J. De Frank and D.W. Ribbons, *Biochem. Biophys. Res. Commun.* **70**, 1129 (1976).
39. J.J. De Frank, Ph.D thesis (1975).
40. W. Reineke and H.-J. Knackmuss, *Biochim. Biophys. Acta* **542**, 412 (1978a).
41. R.Y. Stanier, *J. Bacteriol.* **55**, 477 (1948).
42. A.M. Reiner and G.D. Hegeman *Biochemistry* **10**, 2530 (1971).
43. W. Reineke, W. Otting, H.-J. Knackmuss, *Tetrahedron* **34**, 1707 (1978).
44. J.T. Rossiter *et al., Tetrahedron Lett.* **28**, 5173 (1987).
45. A.E.G. Cass *et al., FEBS Lett.* **220**, 353 (1987).
46. E. Schmidt and H.-J. Knackmuss, *Appl. Microbiol. Biotechnol.* **20**, 351 (1984).
47. S. Dagley, W.C. Evans, and D.W. Ribbons, *Nature (London)* **188**, 560 (1960).
48. D.W. Ribbons and W.C. Evans, *Biochem. J.* **76**, 310 (1960).
49. D.W. Ribbons and W.C. Evans, *Biochem. J.* **83**, 482 (1962).
50. T. Nakazawa, E. Hayashi, *Appl. Environ. Microbiol.* **36**, 264 (1977).
51. R.E. Martin, P.B. Baker, and D.W. Ribbons, *Biocatalysis* **1**, 37 (1987).
52. W. Reineke and H.-J. Knackmuss, *Biochim. Biophys. Acta* **542**, 424 (1978b).
53. K.H. Engesser, M.A. Rubio, and D.W. Ribbons, *Arch. Microbiol.* **149**, 198 (1988).
54. R.W. Eaton and D.W. Ribbons, *Arch. Biochem. Biophys.* **216**, 289 (1982a).
55. R.W. Eaton and D.W. Ribbons, *J. Bacteriol.* **151**, 48 (1982b).
56. R.W. Eaton and D.W. Ribbons, *J. Bacteriol.* **151**, 465 (1982c).

Discussion

Gunsalus: What is the order of abundance of fluorine in the environment? How far do you scale down before you get to fluorine in high concentrations?

Ribbons: Fluorine is the thirteenth most abundant element in crushed rocks.

Gunsalus: We are having more and more trouble with fluorine, especially the very stable chlorofluorocarbons, which damage the ozone layer in the stratosphere.

Ribbons: We can now make fragile molecules and chiral molecules containing fluorine. Of course, the stability of fluorine in molecules of biological interest such as drugs and pesticides is usually considered an advantage.

Approaches to Closed and Open Systems

14

The Fate of Chlorophenolic Compounds in Freshwater and Marine Environments

Alasdair H. Neilson
Ann-Sofie Allard
Per-Åke Hynning
Mikael Remberger
Tomas Viktor
Swedish Environmental
Research Institute
Box 21060
S-100 31 Stockholm
Sweden

Laboratory-based procedures have been developed for assessing the hazard of xenobiotics discharged into the aquatic environment. The authors emphasise microbial reactions under both aerobic and anaerobic conditions, and the procedure is illustrated by application to a range of chlorinated guaiacols, catechols and vanillins. The conclusions from these experiments should be verified by analysis of selected field material. It is not sufficient to consider only the persistence and toxicity of the original compounds; attention should be directed also to metabolites that may be produced in the natural environment. In addition, substantial concentrations of xenobiotics may exist in the sediment phase in forms that are not recoverable by simple solvent extraction. Thus, a significant fraction may also be inaccessible to the relevant microflora. A false view of the persistence of a xenobiotic may emerge if reliance is placed solely on the results of laboratory experiments.

Introduction

A variety of organic chemicals is discharged into the environment, either deliberately, for example, as biocides or as by-products of industrial processes. An environmental hazard assessment or environmental impact statement is, therefore, an integral part of all industrial operations. This should aim at being predictive rather than retrospective, and will generally include suggestions for eliminating or minimizing the impact of these chemicals on the environment in light of current or future technology.

A valid evaluation must include data on both exposure and effect, and the following aspects are normally addressed:

1. *Persistence* under environmental conditions, including both abiotic and biotic processes, although the latter are generally of greater significance, except in special circumstances.

2. *Toxicity*. The effect on any organism but generally restricted to a range of organisms and directed to acute, subacute, and mutagenic effects.

3. *Potential* for bioconcentration, which is of particular concern regarding persistent and poorly degradable compounds.

We have developed an experimental program for environmental hazard assessment[1] that consists of two parts, one devoted to laboratory studies, and the other to an attempt to verify these conclusions on the basis of critical analysis of selected field material. The procedure employs a complementary array of chemical, microbiological, and ecotoxicological methodologies, all of which are necessary. Our research program is aimed at evolving general principles of wide applicability to the problem of environmental hazard assessment; it is not directed specifically to any one kind of ecosystem nor is it applicable only to a limited range of chemical structures.

In this short review, we discuss primarily microbial processes, biodegradation, and biotransformation and concentrate on the results of laboratory investigations.

There are very good practical reasons for employing laboratory studies to examine biodegradation and biotransformation.[2] Among these are the following: (1) virtually any environmental condition can be simulated: temperature, salinity, oxygen tension, substrate concentration; (2) the experiments are reproducible and in many cases permit quantitative analysis of kinetic data; (3) it is readily possible to evaluate the significance of the synthesis of intermediate compounds capable of bringing about metabolic "suicide," or that are potentially toxic to other components of the biota; and (4) it is feasible to systematically investigate concurrent metabolism because under natural conditions microbial populations will seldom be exposed only to low concentrations of a given xenobiotic. Generally, substantial concentrations of natural growth substrates will be accessible, even though these may be relatively recalcitrant to microbial attack.

We have chosen to illustrate the microbiological procedures by describing studies on significant components of bleachery effluents that have been carried out in our laboratory over several years. During "brightening" of pulp produced by the sulphate process, different chlorinating agents are employed, which result in the production of a structurally diverse range of chlorinated organic compounds.[3,4] In the present context, we shall concentrate on microbial transformations of the chlorinated phenolic compounds, chloroguaiacols, chlorocatechols, and chlorovanillins. Because the greater fraction of the effluents from Swedish pulp mills is discharged into the Baltic Sea and the Gulf of Bothnia, our report is directed primarily to these essentially brackish-water habitats. The experiments that we describe have been carried out with pure cultures of aerobic bacteria and with metabolically stable consortia of anaerobic bacteria isolated by enrichment of natural samples of water, soil, or sediment from these brackish-water habitats and a few freshwater habitats.

Microbial Reactions: Aerobic Transformations

Initiatory experiments. Initial experiments[5] used dense suspensions of cells grown on 4-hydroxybenzoate and exposed to relatively high (approximately 50mg/l) concentrations of chloroguaiacols. We observed that substantial concentrations of neutral metabolites were formed; for example, from 3,4,5-trichloroguaiacol, 3,4,5-trichloroveratrole was produced as well as 3,4,5-trichlorocatechol and 3,4,5-trichloro-2,6-dimethoxyphenol (3,4,5-trichlorosyringol). This *O*-methylation reaction was observed also for other chloroguaiacols and some chlorophenols. These observations were of particular interest for two reasons: (1) the chloroveratroles appeared stable to further transformation by the cell suspension, and (2) highly lipophilic metabolites were formed rather than the expected polar compounds. We therefore evaluated the toxicity of the chloroveratroles in the standard zebra fish embryo-larvae test which is used in this laboratory.[6] These metabolites were not only at least as toxic as their precursors, the chloroguaiacols, but induced curvature of the larvae and deformation of the notochord, findings that had not been observed with the chloroguaiacols.[7] Experiments to determine the bioconcentration potential in zebra fish showed that indeed these compounds were accumulated with log BCF values for tetrachloroveratrole comparable to that of 1,1,1-trichloro-2,2,di-(4-chlorophenyl)-ethane (DDT). It was on the basis of all these observations and their putative environmental significance that we began a systematic investigation of the *O*-methylation reaction. These results also underscored the fact that in environmental hazard evaluations, it is not sufficient to address only the fate of the original compound: attention also must be directed to the possibility that metabolites at least as toxic or persistent as their precursors may be synthesized under environmental conditions.[2]

   It was particularly desirable, therefore, to evaluate the following factors: (1) distribution of the organisms in the environment, (2) effect of growth conditions and cell density, (3) influence of substrate concentration, and (4) the specificity of the reaction.

   Distribution of O-methylation capacity: the role of substrate concentration. We established[8] that the capacity for *O*-methylation of chlorophenolic compounds was widely distributed in both gram-positive and gram-negative organisms isolated from the Gulf of Bothnia, the Baltic Sea, and from a few freshwater localities. The yield of the products was strongly dependent on the substrate concentration and for many of the gram-positive organisms, the yield at substrate concentrations of 100μg/l was virtually quantitative. It was important to assess the significance of substrate concentration because the high substrate concentrations (approximately 50mg/l) used in our initial studies were clearly environmentally unrealistic. Therefore we carried out a systematic examination[8] of the effect of substrate concentration, which revealed the following significant facts: (1) the rate of *O*-methylation was not a linear function of the concentration so that the rate at low concentration predicted from experiments carried out at high concentration was much too low, and (2) in the case of 3,4,5-trichloroguaiacol, the nature of the products was determined by the concentration; at low concentration, only the corresponding chloroveratrole was formed, but at higher concentrations, 3,4,5-trichloro-2,6-dimethoxyphenol (3,4,5-trichlorosyringol) and 1,2,3-trichloro-3,4,5-trimethoxybenzene became the dominant products. These results underlined the significance of substrate concentration in determining the fate of xenobiotics in the aquatic environment. The results also underlined the inherent limitations in traditional experiments on biodegradation that generally employ relatively high substrate concentrations in order to detect oxygen consumption, evolution of CO_2, or diminution in concentration of total organic carbon and do not generally carry out specific analysis of the concentrations of the substrate and potential metabolites. The observations made in our study would, therefore, have been overlooked. In discussing the effect of substrate concentration on biodegradability in general, it is worth drawing attention to an interesting and hitherto unresolved issue: The possible existence of a threshold concentration below which rates of microbial reactions are extremely low or negligible.[9]

The growth status of the cells: concurrent metabolism. Natural populations of bacteria will not normally be exposed only to a given xenobiotic and seldom to readily degraded substrates such as carbohydrates or simple carboxylic acids. In addition, although resting cells may indeed dominate natural populations, cell growth is an obligate condition for long-term survival of a population. Therefore, we investigated the occurrence of the *O*-methylation reaction of chloroguaiacols at low substrate concentration (approximately 100μg/l) during growth of reference bacteria, representing gram-positive and gram-negative genera; we used a range of substrates such as gluconate, succinate, betaine, 4-hydroxybenzoate, and vanillate in high concentration (approximately 500mg/l). *O*-methylation took place during growth, and was significant even when only quite low cell densities had been attained.[8] The potential metabolic complexity was revealed in an experiment with vanillate as growth substrate and 4,5,6-trichloroguaiacol as co-substrate. A series of reactions took place whereby de-*O*-methylation of 4,5,6-trichloroguaiacol rapidly took place to the formation of 3,4,5-trichlorocatechol; this compound was then partially and specifically *O*-methylated to 3,4,5-trichloroguaiacol, which was finally *O*-methylated to 3,4,5-trichloroveratrole.

We concluded from this series of experiments that: (1) *O*-methylation could take place in cells growing with a range of structurally diverse substrates, with the nature of the growth substrate playing a significant role in determining the outcome of the reactions, and (2) *O*-methylation would plausibly be expected to be competitive with biodegradation in natural populations of bacteria.

The substrate specificity of O-methylation. It was clearly desirable to assess the extent to which *O*-methylation occurred in a range of halogenated phenols and to assess the significance of the nature of the halogen, the variation among isomers, and the importance of the number of halogen atoms. We investigated the *O*-methylation reaction in a structurally diverse range of both chlorinated and brominated phenolic compounds both in whole cells[10] and in cell-free extracts:[11] these experiments clearly revealed the virtual ubiquity of the *O*-methylation reaction for such compounds and emphasized the significance of both the position and the number of substituents in determining the reaction's rate. Indeed, the relative position of the substituents was at least as important as the degree of substitution.

Verification studies. Although we concluded from these studies that the *O*-methylation of halogenated phenolic compounds was widely distributed and could take place under simulated environmental conditions, it was necessary to assess the environmental relevance and significance of this reaction through critical experiments on field material. This was attempted from two converging directions: (1) from the results of spiking experiments using natural sediments without the addition either of bacterial cells or supplementary carbon sources[12] and (2) by analysis of fish samples from areas putatively contaminated with bleachery discharge.[7] These experiments clearly demonstrated that: (1) populations of bacteria under conditions virtually identical to those occurring naturally, carried out O-methylation of chloroguaiacols and (2) wild fish indeed contained chloroveratroles in liver fat.[7] Additional experiments carried out in a brackish-water mesocosm system treated with 4,5,6-trichloroguaiacol over an extended period of time also confirmed the occurrence of 3,4,5-trichloroveratrole in segments of the biota.[13] It should be noted, however, that laboratory experiments with zebra fish had shown that although chloroveratroles were readily concentrated in the fish, they were also de-O-methylated to the corresponding chloroguaiacols and chlorocatechols that were excreted into the aqueous phase as water-soluble conjugates.[13]

An Environmental Perspective on O-Methylation

Our laboratory investigations using both gram-positive and gram-negative bacteria have clearly demonstrated the occurrence of O-methylation in a structurally diverse range of halogenated phenolic compounds. This reaction has been confirmed with a group of Gram positive organisms in another laboratory,[14] so that there can be no doubt of its ubiquity, at least in the Nordic areas that have been examined. Consistent with these isolations, is the recovery from environmental samples of chlorinated anisoles and veratroles;[7,15] similar compounds have been identified in geographically remote areas.[10] In light of these observations and the fact that the O-methylation activity appears to be constitutive,[11] we have hypothesized that this is probably a universal microbial reaction in the aquatic environment where it may serve as a detoxification mechanism for the organisms carrying it out.[8] In the terrestrial environment, probably fungal O-methylation is at least or more important.[16] We therefore regard O-methylation of halogenated phenolic compounds as a significant alternative to biodegradation; this reaction has been unambiguously demonstrated both in highly chlorinated phenols[17] and guaiacols.[18]

On the basis of these observations, we felt assured of the validity of the conclusions drawn from the laboratory experiments and convinced of the value of the experimental methodology employed.

The Sediment Phase: Binding and Anaerobiosis

In the course of the verification experiments using natural sediment samples,[12] several significant observations were made that altered our perspective on the whole issue of persistence: (1) these sediments were often heavily contaminated with a range of chlorinated guaiacols, catechols, and vanillins, all of which may putatively be assumed to originate from bleachery effluents; (2) chloroveratroles were uniformly absent; (3) there were appreciable differences in the recoverability of the chlorinated guaiacols and catechols by chemical procedures, (4) the partition of all the chlorinated compounds just mentioned between the aqueous and sediment phases strongly favored the latter; and (5) the sediments were frequently rich in organic carbon and highly anaerobic. The last observation suggested a more thorough investigation of the metabolic role of anaerobic bacteria. We hypothesized that the failure to recover chloroveratroles could be due to their ready de-O-methylation under anaerobic conditions. Although this hypothesis was subsequently shown to be correct, the whole issue turned out to be very much more complex.

Anaerobic Bacterial Transformations

Experimental determinants. Although we applied the general principles evolved during work with aerobic organisms, a number of significant alterations had to be introduced:[19] (1) use of an anaerobe chamber and prereduced media, (2) significantly more lengthy periods of enrichment lasting up to one year necessitated by the much slower growth of anaerobic bacteria, (3) use of metabolically stable consortia instead of pure cultures, which would have taken even longer to achieve, and (4) use of sealed glass ampules that simultaneously eliminated problems due to failure to maintain anaerobiosis through introduction of oxygen and possible loss of appreciably volatile substrates or metabolites. Initially we carried out experiments under conditions of "concurrent metabolism;" the growth substrate was employed at concentrations of approximately 500mg/l and the substance being investigated (cosubstrate) was employed at concentrations of approximately 100µg/l.

Experiments have been carried out using consortia obtained by enrichment with a range of substrates, mostly without chloro-substituents, chosen on the basis of their structural resemblance to naturally occurring humus or tannin-like compounds. Results presented here are based on enrichment cultures using 3,4,5-trimethoxybenzoate, 3,4,5-trihydroxybenzoate, 1,3,5-trihydroxy-benzoate, and 5-chloro- and 5-bromovanillin.

De-O-methylation. We concentrated first on the question of the stability of the chlorinated veratroles and guaiacols. It could readily be shown that the veratroles and guaiacols were rapidly de-*O*-methylated to the corresponding chlorocatechols.[19] Although this provided a satisfying rationalization for the failure to recover chlorinated veratroles from sediment samples, it provided at the same time an apparent anomaly in the ability to recover chloroguaiacols. In view of the differential chemical extractability of chloroguaiacols and chlorocatechols to which we have already referred,[20] we have hypothesized that these compounds are "bound" in sediments by different mechanisms: whereas metal cation complexes with Fe^{III} or Al^{III} may be formed from the catechols, these are readily disassociated in contrast to more stable, probably covalent, complexes formed from the guaiacols.[20]

Dechlorination. Initial experiments[19] showed clearly that the chlorocatechols formed from the chloroguaiacols were not stable under anaerobic conditions. They were dechlorinated and apparently, specifically so. Tetrachlorocatechol formed 3,4,6-trichlorocatechol, and 3,4,5-trichlorocatechol formed 3,5-dichlorocatechol. Extensive investigations have now been directed to confirming and extending these observations because they raised a number of significant and hitherto unresolved issues: (1) these experiments suggested that complete dechlorination may not necessarily occur and that the higher congeners may indeed be more readily attacked than the lower ones; (2) the dechlorination was highly specific, because we have never observed dechlorination of a diverse range of chlorinated phenols. We particularly emphasize that these results, which are consistent with data from other laboratories on anaerobic transformations of highly chlorinated aromatic compounds,[21,22] including chlorophenols,[23] seem at variance with the generally accepted view based on results from aerobic degradation of chloroaromatic compounds. Under aerobic condtions the more highly substituted compounds are the most resistant to biodegradation. Collectively, these observations strongly suggest that, despite the lower toxicity of the lower congeners, they may be appreciably persistent under anaerobic conditions. Further experiments have brought to light the existence of other patterns of dechlorination; and that the one chosen depends critically on the growth substrate. Clearly, many unresolved issues remain before any general conclusions can be drawn.

Transformations of aromatic hydroxyaldehydes. Chlorinated vanillins and chlorinated 4-hydroxybenzaldehydes are established constituents of bleachery effluents. Extensive studies have been carried out on their anaerobic transformation. Under growth conditions with high substrate concentrations (approximately 200-500 mg/l), the metabolism of 5- and 6-chlorovanillin, 3-chloro-4-hydroxybenzaldehyde, and 3,5-dichloro-4-hydroxy-benzaldehyde was examined.[24] Whereas the dominant reaction was synthesis of the corresponding carboxylic acids that were generally decarboxylated to the corresponding phenols or catechols, this reaction was accompanied by reductions of the aldehyde groups initially to hydroxymethyl compounds. These derivatives, which were for the vanillins, were subsequently further reduced to methyl compounds. We draw attention to these reactions for a number of reasons: (1) reductions of this type produce metabolites that are significantly different in chemical properties from their precursors and (2) C-methyl catechols may be recoverable from natural samples; indeed we have identified them in sludge samples from an anaerobic reactor treating bleachery effluents.

The Emergence of a Dilemma

An apparent dilemma has emerged from these investigations: the occurrence and, therefore, putative persistence of chloroguaiacols, chlorocatechols, and chlorovanillins in the natural environment. Current evidence on the biodegradability of chloroguaiacols under aerobic conditions and the biotransformation of both chloroguaiacols and chlorocatechols under anaerobic conditions would have suggested that these compounds should not be persistent in the environment. On the other hand, their recoverability from contaminated sediments and the much lower concentrations of their putative metabolites suggests a significant degree of resistance to microbial attack. The simplest resolution of this contradiction would be to propose that these compounds are not readily accessible to the organisms capable of carrying out the reactions observed in laboratory experiments. This in turn suggests that it is not sufficient to assess environmental persistence solely in light of evidence of biodegradability; xenobiotics may have a significantly greater degree of persistence than predicted from the results even of well-designed laboratory experiments. Support for this view comes from the results of a laboratory experiment[20] in which we incubated a naturally contaminated sediment sample under anaerobic conditions at 22° C for up to two years. Analysis showed that: (1) only approximately 20 percent of the chlorinated catechols and guaiacols were degraded, with the remainder recoverable from the sediment; (2) the reactions took place almost entirely within the first four months and then occurred at a negligible rate; and (3) microbial processes were probably responsible for this partial degradation, because samples incubated at 4°C or in the presence of azide at a concentration of 2g/l had undiminished concentrations of the chlorinated phenolic compounds.

We suggest that the question of bioavailability has not been hitherto sufficiently addressed in discussions of the environmental fate of xenobiotics. Under natural conditions, quite appreciable concentrations may remain persistent in the sediment phase, which functions as an effective "sink" for many of xenobiotics over extended periods of time.

A Perspective

Finally, we attempt briefly to place these observations in a wider environmental perspective in which it is essential to consider not only microbial processes but the effect of possible metabolites on other components of the ecosystem.[2]

1. Microbial activity may bring about a variety of transformations whose outcome depends on the substrate concentration, the nature and number of the microbial cells, the accessibility of growth substrates, and the oxygen tension. The possibility for synthesis of metabolites that are more lipophilic rather than more polar than their precursors must be taken into account, and it should be appreciated that metabolites may be more toxic than the initial xenobiotics.

2. Many xenobiotics are accumulated in the sediment phase so that their stability under anaerobic conditions is of cardinal importance. In sediments that are rich in organic carbon, an additional complication arises from the unknown extent to which the xenobiotics are accessible to microbial attack.

Simplistic estimates of exposure concentrations, persistence of xenobiotics, and ecosystem effects that do not take into account the factors just mentioned may lead to seriously false conclusions about the fate and effects of xenobiotics discharged into the aquatic environment.

Acknowledgments

We thank the Research Committee of the National Swedish Environment Protection Board and the Swedish Forest Industry Water and Air Pollution Research Foundation for partial financial support.

References

1. A.H. Neilson, in *Toxic Contamination of Large Lakes Vol. 1*, N.W. Schmidtke, Ed. (Lewis Publishers, Chelsea, MI, 1988), pp. 285-313.
2. A.H. Neilson, A.-S. Allard, and M. Remberger, in *Handbook of Environmental Chemistry Vol. 2* (Part C), O. Hutzinger, Ed. (Springer-Verlag, 1985), pp. 29-86.
3. K.P. Kringstad and K. Lindström, *Environ. Sci. Technol.* 18, 236A(1984).
4. K. Lindström and F. Österberg, *Environ. Sci. Technol.* 20, 133(1986)
5. A.H. Neilson *et al.*, *Appl. Environ. Microbiol.* 45, 774(1983).
6. L. Landner *et al.*, *Ecotoxicol. Env. Saf.* 9, 282(1985).
7. A.H. Neilson *et al.*, *Can. J. Fish. Aquat. Sci.* 41, 1502(1984).
8. A.-S. Allard, M. Remberger, and A.H. Neilson, *Appl. Environ. Microbiol.* 49, 279(1985).
9. B.R. Zaidi, Y. Murakami, and M. Alexander, *Environ. Sci. Technol.* 22, 1419(1987).
10. A.-S. Allard, M. Remberger, and A.H. Neilson, *Appl. Environ. Microbiol.* 53, 839(1987).
11. A.H. Neilson *et al.*, *Appl. Environ. Microbiol.* 54, 524(1988).
12. M. Remberger, A.-S. Allard, and A.H. Neilson, *Appl. Environ. Microbiol.* 51, 552(1986).
13. A.H. Neilson *et al.*, in *Advanced Hazard Assessment of Chemicals in the Aquatic Environment*, L. Landner, Ed. (Springer-Verlag, 1989), in press.
14. M.M. Häggblom, L.J. Nohynek, and M. Salkinoja-Salonen, *Appl. Environ. Microbiol.* 54, 3043(1988).
15. J. Paasivirta *et al.*, *Chemosphere* 16, 1231(1987).
16. J.M. Gee and J.L. Peel, *J. Gen. Microbiol.* 85, 810(1974).
17. D.L. Saber and R.L. Crawford, *Appl. Environ. Microbiol.* 50, 1512(1985).
18. M.M. Häggblom, J.H.A. Apajalahti, and M. Salkinoja-Salonen, *Appl. Environ. Microbiol.* 54, 683(1988).
19. A.H. Neilson *et al.*, *Appl. Environ. Microbiol.* 53, 2511(1987).
20. M. Remberger, P.-Å. Hynning, and A..H. Neilson, *Environ. Toxicol. Chem.* 7, 795(1988).
21. T.N.P. Bosma *et al.*, *FEMS Microbiol. Ecol.* 53, 223(1988).
22. M.D. Mikesell and S.A. Boyd, *Appl. Environ. Microbiol.* 52, 861(1986).
23. B.Z. Fathepure, J.M. Tiedje, and S.A. Boyd, *Appl. Environ. Microbiol.* 54, 327(1988).
24. A.H. Neilson *et al.*, *Appl. Environ. Microbiol.* 54, 2226(1988).

Discussion

Schink: I understand that you did these anaerobic experiments in reduced medium. Did you use sulfide for reduction?

Neilson: Yes, we copied your media exactly. We used prereduced sulfide medium with a gas atmosphere of 90 percent nitrogen plus 5 percent carbon dioxide plus 5 percent hydrogen. Media were degassed under nitrogen, before adding sulfide.

Schink: Did you ever find any formation of mercaptans? With these methylated aromatics, methylmercaptans are sometimes formed as intermediates. We have not so far elucidated the mechanism.

Neilson: We have had no trouble with mercaptans, but we have had serious problems with inorganic sulfur. Whether that is a true metabolic product I am not sure.

Chakrabardy: As somebody who works only with aerobes and therefore has very little understanding of the anaerobes, I have listened with great interest to the description of the ability of anaerobes to degrade, or rather biotransform, all these interesting compounds. It seems to me that the problem arises when you do the experiments with anaerobes using very low concentrations of the substrates. From a practical point of view, there appears to be a really high concentration of these compounds in the sediment phase. If I was working with anaerobes, I would try to understand the enzyme systems you mentioned, specifically the dechlorinases. Various research groups have been working with those dechlorinases, and I would like to understand which enzymes are responsible. How can I increase the yields of a given cell type so that cells would be able to handle higher concentrations of these compounds? Is there any attempt to purify various anaerobes and examine the relevant genes and their regulation?

Neilson: When we examined in detail the *O*-methylation problem, we used substrate concentrations that were environmentally relevant, although when we turned to cell-free extracts, we used much higher concentrations. I agree with you entirely that if you want to look at metabolic pathways, it is convenient to use higher substrate concentrations. For anaerobic bacteria, elucidating metabolic pathways and studying the relevant enzymes is a difficult challenge. It is very difficult to obtain pure cultures, and it may well be that natural systems need syntrophic associations of organisms to carry out the required transformations. If you want to look at environmental persistence, however, there is certainly an advantage, which Dr. Young mentioned also, in using these stable metabolic cultures. We use low concentrations because there is clear evidence that the concentrations in water or in interstitial water of sediments are extremely low. The interstitial concentration in the water phase of sediments has been shown to be reasonably high for a number of neutral organochlorine compounds, but we have never found substantial concentrations of chlorophenolics in the interstitial water of contaminated sediments. Thus, if we are interested in the aquatic sediment phase interaction, we feel that we are justified in using these low concentrations.

Chakrabardy: What I am really trying to find out is how one studies the enzymes that are carrying out these transformations, although I realize that the level of the enzymes in many of these anaerobes may be extremely low. There are well-developed procedures for aerobic bacteria, isolating the total DNA, cutting this with restriction enzymes, and cloning the genes in expression vectors.

Neilson: I think everybody who works with anaerobic dechlorination is trying to obtain pure cultures of bacteria and obtain cell-free extracts to do the kind of study you are discussing.

Chakrabardy: You do not need pure cultures.

Neilson: Maybe not, but it is very difficult to work with the consortia of the type that most of us are working with, and try to make an extract from these mixed cultures. Additionally, most of us working in this area do not have unlimited amounts of cell material. With mixed cultures, approximately 200ml of cell suspension is about maximum that we can produce. We cannot realistically grow more than approximately two liters of culture under normal conditions. I know that Ann-Sofie Allard has worked for two or three years trying to get pure cultures in order to have a more defined system and has not so far been successful. I agree with you philosophically, but I am appalled by the experimental complications.

Omenn: Neilson may have addressed these issues adequately, but there are several others here who work extensively with anaerobes. Is there anyone who wants to embellish the discussion we just had between Dr. Chakrabarty and Dr. Neilson?

Young: I wish to support what Dr. Neilson is saying. The difficulties at this point with mixed cultures and environmental samples are such that to grow liter volumes of the organisms for enzymatic investigations presents a formidable challenge, although there are many people who are trying. Those efforts will, I think, be met with success in the near future. The dechlorinating enzyme from strain DB-5 has been isolated, and its properties were reported at the last American Society for Microbiology meeting. Work on the dechlorinating enzymes is being pursued vigorously. In your aerobic and anaerobic cultures, you found relatively impressive rates, especially for the anaerobes, with activity and effective dechlorination within eight to 10 days. It is not unusual for those of us working with anaerobic systems to incubate them for months before we see activity. In terms of the products formed, were any incubations left longer for observation of eventual loss of these metabolites that you showed?

Neilson: We incubate routinely for up to 90 days. I agree with you entirely that if we had stopped at the times that I showed (approximately 20 days), we would have come to some rather erroneous conclusions on the stability of some of these metabolisms. We have also carried out experimental incubations for up to three years. Because these processes are slow, and because during the initial enrichment series we use many successive transfers, over one or two years, one should be very cautious about drawing conclusions from short-term experiments. I agree with the caution you express.

Anderson: Regarding the long-term experiments, you are incubating for quite extensive times up to a year in sealed ampules. What worries me is because we work with aerobic systems that degenerate once you take them out of the environment, how do you check the survival of your organisms in these systems? Do you make periodic checks as we do with aerobic systems, or are the ampules simply sealed and opened after a year or after the relevant time of incubation?

Neilson: There are two checks we make. First we make checks for viability. More importantly, we make metabolic checks. We add a chlorinated substrate that we know is metabolized in a relatively short period of time, after each 30 or 60 days, and make sure that it is dechlorinated or demethylated at rates that are comparable to those which existed in the original culture. We take this as putative evidence that the organisms are still present and functional. I should mention that the controls lacking cells were totally negative in all of these experiments. We have had troubles with brominated compounds in which the controls have altered during the experimental conditions, but I have not reported data from any of those experiments.

Omenn: You mentioned that there were substantial differences in the susceptibility to dechlorination, particularly of isomeric dichlorocatechols. Because many of us here are interested in dehalogenation reactions, is there any pattern emerging with respect to more substitution patterns and which are the more resistant substitution patterns?

Neilson: I agree it is a very interesting question. We have thought about this quite a bit. We have erected hypotheses about the relative position of substituents and then waited for the next experiment, which proved it was not quite so simple. I would like to be very cautious about drawing general conclusions. There are certain groups of dichlorocatechols that currently seem to be quite resistant to transformation, and the same is true for other groups of organochlorine compounds. However, any attempt to promulgate general rules is exceedingly difficult. It depends on the history of the cells, on the substrate used for the enrichment, and on the substrate you are investigating.

Salkinoja-Salonen: You showed that the concentration of the chlorinated substrates is very important. As determinants of the reactions that may occur, what is the role of carbon sources used as sources of energy? If you have low or high concentrations of growth substrates, does that have a bearing on the relative degree of hydroxylation or O-methylation of chlorophenolic compounds?

Neilson: We have never systematially investigated the effect of the concentration of the growth substrate on, for example, methylation. In concurrent metabolism experiments, we have used concentrations on the order of hundreds of milligrams per liter, which would support bacterial growth; I do not know what would happen if these growth substrates were present at low concentrations. We have looked at the transformations during growth of cultures. Even at very low substrate concentrations where the cell density is 10^4 to 10^5 cells per ml, you get very effective biotransformation. Under those conditions, the amount of substrate that has actually been metabolized for growth must be low. Without really investigating the issue systematically, we concluded that this was unlikely to be a major bottleneck in natural situations.

Salkinoja-Salonen: This may be an important issue in situations where one has to decide whether to treat a chlorophenolic waste stream alone or to mix it with readily degraded substrates. For instance, there are several instances where biodegradation is claimed for effluents discharged directly to domestic sewage plants, whereas what had been achieved was biomethylation.

Neilson: I agree with you on the dangers of extrapolating data from the kinds of experiments we have done, which are related to the natural environment to wastewater treatment systems. These are very different metabolic situations, both with respect to the mixture of compounds that are to be metabolized, and to the very different range of concentrations of compounds that are available for growth. Probably insufficient attention has been devoted to the significance of neutral metabolites.

15

Hazardous Waste Degradation by Wood Degrading Fungi

John A. Glaser
United States Environmental Protection Agency
Risk Reduction Engineering Laboratory
26 W. Martin Luther King Dr.
Cincinnati, OH 45268

The persistence and toxicity of many hazardous waste constituents indicate that the environment has a limited capacity to degrade such materials. The presence and competence of degrading organisms significantly affects our ability to treat and detoxify these hazardous waste chemicals. Competence is often specified by the ability of the organism(s) to convert toxic chemicals to nontoxic entities, most desirably to carbon dioxide. A wood-degrading fungus, *Phanerochaete chrysosporium*, has been investigated to determine its role as a degrader of toxic waste materials. Due to the organism's widely recognized ability to degrade lignin, a persistent biogenic polymer, and the nonspecific enzyme systems supporting such activity, this fungus was thought to have great promise as a toxic waste degrader.

Introduction

Detoxification of hazardous waste is increasingly important to the reduction of the risk associated with such waste. The potential of biological means to detoxify hazardous waste is beginning to be recognized. Environmental compatibility and lower costs are inducements that permit bioremediation technology to compete more effectively for site cleanup considerations. Biological detoxification has excellent credentials in applications to industrial and municipal wastestreams but is underdeveloped for treatment of toxic and/or hazardous waste chemical mixtures found at contaminated sites.

Wood Treatment Industry Waste[1]

A major hazardous waste problem confronting authorities in the United States is the waste associated with the wood treatment industry. An estimate of some 700 existing wood treatment sites requiring eventual remediation serves to emphasize the need for reliable remediation technology. Depending on the age of a facility, three successive technologies relating to treatment of the following compounds have contributed to the accumulated waste: creosote, pentachlorophenol, and copper chromated arsenite. Each of these technologies presents its special conditions for cleanup. Creosote, derived from coal tar production, usually contains a host of compounds that range from low molecular weight, volatile aromatic compounds to polyaromatic species, including smaller quantities of aromatic nitrogen bases and an array of phenolic compounds. Diesel or fuel oil fractions were used as diluents of the creosote mixture in the wood treatment processing steps. The lower vapor pressure components of this mixture contribute to the residuals found at such sites. Pentachlorophenol, a potent fungicide, is a major contaminant at wood treatment sites and exhibits significant toxicity towards microflora. The analysis of wastes derived from this technology has identified other potentially toxic components. For our current development efforts, we have focused narrowly on a significant portion of the waste, including major contributors that are polycyclic aromatic compounds and phenols. It is necessary to limit the scope of contamination treatable by this technology to permit the development activity to be achievable in a reasonable time frame. Treatment technology developed in this program will also be useful for coke oven property and town gas site remediation efforts.

Fungi Versus Bacteria[2]

Microorganisms are known to possess a variety of detoxification skills.[3] Xenobiotic chemical pollutants generally do not provide sufficient energy to sustain many microorganisms. The biological degradation of such substrates occurs as part of a cometabolic activity, where the organism's growth is maintained by specific substrates, and the detoxification occurs as a supplemental activity. Many bacteria and fungi can accomplish simple transformations on organic substrates but often fail to complete the conversion of the toxicant substrate to carbon dioxide or generate a toxic intermediate that can impair the growth of microorganisms. In the case of pentachlorophenol, many bacterial strains are intolerant of small concentrations of this compound.[4] The use of bacterial communities can combine the use of many species; where the abilities of one species supplant the inadequacies of another. Because the collective action of these communities is important to treatment success, protection from environmental effects that may adversely affect the communities is crucial to the treatment technology.[5]

Fungi have not been investigated to any extent for use as degraders of waste materials until recently.[6] Sewage treatment operations steered clear of filamentous fungi due to processing problems and the possibility that such fungi may be pathogenic. Exceptions to these generalizations do exist.[7] A wood-rotting basidiomycetes, *Trametes versicolor*, was studied 25 years ago in an attempt to quantify its ability to degrade chlorinated phenols.[8] Wood preservative chemicals have been found to be degraded by fungi.[9,10]

Selection of Fungi

Phanerochaete chrysosporium is a filamentous, white, wood-rotting fungus that has been classified as a member of the Hymenomycetes subclass of Basidiomycetes.[11] Fungi are eukaryotic, that is, they possess a nuclear membrane; as microorganisms they are considered to be plantlike, despite lacking chlorophyll and photo-synthetic abilities, which distinguishes them from bacteria.[12]

P. chrysosporium, characterized by fast growth and easy repro-ductive cycles, degrades an extensive list of hazardous waste constitu-ents under laboratory conditions. This ability to degrade hazardous pollutants appears to correlate well with the fungus's ability to degrade lignin, a complex natural polymer, composed of phenyl-propane units, that is resistant to decay by many microorganisms. The lignin-degrading ability has been attributed to a complex mixture of enzymes secreted by the fungus to the extracellular medium. The enzymes are peroxidases that utilize hydrogen peroxide from comple-mentary enzyme systems to perform the initial oxidative conversion of pollutant substrates.

Some of the more common substructures of lignin resemble the chemical structure of many persistent organic compounds contami-nating the environment. This structural similarity gave sufficient reason to pursue application *P. chrysosporium* to the biodegradation of hazardous waste constituents.[13]

Wood-Degrading Fungi's Carbon-Degrading Abilities,

White rot fungi are primary wood degraders in nature.[14] They excel compared with brown rot fungi, in their ability to recycle carbon of wood origin. The naturally occurring polymers of cellulose and lignin are degraded by these fungi, forming the major sources of carbon to assist fungal growth. Lignin is by far the more difficult to degrade due to its composition as a heteropolymer formed from the cross-linking of three precursor cinnamyl alcohols; cannot serve as the sole carbon source for growth of *P. chrysosporium*.[15] The fungus must be able to switch its ability to degrade these various polymers as the concentration of polymer varies with the composition of the wood. The degrading ability of nonmutant strains of *P. chrysosporium* is controlled by the absence of certain nutrients. Nitrogen deficiency is generally used to induce this secondary metabolic cycle of lignin utilization.[16]

The enzyme systems responsible for the initial attack on lignin require unusual abilities due to the complexity and resistance of the lignin structure. The 600,000 to 1,000,000 dalton size range for lignin is far too large to enter the cells of microorganisms by known transport systems. An enzyme system permitting the microorganism to overcome this limitation would most likely be extracellular, nonspecific (due to the heterogeneity and large molecular weight of the substrate), and resistant to protease destruction. It is important to realize that the ability of *P. chrysosporium* to degrade lignin by these extracellular enzymes occurs in a secondary metabolic cycle. The fungus uses cellulose as its primary growth substrate, but when large quantities of lignin are encountered or certain nutrients are not present, the secondary metabolic cycle is entered.[17]

Extracellular Oxidative Enzymes

The extracellular lignin-degrading enzymes serve to fragment lignin into pieces that can be assimilated by the fungus. This conceptualization of degradation activity stresses the importance of the individual enzyme's wide range of activity and function. The intracellular enzyme components complete the conversion of the lignin fragments into carbon dioxide.

Lignin cleavage reactions are catalyzed by a hemoprotein ligninase.[18-20] Hydrogen peroxide is consumed in this reaction that degrades lignin, indicating a peroxidative mechanism. The activity of the lignin peroxidase isozymes enables the oxidation of a variety of aromatic substrates to radical cation intermediates.[21] Depending on the radical cation's structure, it may act as an oxidant, an electron shuttle, or an intermediate that collapses to oxidized product.

Recent work has differentiated the extracellular ligninase mixture into two discrete categories of lignin peroxidase isozymes and manganese dependent peroxidase isozymes. The oxidation-reduction potentials of lignin peroxidase isozymes H1, H2, H8, and H10 have been determined by potentiometric titration.[22] The isozymes have potentials of $-142mV$, $-135mV$, $-137mV$, and $-127mV$ respectively, versus standard hydrogen electrode. The manganese dependent peroxidase isozymes, H3 and H4, have been found to have redox potentials of –88mV and –93mV, respectively versus the standard hydrogen electrode. The midpoint potential of isozymes H1 and H4 indicates that the reductive half-reaction converts the ferric lignin peroxidase to ferrous form. The redox cycle of the lignin peroxidase isozymes has been formulated as the two-electron oxidative conversion of the native state iron(III) enzyme to compound I iron(IV) cation radical by reaction with a single molecule of hydrogen peroxide. The compound I state is reduced to a compound II iron(IV) noncharged state through a single electron transfer, and finally the compound II state is reduced back to the native enzyme state.[21]

The generation of hydrogen peroxide has been attributed to four different enzymes: glyoxal oxidase,[23] glucose oxidase,[24,25] pyranose-2-oxidase,[26,27] and methanol oxidase.[28] The glucose oxidase enzyme, now rivaled by the glyoxal oxidase enzyme, has been considered the major contributor to hydrogen peroxide production. The glucose oxidase has been located in unique periplasmic microbodies, whereas the glyoxal oxidase appears to be a completely extracellular enzyme system.

Stoichiometries of product formation, as well as hydrogen peroxide and oxygen uptake, are consistent with a radical pathway.[18] These results established the one-electron oxidative mechanism as the primary extracellular oxidative pathway for *P. chrysosporium*.

It has been shown that *P. chrysosporium* produces at least 10 extracellular hemoproteins; roughly half have ligninase activity.[29] The heterogeneity among the various extracellular proteins produced by *P. chrysosporium* points to possible functional differences important to pollutant degradation. A study comparing the ligninase activity of the separated ligninases with a corresponding ability to oxidize 2,4,6-trichlorophenol amply shows that ligninolytic activity of the individual enzymes is a poor predictive base to estimate the enzyme's ability to oxidize alternative substrates.[30] The phenoloxidase activity of the enzymes was observed to be an order of magnitude lower than the ligninase activity. Furthermore, poor lignin-oxidizing enzymes were shown to be among some of the better phenoloxidase enzymes. The direct application of these enzymes to treatment technology has been enhanced through other recent applications in the literature.[31]

Life Cycle of *Phanaerochaete Chrysosporium*

To adequately harness the striking abilities of the wood-rotting fungi, it is necessary to understand both their life cycle and morphological forms to optimize a fungal treatment process. The life cycle of Hymenomycetes fungi is characterized by many structures formed during vegetative, sexual, and asexual reproductive phases.[12]

The fungal mycelium, a mass of interwoven filamentous hyphae, is usually submerged in growth medium when cultured in liquid. The mycelium passes through three distinct stages of development. The primary mycelium growth phase is not vigorous. Once secondary mycelium is formed, subsequent growth is frequently different from the primary mycelium. As the mycelium tissues organize and specialize, the tertiary phase is initiated. Secondary and tertiary mycelia comprise the vegetative segment of the life cycle. The vegetative phase is the longest and dominant growth phase. The highest concentration of extracellular enzymes is secreted during the vegetative phase. Eventually, the tissues of the tertiary mycelium differentiate into fruiting bodies that are shed, depending on environmental conditions. Asexual reproduction with continued maintenance of current degrading abilities can occur anytime during the vegetative growth phase. *P. chrysosporium* produces asexual spores prolifically and at all stages of the life cycle.[32]

Degradation Studies of Waste Constituents

An expanding list of hazardous waste organic chemicals have been shown to be degraded to carbon dioxide by the *P. chrysosporium* fungal strain through the use of radiorespirometry. In the case of 1,1,1-trichloro-2,2-bis(p-chlorophenyl)ethane(DDT), it appears that ligninolytic conditions are not necessary for the fungus to degrade this substrate.[33,34] There may may be additional instances of organic substrates not requiring ligninase for breakdown. The search for other organic hazardous waste substrates not requiring ligninolytic conditions is under investigation by several researchers.

Radiorespirometric studies of the degradation of [U-14C] pentachlorophenol in aqueous media and under ligninolytic conditions have indicated that the substrate was rapidly converted to carbon dioxide.[35] Enzyme studies showed that pentachlorophenol is converted to 1,4-tetrachlorobenzoquinone by the fungus.[30] The quinone was difficult to quantify due to its propensity to form charge transfer complexes with cellular materials. Further metabolic pathway elucidation of the is in progress. Several aromatic hydrocarbons, benzo[a]anthracene, pyrene, anthracene, benzo[a]pyrene, and pyrelene (constituents of creosote), were converted to carbon dioxide by the fungus in liquid culture.[19,20] This latter finding serves to differentiate the fungus from bacterial species, because few bacteria have the ability to utilize the higher molecular weight aromatic polycyclics.

Contaminated Liquid Treatment Technology Development

A water treatment process(*MyCOR*—Mycelial Color Removal), utilizing *P. chrysosporium*, has been investigated for use as a decolorization process for Kraft pulp liquor.[36] Continued work with this technology has been expanded to the soluble fraction of organic components associated with the wood treatment industry. The patented reactor is a specifically designed rotating disk reactor that accommodates the specific growth needs of the fungus. Because the fungus does not adhere to a surface as do bacteria, the reactor was modified to permit attachment of fungal biomass to the disks. Results derived from bench scale operation show that the fungus in this reactor will degrade 250ppm pentachlorophenol in water to 5ppm in eight hours.[37] Subsequent research has shown that chlorinated phenols and guaiacols can be effectively degraded by *P. chrysosporium*. Using pure organics in water, approximately 60 percent of the phenols and guaiacols could be degraded in 3 to 4 hours.[38] Methylation of the phenols occurred in addition to degradation. Roughly 10 to 20 percent of the phenol concentration was converted to anisole. Methyl ether formation has also been observed with other fungi too in their degradation of pentachlorophenol.[39] Methyl ethers are known to be good substrates for *P. chrysosporium*, so their formation only indicates slower degradation kinetics for pentachlorophenol.

Pink water associated with munitions production is adequately treated in the process just described.[40] Degradation of 2,4,6-trinitrotoluene and 2,4- dinitrotoluene in concentrations of 150ppm in water occurs in an eight-hour treatment period. For each case, several additional doses were degraded with the same efficiency. The continued ability to remove the contaminants from the water phase was interpreted to indicate that the fungus continues to degrade the contaminants and that contaminant loss is not merely an adsorption phenomenon.

Activities to bring this process to pilot scale have been pursued at the Cincinnati Environmental Protection Agency Testing and Evaluation Facility. We are critically evaluating the operations of the reactor to determine the optimal conditions. Mass transfer of substrate, oxygen uptake, and quantity of growth substrate(s) are items selected for early control status. Control of biofilm growth through the use of alternate carbon substrates is under investigation. The relative activities of the hydrogen peroxide generating enzymes are crucial to this evaluation. Published activities for the various enzymes have guided our selection of candidate carbon substrates for testing.

Reactor behavior is currently monitored by means of Kraft pulp liquor decolorization treatment. Adherence of the fungus to the high density polyethylene disks of the pilot scale unit is very good. Control of the biofilm thickness is important to the lifetime of the reactor for several reasons: biofilm mechanical characteristics, biofilm oxygen uptake, and the risk that thicker biofilms may lead to anaerobic zones on the disks that the organism cannot tolerate.

Surrogate wastestreams containing creosote chemicals and pentachlorophenol will be fed to establish initial operating conditions, which then will be optimized. Reactor performance will be determined through the use of leachate or contaminated groundwater collected from contaminated wood-treating sites.

Soil Detoxification Technology Development

The general success of liquid phase biodegradation studies with the fungus stimulated speculation that this microorganism may be an appropriate candidate for the treatment of contaminated soils. Attempts to inoculate environmental matrices with nonnative microorganisms have met with varying degrees of success.[41] The elucidation of optimal practices leading to successful inoculation of contaminated environmental materials remains to be discovered.[42] At the outset of this research, *P. chrysosporium* was not known to inhabit the soil. Due to this general lack of knowledge of the habitat, a rather cautious research effort was initiated to determine the ability of the fungus to inhabit and thrive in the soil. Early work indicated that *P. chrysosporium* did not grow well in non-sterile soils; this may be attributable in part to ineffective competition with the indigenous microflora, because the soil is not the normal habitat of *P. chrysosporium*. Lately, it has been found that growth within the soil can be accomplished through the use of larger quantities of inoculum.[35,43-45]

Three well-characterized soils (topsoil and subsoil) were used in this work (Table 1). We evaluated the effect of soil type, pH, temperature, and water potential on the growth of *P. chrysosporium* in three sterile soils in a factorial experiment. Soils were sterilized by fumigating with methyl bromide to avoid confounding effects from native microflora. Growth of the fungus was evaluated at five soil temperatures ranging from 25 to 39°C and four water potentials ranging from −0.03 to −1.5 mPa. The extent of growth was determined by measuring the amount of ergosterol that could be extracted from two subsamples of the soil from each test at the end of a two-week incubation period and reported as micrograms of ergosterol per gram of soil.[46,47]

Table 1
Physical and Chemical Characteristics of Test Soils

Macro Features			
Soil Type	Batavia	Marsham	Xurich
Texture	silty clay–loam	sandy loam	sandy loam
Horizon	Bt2	A	A
Cation exchange Capacity (meq/100g)	17	38	14
Base Saturation (%)	29.5	66.4	24.0
pH	5.4	6.8	7.1
Organic matter(%)	0.5	12.0	39.0
Nitrogen(%)	0.05	0.46	0.18
Trace Constituents (ppm)			
Calcium	1950	4900	1675
Magnesium	850	1650	640
Potassium	145	90	80
Phosphorus	75	17	17
Boron	0.6	1.3	0.8
Manganese	12.5	9.0	77.5
Zinc	1.9	12.2	6.4
Sulfur	9.7	11.3	3.9

Growth of the fungus was the greatest in the Marsham soil, intermediate in the Xurich soil, and least in the Batavia soil. The same trend was observed when a visual assessment system of growth was used. Soil water potential had a significant effect on the growth of the fungus. As the soil water potential was increased (corresponds to decrease in soil water content), fungal growth decreased. Water potential is another easily controlled soil factor.[48] Growth of the fungus was unaffected as temperature was increased from 25°C to 35°C but significantly decreased at 39°C. These results do not agree with earlier work using the visual growth estimation technique. The difference may be attributable to an increase of sporulation by the fungus at the soil surface with increased temperature, leading to a biased measurement of growth. Soil temperatures under field conditions can be controlled by selecting the normal warm months for operation and by using soil solarization. Biomass accumulations as well as growth habit of *P. chrysosporium* were greatly influenced by soil type (see Table 1).

Growth Measurement

The measurement of growth has presented major problems for this area of study. Assessment of growth in the early stages of these studies was done by means of visual estimation on a ranking basis. Due to the three-dimensional growth patterns of the fungus in a solid substrate such as soil, it was necessary to find a more reliable means to determine the extent of fungal growth. The normal means of assessing growth in bacterial systems have no application to the present study. Based on work investigating the infestation of cereal grains by fungi, a mycosteroid, ergosterol (ergosta-5:6,7:8,22:23-trien-3-ol), has been employed as a quantitative means to determine growth of the fungus.[49] It has been shown to correlate well with the visual estimation technique.

The application of the fungus to soil treatment is focused on the remediation of wood treatment sites. Target pollutants identified for treatment at these sites are pentachlorophenol(PCP) and the major aromatic hydrocarbon contaminants found in creosote(naphthalene, anthracene, and phenanthrene). Creosote has been extensively characterized, and new substrates will be added to the mixture when deemed necessary.[50]

PCP has been reported in the literature as subject to degradation by the fungus.[51] This literature study lacked a complete material balance of substrate and conversion products. Thus, we studied the degradation of ^{14}C[UL]-pentachlorophenol over an eight-week period in the three soils. Mineralization, volatile losses, extractable PCP in the soil, and soil residuals containing bound PCP and transformed products were measured to develop a tight material balance.[52] A very small percentage of the total ^{14}C was accounted for by mineralization and volatilization. Both mineralization and volatilization were significantly greater in inoculated than in noninoculated cultures of the three soils. The extractable quantities of PCP were greatly reduced by inoculation with *P. chrysosporium*. The greatest rate of PCP removal due to fungal activity was found with the Marsham soil.[45] Extractable PCP after 14 days was approximately 2ppm of the original 50ppm spiked amount; that was reduced to roughly 1ppm after an additional 14 days of treatment. Decreases of PCP concentration in the soils of the control tests are attributable to several potential causes: abiotic avenues of degradation or loss, irreversible binding to the soil, or degradation due to the regrowth of native organisms.

The degradative ability of the fungus in the soil has been evaluated through measurement of evolved labeled carbon dioxide. Disappearance of the parent compound was monitored by gas chromatography or high-pressure liquid chromatography techniques. Separation of the soil into solvent extractable, humic acid, fulvic acid, and humin fractions permitted material balance evaluations.[53] The fate of ^{14}C-PCP in the soil was determined by analysis of the recoverable carbon label from: an organic extractable fraction, the soil organic matter (humic and fulvic fractions), and the nonextractable humin fraction. Combustion analysis was used to assay the amount of ^{14}C associated with humic and fulvic acid fractions and the nonextractable humin fraction.

The percent of total ^{14}C recovery ranged from 55 to 84 percent over a 56-day period for the Marsham soil tests. Volatilization losses were less than 3 percent for the three soils. There was a significant amount of labeled carbon activity associated with nonextractable fractions, indicating that there is possibly incorporation in the soil material of the pollutant substrates during its metabolism. Bollag[54] has shown the possible polymerization reactions between PCP and soil chemicals such as syringic acid. Polymeric forms of a series of pollutants were constructed by Haider and Martin,[55] who showed that *P. chrysosporium* would degrade these higher molecular weight materials but at a slower rate than the parent pollutant substrate. A more recent study shows that *P. chrysosporium* can degrade humic acid materials.[56]

Future research in the soil application will include small-scale treatment of selected pollutants at environmentally significant concentrations, the evaluation of amendments on primary and secondary metabolism, and the delivery of oxygen within the soil to the growing fungus.

Acknowledgments

The much of the treatment technology research reported in this paper has been supported by programs of the U.S. Environmental Protection Agency. Research groups at the U.S.D.A. Forest Products Laboratory, the State University of New York at Syracuse, North Carolina State University, the University of Cincinnati, and the U.S. Environmental Protection Agency have contributed to this report.

References

1. U.S. Department of Agriculture. *The Biological and Economic Assessment of Pentachlorophenol, Inorganic Arsenicals, Creosote, Vols 1 and 2* (Technical Bulletin 1658-I and 1658-II), 1980.
2. D.M. Griffin, in *Bacteria in Nature, Vol. 1*, E.R. Leadbetter and J.S. Perlmutter, Eds. (Plenum, New York, 1985), pp. 221-255.
3. M. Wainwright, *Trans. Br. Mycol. Soc.* **90**, 150 (1988).
4. V.D. Kozak *et al.*, *Reviews of the Environmental Effects of Pollutants: XI. Chlorophenols* (United States Environmental Protection Agency, EPA-600/1-79-012, 1979), pp. 260.
5. J.H. Slater and D. Lovatt, in *Microbial Degradation of Organic Compounds*, D.T. Gibson, Ed. (Marcel Decker, New York, 1984), pp. 439-485.
6. D.C. Eaton, *Enzyme Microb. Technol.* **7**, 194 (1985); J.A. Bumpus *et al.*, *Science* **228**, 1434 (1985).
7. J.-M. Bollag, *Crit. Rev. Microbiol.* **2**, 35 (1972).
8. H. Lyr, *Phytopathol. Z.*, **47**, 73 (1963).
9. C.G. Duncan and F.J. Deverall., *Appl. Microbiol.* **12**, 57 (1964).
10. H.H. Unligli, *Forest Prod. J.* **18**, 45 (1968).
11. H.H. Burdsall and W.E. Eslyn, *Mycotaxon.* **1**, 123 (1974).
12. J.W. Deacon, *Introduction to Modern Mycology* (Blackwell Scientific Publications, Oxford, England, 1984), pp. 1-24.
13. J.A. Bumpus and S.D. Aust, *BioEssays* **6**, 166 (1987).
14. A.D.M. Rayner and C. Boddy, *Fungal Decomposition of Wood—Its Biology and Ecology* (John Wiley & Sons, New York, 1988).
15. T.K. Kirk and M. Shimada, in *Biosynthesis and Biodegradation of Wood Components*, T. Higuchi, Ed. (Academic Press, New York, 1985), pp. 579-605.

16. T.K. Kirk, in *Microbial Degradation of Organic Compounds*, D.T. Gibson, Ed. (Marcel Dekker, New York, 1984), pp. 399-438.

17. T.K. Kirk and R.L. Farrell, *Ann. Rev. Microbiol.* **41**, 465 (1987).

18. K.E. Hammel *et al.*, *J. Biol. Chem.* **260**, 8348 (1985).

19. K.E. Hammel, B. Kalyanaraman, and T.K. Kirk, *Biol. Chem.* **261**, 16948 (1986).

20. S.D. Haemmerli *et al.*, *J. Biol. Chem.* **261**, 6900 (1986).

21. J.M. Palmer, P.J. Harvey, and H.E. Schoemaker, *Phil. Trans. R. Soc. London* A **321**, 495 (1987).

22. C.D. Millis *et al.*, *Oxidation-Reduction Potentials and Ionization States of Extracellular Peroxidases From the Lignin-Degrading Fungus* Phanerochaete chrysosporium. (Abstracts, Fourth International Conference—Biotechnology in the Pulp and Paper Industry, Raleigh, N.C., May 16-19, 1989) p. 139.

23. P.J. Kersten and T.K. Kirk, *J. Bacteriol.* **169**, 2195 (1987).

24. R.L. Kelley and C.A. Reddy, *J. Bacteriol.* **166**, 269 (1986).

25. R.L. Kelley and C.A. Reddy, in *Methods in Enzymology, Vol. 161, BIOMASS Part B, Lignin, Pectin, and Chitin*, W.A. Wood and S.T. Kellogg, Eds. (Academic Press, Inc., New York, 1988), pp. 307-315.

26. K.-E. Eriksson *et al.*, *Appl. Microbiol. Biotechnol.* **23**, 257 (1986).

27. J. Volc and K.-E. Eriksson, in *Methods in Enzymology, Vol. 161, BIOMASS Part B, Lignin, Pectin, and Chitin*, W.A. Wood and S.T. Kellogg, Eds. (Academic Press, Inc., New York, 1988), pp. 316-321.

28. K.-E. Eriksson and A. Nishida, in *Methods in Enzymology, Vol. 161, BIOMASS Part B, Lignin, Pectin, and Chitin*, W.A. Wood and S.T. Kellogg, Eds. (Academic Press, Inc., New York, 1988) pp. 322-326.

29. T.K. Kirk *et al.*, *Enz. Microb. Tech.* **8**, 27 (1986).

30. K.E. Hammel and P.J. Tardone, *Biochemistry* **27**, 6563 (1988).

31. J.R. Shannon and R. Bartha, *Appl. Environ. Microbiol.* **54**, 1719 (1988).

32. M.H. Gold and T.M. Cheng, *Arch. Microbiol.* **121**, 37 (1979).

33. A. Kohler *et al.*, *Appl. Microbiol. Biotechnol.* **29**, 618 (1988).

34. J.A. Bumpus and S. Aust, *Appl. Environ. Microbiol.* **53**, 2001 (1987).

35. R.T. Lamar, J.A. Glaser, and T.K. Kirk, *Use of White-Rot Fungi to Remediate Soils Contaminated with Wood Preserving Waste.* (Abstracts, Fourth International Conference Biotechnology in the Pulp and Paper Industry, Raleigh, N.C., May 16 19, 1989) p. 82.

36. H.M. Chang *et al.*, U.S. Patent No. 4, 554, 075 (1985).

37. T.W. Joyce *et al.*, in *Chemical and Biochemical Detoxification of Hazardous Waste*, J.A. Glaser, Ed. (Lewis Publishers Inc., Ann Arbor, Mich.), in press.

38. H. Guo *et al.*, *Degradation of Chlorinated Phenols and Guaiacols by the White-Rot Fungus* Phanerochaete chrysosporium. (Abstracts, Fourth International Conference—Biotechnology in the Pulp and Paper Industry, Raleigh, N.C., May 16-19, 1989) p. 69.

39. A.J. Cserjesi and E.L. Johnson, *Can. J. Microbiol.* **18**, 45 (1972).

40. J.L. Popp and T.K. Kirk, *Studies on the Oxidation of Methoxybenzenes by Manganese (III) and the Manganese-Dependent Peroxidase of* Phanerochaete chrysosporium. (Abstracts, Fourth International Conference—Biotechnology in the Pulp and Paper Industry, Raleigh, N.C., May 16-19, 1989) p. 149.

41. B.R. Zaidi, G. Stucki, and M. Alexander, *Environ. Toxicol. Chem.* **7**, 143 (1988).

42. R.M. Goldstein, L.M. Mallory, and M. Alexander, *Appl. Environ. Microbiol.* **50**, 977 (1985).

43. R.T. Lamar *et al.*, in *Land Disposal, Remedial Action, Incineration and Treatment of Hazardous Waste*. Proceedings of the 13th Annual Hazardous Waste Symposium, EPA/ 600/9-87/015 (U. S. Environmental Protection Agency, Cincinnati, Ohio, 1987), pp. 419-429.
44. R.T. Lamar *et al.*, in *Chemical and Biochemical Detoxification of Hazardous Waste*, J.A. Glaser, Ed. (Lewis Publishers, Ann Arbor, Mich., 1990).
45. R.T. Lamar, J.A. Glaser, and T.K. Kirk, *Fate of Pentachlorophenol(PCP) on Soils Inolculated with the White-Rot Basidiomycete Phanerochaete chrysosporium: Mineralization, Volatilization, and Depletion of PCP*, manuscript in preparation.
46. S.E. Matcham, B.R. Jordan, and D.A. Wood, *Appl. Microbiol. Biotechnol.* **21**, 108 (1985).
47. L.M. Seitz *et al.*, *Phytopathology* **69**, 1202 (1979).
48. L.E. Sommers *et al.*, in *Water Potential Relations in Soil Microbiology*, SSA Special Publication Number **9** (Soil Science Society of America, Madison, Wis., 1981), pp. 97-117.
49. J.D. Weete and D.J. Weber, *Lipid Biochemistry of Fungi and Other Organisms* (Plenum Press, New York, 1980).
50. F.H.M. Nestler, *U.S. Department of Agriculture Forestry Service Research Paper* FPL 195. U.S. Department of Agriculture, Forestry Service, Forest Products Laboratory, Madison, Wis.
51. J.A. Bumpus, *Appl. Environ. Microbiol.* **54**, 2885 (1988).
52. J. Mayaudon, in *Soil Biochemistry, Vol. 2*, A.D. Mclaren and J. Skujins, Eds. (Marcel Decker, New York, 1971), pp. 202-256.
53. F.J. Stevenson, *Humus Chemistry, Chap. 2*, (Wiley, New York, 1982) pp. 26-54.
54. J.M. Bollag and S.Y. Liu, *Pest. Biochem. Physiol.* **23**, 261 (1985).
55. K.M. Haider and J.P. Martin, *Soil Biol. Biochem.* **20**, 425 (1988).
56. R. Blondeau, *Appl. Environ. Microbiol.* **5**, 1282 (1989).

Discussion

Salkinoja-Salonen: Just to clarify it went too fast for me. What was the degree of mineralization to carbon dioxide you got with the pentachlorophenol.

Glaser: Two percent.

Salkinoja-Salonen: So I was right. Two percent in about 28 days.

Glaser: No, two percent in about two months.

Salkinoja-Salonen: Then I was right, much more of your pentachlorophenol dissapeared. So you concluded that it has been bound to humic matter?

Glaser: That is right.

Salkinoja-Salonen: Then I would like to ask, how do you extract your pentachlorophenol from soil? Was the extraction scheme an organic solvent that is a hydrophilic miscible solvent or immiscible solvent?

Glaser: It contained both a hydrocarbon and something that wetted the soil to pull the pentachlorophenol out. I will have to check to tell you exactly what the extraction solvent was but we looked into that.

Salkinoja-Salonen: Our experience is with unknown poorer solvents you will not do much with soil especially after you added pentachlorophenol in soil but a week or a month later you will not get it out any more.

Glaser: I would agree with you. Our recovery of labeled material points that we have been fairly efficient in our monitoring studies. Our studies were isotope dilution experiments so that we had a lot more material in the soil then we could actually buy isotopically labelled. We also monitored our ability to recover it from the soil. Our total recovery of the labelled material was of the order of 80 percent.

DeFrank: Obviously, you are primarily interested in degradation of xenobiotics that is the major problem in this area. Are you aware of any experimental work using *phanerochaete* or the lingninases with biologically derived toxic materials like aflatoxins or non-proteinacous toxins.

Glaser: No I am not. I am not at all familiar with any applications. Let me give you some idea of the fungus. It appears in its biomass to be almost immune to some of the very toxic materials that we have tested. We have loaded lots of reactor systems with pentachlorophenol and have seen no adverse consequences to the biomass. Whether it is an issue that it actually adheres for some period to the biomass and then is eventually degraded we do not know but some studies leading into answers to these questions are underway.

Eveleigh: How competitive is this organism in the soil? I can quote a dismal example, in New Jersey where by they went composting and the result was *Aspergillus fumigatus*, which is actually a kind of a mild pathogens of humans for compromise people. I think it is all very elegant but I also see the selection of basidomycete white fungi if there could be something on competitiveness as well.

Glaser: Well, we looked into the competitiveness. We were concerned initially. We were of the mind that we could actually work into part of our treatment scheme fumigation of the plot before we actually treated it. Well, this alternative was viewed very dimly, in spite of the fact that fumigation is used nation-wide in forestry nurseries right now. So we backed off from that position and actually looked to see what was required to put in it non-sterile soils and the answer is that we have to put in about three times the amount of innoculum to successfully innoculate non-sterile soil.

Chakrabarty: Does phanerochaete need hydrogen peroxide to degrade pentachlorophenol or other chlorophenols?

Glaser: That is an experiment that we are doing right now. In light of the fact that the DDT situation that has come up. The work of Hammel, was done specifically with the enzymes showing the conversion of the phenol to the quinone.

Chakrabarty: Did you use any hydrogen peroxide?

Glaser: No we did not.

Chakrabarty: It did it without hydrogen peroxide?

Glaser: The fungus has its own system to generate hydrogen peroxide. It may be glucose oxidase or it may be glyoxal oxidase that are hydrogen peroxide generators for the organism.

Chakrabarty: Did you use glucose? Does it cause any ecological problem if you dump a lot of glucose in a field?

Glaser: We used glucose. Yes, we are backing off from the use of glucose we would rather use glyoxal oxidase and use the substrates that glyoxal oxidase finds useful to it.

Bedard: Is this work that you are describing all being done at your lab in Cincinatti?

Glaser: No, I did not mean to imply that, the soil work is done in conjunction with T. Kent Kirk at Forest Products Laboratory, the scale-up of the RBC is done specifically in Cincinatti.

Bedard: What does RBC mean?

Glaser: Rotating biological contactor it is, in other words, a series of discs on which grow the biofilm for treatment. We have another component to the RBC work that is the Ho Min Chang and Tom Joyce group at North Carolina state. Ken Hammel, as I have mention several times, has done much of the enzyme work.

Bedard: Thank you.

Janssen: You apparently achieved in specifically establishing this fungus in the biological contactor. Did you undertake any specific measures to obtain that establishing of the fungus in the reactor and was it indeed a the dominating organism in the system?

Glaser: Good question. You cannot put the fungus into a waste stream where you have competitors to the fungus. We can grow it up on Kraft liquor for instance. The Kraft liquor coming out of E1 and you can grow it up from spores at that stage but you cannot grow it up out of primary effluent from a mixed liquor wash plant. There are too many predators and competitors for the fungus under those circumstances. We grow it up and once it is proficient and established in a biofilm we expose it to waste.

16

Solid Waste Biodegradation by Anaerobic Digestion:
A Developing Technology in Europe

correspondence
Franco Cecchi
*Department of
Environmental Science
University of Venice
Dorsoduro 2137
30123 Venice
Italy*

Joan Mata-Alvarez
*Department of Chemical
Engineering
University of Barcelona
C. Martii Franques 1
pta.6-08028 Barcelona
Spain*

Using data available in recent literature, we present the state of the art in the field of anaerobic digestion of municipal solid waste in Europe at the research, development, and commercial level. A comparative analysis of the results takes into account the ultimate biogas production and the kinetics of the substrate utilization to evaluate the performance obtainable with differently collected organic fractions of municipal solid waste. An approach to the stability process control through the reactor supernatant recirculation is presented. The pH and the CO_2/CH_4 ratio are modeled as stability process parameter indices. Our conclusions outline the fields where further work must be carried out in the near future.

Introduction

Final disposal of municipal solid waste (MSW) is an open question today. The sector operators have two main possibilities from which to choose:

1. To favor the massive disposal techniques in sanitary landfills or by incineration; or
2. To choose technologies that can reduce the environmental impact and recover energy and materials.

From the management point of view, the first approach seems very simple and does allow energy recovery with biogas collection from a landfill or by adapting incinerators with heat and electricity recovery. However, this approach leaves the organic fraction biological cycle open, making the soil humus content worse. This choice may seem to reflect an intention to defer an account that has to be paid. Furthermore, one of the major environmental problems today is the impoverishment of the organic fraction in the soil.

The second approach is in greater harmony with the biological cycles. The refuse is collected and sorted into three main fractions: inert, combustible, and putrescent organic fraction.

The inert fraction, after separation and recovery of ferrous materials, is disposed of in landfill sites, thus presenting fewer environmental problems in comparison with massive disposal and requiring less landfilling volume. The combustible fraction, which presents a calorific value that is two to three times higher and of more constant quality than the raw refuse, is burned in smaller and easier controlled incinerator plants equipped with the energy recovery section. The putrescent organic fraction is anaerobically digested and/or aerobically composted before being utilized on agricultural soil.

Together with both the final disposal strategies, we may consider the separated collection of the sorted organic fraction of MSW. There are, in fact, many towns in which this part of the refuse can be separately collected before mixing and pollution with other refuses; moreover, its amount is not negligible.[1] The separately collected organic fraction of MSW can be treated to produce "green-compost" or "green-biogas" that has very high performance or can easily be integrated with other environmental technologies, producing very important energy savings.[2] Figure 1 presents two strategy schemes that consider the second approach to the final disposal of MSW.

This paper has three goals. First, we present the state of the art in the field of biomass and energy from waste in the context of the work carried out in Europe in the anaerobic digestion of the organic fraction of municipal solid waste at research, development, demonstrative, and commercial levels. Particular emphasis is paid to the results obtained during five years of research carried out through a close

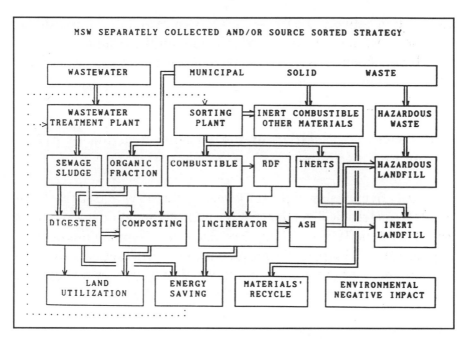

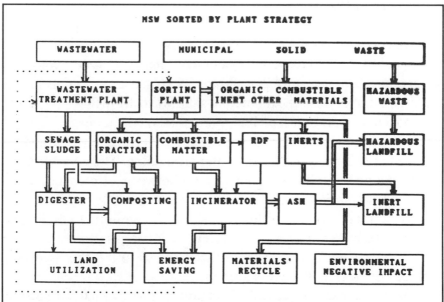

Figure 1. Integrated strategy on the MSW final disposal. A, source sorted and or separately collected strategy; B, MSW sorted by plant strategy; (====) main flow, (——) alternative flow.

cooperation between the University of Venice and the University of Barcelona; second, we compare critically all the results presented. Finally, we consider some aspects connected with monitoring and process stability control.

The Anaerobic Digestion of the Organic Fraction of MSW: European Experience

Only over the last eight to 14 years have MSW alternative treatments by anaerobic digestion received serious attention in Europe. In fact, since June 1978 the Council of European Communities decided to grant financial support for projects in the field of alternative energy sources and energy savings. Biomass and energy from waste was a part of the program.

Commercial Plants

A commercial plant in Bellaria, Italy, is treating a mixture of sewage sludge and the organic fraction of municipal solid waste. The plant consists of a sorting line (80 ton MSW per day), which selects the organic fraction of the municipal solid waste from the other refuse components (inert, combustible, and metals), two conventional digesters ($850m^3$ each) mixed with a gas recycling system, and an engine for electricity and warm water production. The concentration of the sludge fed to the digesters ranges between 11 percent and 12 percent total solids, and the mean organic loading rate value is 8kgTVS (total volatile solids)/(m^3·day). The minimum hydraulic retention time used is equal to 10 days. The biogas produced is 1.5 million m^3/year; 25 percent is utilized for warming the digesters, whereas the rest at present is burned.

In Italy, Snamprogetti SpA is building a plant with four digesters for the Municipality of Bergamo. This plant will be able to handle 38 tons per day of organic fraction of municipal solid waste (TS basis) mixed with sewage sludges in thermophilic conditions. Other plants are being designed for the Verona area (500 tons per day),[3] and for an area called "CITA" (400,000 equivalent inhabitants, EI). Both of these plants are in the Veneto region and are part of integrated systems of technologies. Other plants in Italy are being planned for Asti (Piedmont region), Empoli (Tuscany region), Caltanisetta (Sicily region).

In France, there are several plants under construction or in the planning phase that apply the dry fermentation VALORGA technology. They are: Foix [30,000 tons/years (t/y)]; Dunkerque (100,000 t/y); Doulons (40,000 t/y); Lorient (40,000 t/y); Saint Brieuc (35,000 t/y); Nimes (88,000 t/y); and Jueret (30,000 t/y).[4] A further commercial plant has been running in France since June 1988 at Amiens. This plant, with a total reactor volume of 2400m,[3] has been designed for operation under thermophilic conditions (VALORGA process).[5]

In Finland, the DN-BIOPROCESSING LTD is working to construct an anaerobic digestion plant with a fermentation technology called WABIO-Process.[6] The WABIO-Process is an aerobic-anaerobic fermentation treatment system, with composting and the anaerobic digestion units. The organic fraction of MSW, sewage sludge, and other organic wastes are mixed and homogenized in the compost unit. This step increases the temperature of the organic mixture. The heated wastes are then fed to the biogas reactor. The digested material is pressed dry, and the pressing liquid is recycled in the process.

The WABIO-Process data are the following: specific biogas production rate 0.38 to $0.47 m^3/kgTVS$; methane content in the biogas approximately 60 percent; retention time 20 to 28 days; process temperature 30° to 50°C.

Demonstrative and Development Plants

A demonstration plant has been constructed at Broni, Italy, with EEC economic support[7] (digester volume = $2000 m^3$). The feed of the digester is a mixture of the organic fraction of MSW and sewage sludge, with a mixing ratio of 1:6.3 MSW:sewage sludge (w/w). The digester performance reported was 0.43 to 0.53m³ biogas/kgTVS (1.3 to 1.6m³CH₄/(m³·day)) when the organic loading rate to the digester was 5kgTVS/(m³·day) and the hydraulic retention time 10 days. The feed concentration was 10.7 percent total solids(TS), and the concentration inside the digester seven percent to eight percent TS.

A plant that can be considered both demonstrative (in terms of scale) and developmental is that of La Buisse (France). This was built by VALORGA. The plant comprises four sections: the crushing and sorting section, where the organic fraction of the refuse is sorted from ferrous magnetic metals and shredded: the digesting section, where the organic fraction of MSW is digested (the retention time is more than 15 days); and the finishing and biogas utilization sections, where the digested liquor is dewatered, solid is recovered as humus, and the biogas is stored and utilized.

The VALORGA process can be classified as a dry fermentation process because the shredded organic fraction of MSW is only diluted to a total solids content of about 35 percent before feeding and fermentation under mesophilic conditions. The digester is fed semi-continuously. After the reactor has been fed, gas production increases the digester pressure, which permits the digested residue outlet. A sudden release of the pressure occurs when a value of 500mbar is reached, and gas recycling system permits mixing of the digester. Design characteristics of the digester and some operating conditions are available from the literature,[7,8] both for the demonstrative mesophilic plant and the thermophilic laboratory system. These can be summarized as follows. In mesophilic conditions, the pilot plant loaded at 13.7kgTVS/(m³·day) yields 4 m³biogas/(m³·day), with 65 percent methane [maximum value 7 m³/(m³·day)], and the specific gas production rate was 0.35m³/kgTVS. In the laboratory plant, thermophilic conditions at 12 and 9 days, retention time and 16.5 and 18 to 20kgTVS/(m³·day) organic loading rate were tested; the performance obtained was 6.0 and 6.5 to 8.0m³/(m³·day) 55 methane percent, respectively, and the specific gas production rate was 0.36 and 0.39m³/kgTVS.

In development of dry fermentation processes, the work carried out by ARBIOS S.A. together with the University of Ghent (Belgium) at laboratory and pilot plant level[7,9,10] must be considered. In their "Dranco Process," anaerobic treatment of the organic fraction of household refuse takes place in an intensive reactor during a period of 12 to 18 days. This step is followed by a postdigester with a retention time of two to three days. Both steps take place at the same operating temperature and concentration of solids. The residue digested is dewatered, and the liquid separated is used to correct solid concentration of raw incoming matter. In this manner, no wastewater is produced. On the other hand, the cake is dried to 45 percent to 55 percent total solids. Engines running on the biogas produced provide electricity and waste heat. Fifty percent of the electricity produced is used for the plant, and fifty percent can be sold. The waste heat is utilized to heat the digester and to dry cake solids. Mesophilic and thermophilic conditions were studied at pilot and laboratory level. The organic loading rates were 14.2 to 18.7kg COD/$(m^3 \cdot day)$ in the laboratory plant and 21.3kgCOD/$(m^3 \cdot day)$ in the pilot plant; 4.8 to 5.9m^3/$(m^3 \cdot day)$ biogas were produced in mesophilic conditions and 5.2 to 6.8 in thermophilic ones in the laboratory unit. Working with the pilot plant under mesophilic conditions, the yield was 5.2 m^3/$(m^3 \cdot day)$; the methane content in the gas was always approximately 50 percent.

In West Germany, Klein and Rump[11] performed laboratory and demonstration tests on dry fermentation and designed a pilot plant to handle five tons per day. In this KWU-Fresenius process, as in the dry fermentation processes previously described, no water has to be added to the 40 percent total solids feed (half of which is organic matter), and approximately two or three times as much energy is generated as is required to operate the process. Organic loading rates from 3.3 to 10kgTVS/$(m^3 \cdot day)$ were tested. Gas production rates were 1.7 and 5.0m^3/$(m^3 \cdot day)$ respectively; the specific yield was 0.5m^3/kgTVS, and the methane content in the biogas was around 60 percent.

The process called "BIOMET"[12] has recently been studied at pilot scale in Sweden. This is a codigestion process; the percentage of sewage sludge mixed with the organic fraction of municipal solid waste is only 15 percent TS basis. The BIOMET process was studied in a 20m³–reactor stirred by a rotatory grid device. The feed concentration was within the range of conventional reactors (seven percent to 10 percent TS). During a one-year period, two experiments were performed at 27 and 19 days hydraulic retention time. At 27 days, retention time, the organic loading rate was 1.6kgTVS/(m³·day), the gas production 0.8m³/(m³·day) (57 percent methane), and the specific gas production rate 0.51m³/kgTVS. At 19 days' retention time, the organic loading rate was increased to 2.6kgTVS/(m³·day), the gas yield increased to 1.1m³/(m³·day) (53 percent methane), and the specific gas production rate decreased to 0.43m³/kgTVS.

A two-phase anaerobic digestion process of the organic fraction of municipal solid waste was studied in Europe by Hofenk *et al.*[13] within the framework of the EEC grants. The work was carried out with the aim of developing a new process for the anaerobic digestion of solid organic waste with biogas and compost as final products. The experiments were carried out both at laboratory and pilot plant levels. In particular, the latter tests were carried out with two stages of batch digesters: the first was composed of five 60m³ liquefactioning reactors, and the second of a 10m³ upflow anaerobic sludge bed reactor (UASB) methane reactor. The substrate used in the experiments was obtained by a sorting plant. The screened fraction smaller than 40mm was considered organic matter; however, this fraction still contained about 50 percent inorganic matter. With a solid retention time of four or six weeks, 58 percent and 69 percent of the volatile solids added to the plant were converted, respectively. The authors encountered some operating problems when too fine a material was used in the first phase reactor (leachate problems) and with heavy granules after several runs in the UASB reactor. The optimal organic loading rate to the second phase digester was 25kgCOD/(m³·day). The authors concluded that the process can be considered technologically feasible, but an economic feasibility is more complex and has to be judged for any given situation. They also noted that no difference in gas yield between the one-stage and the two-stage system could be established.

Research Activity

There are several research groups in Europe that have worked or are working on the anaerobic digestion of municipal solid waste. Numerous results considering polysubstrate mixture containing the organic fraction of municipal solid waste are reported in the literature. The latter will not be considered in this paper if the portion of the MSW in the substrate is not relevant. We present here results considering together those obtained by Pauss *et al.,* [14] Catholic University of Louvain (Belgium); Marty *et al.,*[15] University of Aix Marseille (France); Le Roux *et al.,*[16,17] Warren Spring Laboratory, Stevenage (United Kingdom); Glauser *et al.,*[18] University of Neuchatel (Switzerland); and, separately, the authors' experiences.

The Experiences of the Universities of Venice and Barcelona

Since 1983 the University of Venice has set up, in cooperation with the municipality of Treviso city, an experimental station[19] where studies of the anaerobic digestion of solid wastes are carried out following the second strategy for the final disposal of the organic fraction of the municipal solid waste outlined in the introduction and illustrated in Figure 1, A. In particular, the obtainable performances from the anaerobic digestion process of the following substrates were investigated under mesophilic conditions: primary sewage sludge; primary and secondary sewage sludges; primary and secondary sewage sludge mixed with separately collected organic fraction of municipal solid waste; primary sewage sludge mixed with source-sorted organic fraction of municipal solid waste; source-sorted organic fraction of municipal solid waste; separately collected organic fraction of municipal solid waste; and organic fraction of municipal solid waste sorted by plant.

Digestion of the organic fraction of municipal solid waste sorted by plant also was studied under thermophilic conditions. Complementary works on process monitoring and control and on particular aspects of the digestion process were carried out. These studies included the fate of the particulate matter fed to the digester;[20] effects of external factors such as temperature and changes in the quality of the organic matter on digestion performance;[21] process stability in relation to process monitoring and recovery from digester failure conditions;[22,23] behavior of the digester when going from mesophilic to thermophilic conditions,[24] and when going from digesting only sewage sludge to 80 percent separately collected organic fraction of municipal solid waste.[25]

Given the aim of this paper, only the data related to the anaerobic digestion of the organic fraction of municipal solid waste will be considered, leaving the digestion and co-digestion of sewage sludges for discussion elsewhere. Moreover, the kinetic aspects of the process will be considered in the companion paper presented by Mata and Cecchi.[26]

Operating under mesophilic conditions between 9 and 25 days retention time and feeding the digester with a constant substrate concentration equal to 64 to $66 kgTVS/m^3$ (corresponding to 2.1 to $6.9 kgTVS/[m^3 \cdot day]$ organic loading rate), the performances obtained digesting source-sorted organic fraction of municipal solid waste ranged between 1.3 to $3.6 m^3/(m^3 \cdot day)$ gas production rate and 0.63 to 0.53 specific gas production rate $(m^3/kgTVS)$; the methane percentage in the gas was 63 to 56.[27] For the separately collected organic fraction, the results obtained were similar; with an organic loading rate of 4.5 to $5.0 kgTVS/(m^3 \cdot day)$, the gas production rate expected is 2.9 to $3.2 m^3/(m^3 \cdot day)$, 60 percent methane, and the specific gas production rate is $0.65 \ m^3/kgTVS$. These data are derived from the experimental results obtained by digesting the separately collected organic fraction of MSW and sewage sludge with a feeding ratio of 80:20 TS basis.[28,29]

When the organic fraction of the MSW is sorted by plant, the quality of the digestible matter decreases as does the digester performance. The mesophilic anaerobic digestion of the organic fraction sorted by the industrial plant of S. Giorgio di Nogaro (Italy) was studied at the University of Venice for ten months.[30] Over this period,

Table 1
Mean Process Parameters and Performance of a Reactor Treating Organic Fraction of MSW Sorted by Plant[31]

Conditions	Mesophilic	——————— Thermophilic ———————			
Reactor Temp., °C	35.8	55.0	54.8	54.3	51.5
HRT/SRT, days	14.5	14.5	11.5	8.5	6.1
OLR, kgTVS/(m³·day)	7.5	5.9	8.0	12.0	20.0
GPR, m³/(m³·day)	1.4	2.5	2.8	3.5	4.7
SGPR, m³/kgTVS	0.20	0.43	0.35	0.28	0.23
Methane, percent	52	61	60	53	57

two steady-state conditions were reached, and the performance of the digester was not excellent. In particular, when the organic loading rate was 4.1 and 6.8 and the hydraulic retention time approximately 16 days, the gas production rates were 0.9 and 1.6m³/(m³·day), respectively; the specific gas production rate was constant at 0.23m³/kgTVS; and the methane in the gas was 63 percent and 51 percent.

Passing from mesophilic to thermophilic conditions, the digester performance obtained with the organic fraction of the MSW sorted by the plant of S. Giorgio di Nogaro increased remarkably.[31]

The preliminary results of these experiments are summarized in Table 1. From the data shown in Table 1, it is possible to see that passing from mesophilic to thermophilic conditions, when the digester hydraulic retention time is approximately 14 to 15 days and the organic loading rate 6 to 7 kgTVS/(m³·day), the increasing of the gas production rate (GPR, m³/(m³·day) is approximately 80 percent, and the specific gas production rate (SGPR, m³/kgTVS) is 115 percent. Moreover, if the methane production is considered, these percentages become 110 and 150, respectively. Further interesting conclusions supported by the data of Cecchi *et al.*[30] in thermophilic conditions are: 11 to 12 days is the optimum retention time when the aim of the process is maximum volatile solid removal, and six to eight days' retention time is the best operative condition when the aim is the production of a large amount of gas.

These results contrast with those reported by Glauser et al.,[18] De Baere,[9] and De Baere and Vestraete[10] who found a 10 percent upgrading only. Even if the data obtained by Cecchi et al. [31] do not agree with those of Glauser and De Baere, more than a year of experiments under controlled thermophilic conditions confirm the consistency of the experimental data collected.

Other Experiences

Pauss et al.[14] used hand-selected municipal solid waste, so the organic fraction contained no indigestible portion (for example, plastic, wood, and so forth). Their digesters were laboratory scale completely stirred tank reactors, which were operating at mesophilic conditions (35°C) with hydraulic retention time/sold retention time (HRT/SRT) values between 14 and 20 days. The concentration of the feed was maintained between 30 and 56gTVS per liter. In these conditions and with an organic loading rate from 1.0 to 4.0kgTVS/ $(m^3 \cdot day)$, the methane production rate was 0.55 to 1.37 $m^3/(m^3 \cdot day)$, and the specific rate was 0.35 to 0.43m^3/kgTVS.

The experiments of Marty et al.[15] were carried out using a substrate containing different concentrations of total solids in the range of the dry digestion process (from 250 to 400g TS per liter). The 60-liter digester was operating at 55°C and between eight and 30 days of HRT/SRT. The organic fraction of MSW fed to the reactor was sorted by plant. The digester performance registered in the range of the organic loading rate of 3.9 to 23.5kgTVS/$(m^3 \cdot day)$ and was 1.6 to 5.6m^3biogas/$(m^3 \cdot day)$, with 60 percent medium percentage of methane in the biogas.

In the United Kingdom, some work was carried out at the Warren Spring Laboratory.[16,17] Le Roux et al. [16,17] studied the anaerobic digestion process of sorted household waste derived from the physical sorting plants of Stevenage and Doncaster at laboratory level. The fractions of the municipal solid wastes processed were 20 percent by weight of the original refuse and consisted largely of paper and vegetable materials. Tests were carried out first in two-liter batch culture bottles and in semicontinuous fermenters[16] and then in a fixed-bed reactor.[17] The semicontinuous laboratory scale plant (3-liters volume) was operating between 16 and 100 days of HRT/SRT. Temperature checked was 30°C, but measurements were carried out also at 34° and 36°C. The feed concentration was between 104 and 660 grams per liter. The reactor was loaded at 2.3 to 3.9kgTVS/(m^3·day); the gas production rate was 0.93 to 1.83m^3/(m^3·day), with 60 percent to 65 percent methane in the biogas; and the specific yield was 0.27 to 0.29m^3/kgTVS.

Glauser *et al.*[18] have carried out a very interesting and exhaustive study on the topic. They used minidigesters (20-liter glass balloons) and microdigesters (100-ml serum flasks). Furthermore, a pilot scale digester (15m^3) is reported to be under construction. Both thermophilic and mesophilic conditions were checked by these workers. The effects of pretreatments and two-stage digestion were studied using a mix of sewage sludge and the organic fraction of municipal solid waste. Regarding this latter substrate, two types of experiments were carried out: one with the hand-sorted organic fraction of municipal household corrected with ammonia because of the unfavorable C/N ratio of the substrate, and the other with the organic fraction of municipal solid waste sorted by plant. However, the results published on this part of the work are not sufficient to be discussed here. The conclusion that the authors reached was essentially that further research is needed towards an optimization of the pilot and industrial levels. The main question remains unanswered regarding the choice of the temperature range used and, with regard to the two-stage processes, the question is whether the benefits obtainable make building a more complicated system worthwhile.

Comparison of the European Experiences

The aim of this part of the paper is to compare the results previously summarized. Only data concerning the mesophilic condition will be considered, because those obtained in thermophilic conditions present large discrepancies and require more experimental work such as that currently in progress at the experimental station of the University of Venice.

Because of the complexity of the wastes studied, mainly due to different collection systems, very dishomogeneous results have been obtained. In order to establish a general rule to understand the different data given in the literature, it is interesting to look in detail at the biodegradability and the kinetic degradation of complex substrates. In fact, for a given waste, the maximum amount of biogas or methane, the so-called ultimate biogas/methane yield[32] (GO [feed ultimate biogas production rate]/BO [feed ultimate methane production rate], m^3/kgTVS), could not actually be obtained because the conversion depends on the operative reaction time.

Degradation Model

Some general relationships regarding the biodegradation in a CSTR-type digester will be deduced to help the discussion of the results. If the steady-state conditions are assumed, the gas/methane balance will be the following:

$$GPR \quad = \quad Q\ TVSf\ GO\ -\ Q\ TVSr\ GO^* \qquad (1)$$

$$MPR \quad = \quad Q\ TVSf\ BO\ -\ Q\ TVSr\ BO^* \qquad (1a)$$

These equations can be arranged, dividing for the organic loading rate (Q TVSf), in:

$$SGPR \quad = \quad GO\ -\ (1 - fTVS)\ GO^* \qquad (2)$$

$$SMPR \quad = \quad BO\ -\ (1 - fTVS)\ BO^* \qquad (2a)$$

where GPR/MPR is the gas/methane production rate; TVSf the total volatile solid content in the feed; TVSr the total volatile solid content in the reactor; GO/BO and GO^*/BO^* the ultimate gas/methane yield of the feed and the effluent respectively; SGPR/SMPR the specific gas/methane production rate; and fTVS the fraction of total volatile solid removed in the digester.

If a first order model is assumed for the substrate utilization, the specific gas/methane production rate can be written as dependent on the substrate biodegradability (GO/BO) and on the kinetic constant k.

$$SGPR = \frac{GO}{1 + 1/(k\,HRT)} \tag{3}$$

$$SMPR = \frac{BO}{1 + 1/(k\,HRT)} \tag{3a}$$

GO/BO and k are intrinsic properties of the waste; thus, the only operative way to increase the yield is to increase the HRT. This latter equation assumes that the system studied reaches biological equilibrium and that washout of microorganisms is avoided. Equations (3) can be used to evaluate the biodegradation achieved at a given HRT. The following ratio represents the efficiency of the biological process:

$$f_B^* = \frac{SGPR}{GO} = \frac{SMPR}{BO} = \frac{1}{1 + 1/(k\,HRT)} \tag{4}$$

*f_B=biodegradation achieved

The organic loading rate applied to a digester is generally expressed as KgTVS/(m³·day) (OLR=TVSf/HRT) but, considering the previous discussion, it would be preferable to consider the portion of the volatile solids that really can be converted to biogas and define the real organic loading rate. Thus, the following expression can be used:

$$OLRr = OLR\,GO = TVSf\,GO\,0.5\,/\,HRT \tag{5}$$

Table 2

Operative Conditions and Performance Obtained When SS-OFMSW, MS-OFMSW, and SC-OFMSW are Digested Under Mesophilic Conditions

Waste	MS-OFMSW		SS-OFMSW			SC-OFMSW *	**
OLR, (kg TVS/m³·day)	4.1	6.8	2.1	3.2	4.2	3.9	4.5
HRT, (day)	16.2	15.6	25	17.8	13.6	14.5	14.5
CH_4, (percent)	63.4	50.6	63	61.5	62.5	61	57
Kinetic constat, (d⁻¹)	0.374	0.432	2.95	2.62	3.53	2.2	2.9
SGPR, (m³/kg TVS)	0.230	0.23	0.633	0.625	0.636	0.660	0.750
SMPR, (m³ CH_4/kg TVS)	0.145	0.114	0.399	0.384	0.398	0.403	0.428
GO, (m³/kg TVS)	0.267	0.264	0.642	0.638	0.649	0.681	0.768
BO, (m³ CH_4/kg TVS)	0.169	0.131	0.404	0.393	0.406	0.415	0.438
Biodegradation f_B, (%)	85.8	87.1	98.6	97.9	98.0	97.0	97.7

*80 percent SS-OFMSW + 20 percent SS (TS basis)
**100 percent SS-OFMSW, value obtained extrapolating data regarding 0, 25, 50, and 80 percent SS-OFMSW[29]

which takes into account the degradable fraction of the volatile solids fed to the digester. The constant 0.5 converts the m³ biogas into grams of carbon, and OLRr ("real") is expressed as gC/(m³·day).

Comparison Between Source Sorted, Mechanically Sorted, and Separately Collected Organic Fraction Municipal Solid Waste

Data from the Treviso digester. The most notable difference is the quality of digesters' feed; when source sorted OFMSW (SS-OFMSW) and OFMSW sorted by plant (mechanically sorted: MS-OFMSW) are compared, the large amount of inert solids and slowly digestible materials is in the latter. The physical aspect (presence of small pieces of glass, wood, paper, plastic, and so forth) explains this difference. These materials are not present when the refuse is source sorted and as a consequence, the biodegradability in this case is much higher. The anaerobic digestion of both types of OFMSW has been studied and reported.[27,30] From the data in Table 2 it is possible to compare the performances obtained at different operative conditions. Yields are much better when SS-OFMSW is used. Under similar

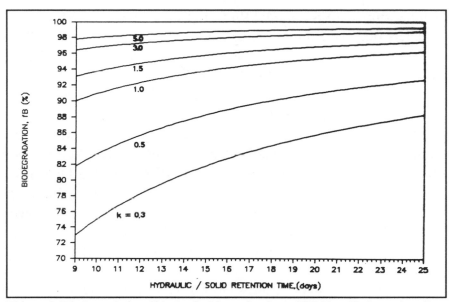

Figure 2. Biodegradation (f_B) obtainable as funtion of HRT and k (equation 4). The values of k are chosen inside the characteristic range for MS-OFMSW and SS-OFMSW.

conditions (HRT=15 days and OLR=4 kgTVS/m^3·day), TVS removal and specific gas production rates are nearly three times larger. The first-order kinetic constant k, estimated through the profiles of biogas production observed during one feed and the subsequent one,[30,33] are also quite different. The biodegradation rates are almost 10 times larger when the substrate is SS-OFMSW. The kinetic constants do not vary greatly with the different conditions tested (using the same substrate) and thus confirm the validity of the first order model used in the development of equations (3) and (4). The biodegradation achieved, expressed in terms of f_B (equation 4), is very high using SS-OFMSW. Digesting MS-OFMSW, similar performances are not obtained even if high values for f_B are reached. This can be due to the large operative HRT used. In fact, to achieve the same f_B with both the wastes, HRT should be approximately ten times larger treating MS-OFMSW. Figure 2 shows the plots of equation 4 for values of k comprised between those of OFMSW-SS and OFMSW-MS, demonstrating the HRT influence on the biodegradation term.

It is important to point out that the f_B is much more descriptive than the simple TVS removal. In fact, TVS removal, which is very often reported in the literature, does not indicate the efficiency of the process, because it is strongly dependent on the biodegradability of the volatile solids entering the digester.

Data from the terni digester. The third set of data reported in Table 2 comes from the experiments carried out at Terni.[28,29] Table 2 summarises the results obtained when the digester feed was 80:20 percent TS basis separatelycollected OFMSW (SC-OFMSW): sewage sludge (SS) and data extrapolated for 100 percent SC-OFMSW. As can be seen, the ultimate gas/methane yield of the mixture is very high; accordingly, so are the percentages of biodegradation achieved (f_B). One hundred percent SS-OFMSW SGPR valueis larger than that of SS-OFMSW; this is a consequence of the higher biodegradability of this type of waste (collected from restaurants, canteens, fruit and general vegetable markets, and so forth). The k value evaluated for a 100 percent SS-OFMSW is a little smaller than that of SC-OFMSW. However, this difference is negligible as far as its effect on f_B is concerned, as can be seen from the plots in Figure 2.

Other data from the literature. Data from the literature generally lack homogeneity in conditions of measurement, units, and so forth[34] Besides, there are not kinetic values to perform an analysis like the one carried out previously. Nevertheless, a collection of data is presented in Table 3. For the OFMSW sorted by plant (non–precomposted), a kinetic constant of 0.6 d^{-1} has been assumed, taking into account the SGPR/SMPR values (Table 2) and the discussion presented in reference 35. The ultimate gas/methane yields are relatively high with respect to those reported in Table 2, but this is not surprising because the quality of a substrate depends very much on the sorting process and on the precomposting process (if it exists at all). The waste coming from the S. Giorgio di Nogaro plant (MS-OFMSW, Table 2) was previously precomposted; thus, its gas/methane yield potential is reduced. This value is comparable with that of the Dranco process in which precomposted MSW are digested. A parallelism of TVS removal, biodegradability, and percentage of biodegradation achieved can be observed by comparing the results presented in Table 3.

Data from the University of Louvain[14] present a relatively high

Table 3
Operative Conditions and Performance Obtained by Various Authors Operating Under Mesophilic Conditions

Waste Process (Ref.)	MS-OFMSW+SS (80:15) Biomet[12]		MS-OFMSW Valorga[8]	MS-OFMSW Dranco[9,10]		MS-OFMSW KWU Fres.[11]	
OLR, (kg TVS/m^3·day)	2.6	1.6	13.7	12	15	10	3.3
HRT, (day)	19	26	15	18.5	21	10	10
CH$_4$, (%)	53	57.5	65	55	55	59	60
Kinetic constant, (d^{-1})	0.6	0.6	0.6	0.6	0.4	0.6	0.6
SGPR, (m^3/kg TVS)	0.430	0.510	0.354	0.47	0.294	0.500	0.500
SMPR, (m^3 CH$_4$/kg TVS)	0.230	0.290	0.230	0.26	0.187	0.300	0.300
GO, (m^3/kg TVS)	0.468	0.542	0.393	0.512	0.329	0.583	0.583
BO, (m^3 CH$_4$/kg TVS)	0.211	0.308	0.256	0.282	0.181	0.350	0.350
Biodegradation f$_B$ (%)	91.9	94.0	90.0	92.3	89.4	85.8	85.8

Wastes Process (Ref.)	HS-OFMSW Louvain[14]					MS-OFMSW Warren[16,17]			
OLR, (kg TVS/m^3·day)	1.5	1	2	4	4	2.9	3.9	3.9	3.9
HRT, (day)	16	20	14	14	14	23	21	33	33
CH$_4$, (%)	–	–	–	–	–	62.5	62.5	62.5	62.5
Kinetic constant, (d^{-1})	4	3	3	3	3	0.6	0.6	0.6	0.6
SGPR(m^3/kg TVS)	–	–	–	–	–	0.43	0.47	0.43	0.45
SMPR(m^3 CH$_4$/kg TVS)	0.393	0.390	0.43	0.43	0.35	0.27	0.29	0.27	0.28
GO, (m^3/kg TVS)	–	–	–	–	–	0.461	0.507	0.452	0.473
BO, (m^3 CH$_4$/kg TVS)	0.398	0.397	0.44	0.44	0.36	0.29	0.313	0.284	0.294
Biodegradation f$_B$ (%)	98.6	98.4	97.7	97.7	97.7	93.2	92.6	95.2	95.2

The second set of the Dranco process data are referred to pre-composted refuse.

biodegradability that is explained because the OFMSW, was selected by hand (HS-OFMSW). Thus, the values of the kinetic constant k do not influence the process yields as dramatically as in the previous case of MS-OFMSW, and 3 d^{-1} can be considered.

A general comparison of all the data is not an easy task. However, in Figures 3 and 4 these results are reported as a function of the f$_B$ versus OLRr and SMPR versus OLRr. The plots permit the conclusion that three areas of digester performance can be compared. The first area, characteristic of the SS-OFMSW, SC-OFMSW, and HS-OFMSW, gives the best digester performance (SMPR = 0.4m^3/

kgTVS, f_B = 98 percent); the second area refers to the non–precomposted MS-OFMSW (MS-OFMSWf), with the following characteristic performance: SMPR = 0.28, and f_B = 91 percent; the third area refers to the data obtained with MS-OFMSW precomposted (MS-OFMSWc), which shows that this kind of refuse obtained the worst performance (SMPR = 0.15, and f_B = 86 percent).

Table 4 was obtained by considering the typical characteristics of each substrate, the optimum retention time under mesophilic conditions (14 days), and the maximum total solid concentration that can be applied to a digester (35 percent TS).[36] This table clearly shows that choice of the source-sorted strategy, together with the separately collected one, is best, not only for the higher performance that could be obtained in the digester but also because the reactor that can be chosen in this case is the simple conventional reactor. The solid concentration inside it is, in fact, low enough to avoid any particular mixing problem. Furthermore, according to the scheme of Figure 1A, the best results could be obtained with the other technologies involved in the integrated plant solution.

The Management of the Process Stability

The stability of the process is an important aspect in treating the organic fraction of the MSW because the reactor has to be managed at the maximum of its performance in order to obtain good results. Digester stability is generally monitored by parameters such as pH, volatile fatty acids, (VFA), alkalinity, and composition of the gas produced. These are closely related to the buffering potential of the digester, which is often estimated from the alkalinity measurement. All the stability parameters are related; however, knowledge of only one of them is insufficient to assess the stability of the process.[22,37]

One requirement for routine monitoring methods is simplicity so that, in a limited time and without sophisticated laboratory techniques, any digester upset can be detected and failure prevented. Unfortunately, this is not so easy. However, as far as the digestion of

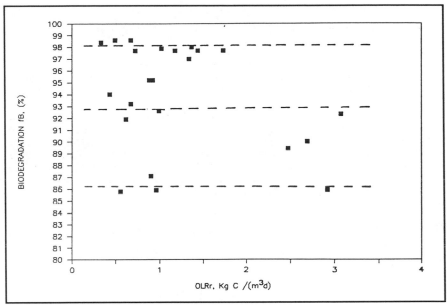

Figure 3. Comparison in terms of OLRr versus f_B of the results of the literature obtained under mesophilic conditions.

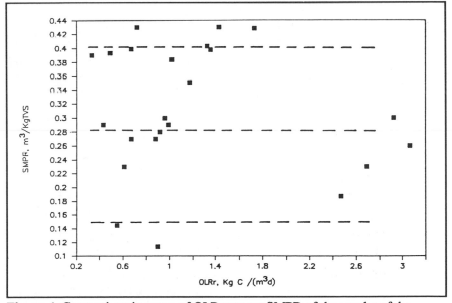

Figure 4. Comparison in terms of OLRr versus SMPR of the results of the literature obtained under mesophilic conditions.

Table 4
Obtainable Performance Feeding a Digester With Differently Collected OFMSW

Waste	Feed			Digester	OLRr,max	k	GO/BO	SGPRmax/	GPRmax/
	TS	TVS	IS	TS g/Kg	KgC/(m³·day)	d⁻¹		SMPRmax	MPRmax
		g/Kg			[OLR:KgTVS/(m³·day)]		m³/KgTVS	m³/KgTVS	m³/(m³·day)
SS-OFMSW	200	176	24	80	6.9 (12.6)	3	0.63/0.40	0.62/0.39	7.8/4.9
SC-OFMSW	163	148	15	42	5.8 (10.6)	3	0.75/0.43	0.73/0.42	7.7/4.5
MS-OFMSWf	350	207	143	247	8.1 (14.8)	0.6	0.45/0.28	0.40/0.25	5.9/3.7
MS-OFMSWc	350	154	196	308	6.0 (11.0)	0.4	0.29/0.16	0.25/0.14	2.8/1.5

TS=Total solids; TVS=Total Volatile Solids; IS=Inert Solids

the organic fraction of MSW is concerned, the pH and CO_2/CH_4 ratio have been proved to be good enough monitoring parameters. This approaches the ideal monitoring technique because it is simple and does not require expensive equipment to perform the analyses. In addition, these parameters are sensitive enough to indicate the digester upset.

In this part of the paper we present two examples that look at the response of these parameters to monitor process disturbances. A method of improving digester stability based on increasing the alkalinity of the system is also presented and modeled, considering the pH and the CO_2/CH_4 ratio as stability process parameter indices.

pH and CO_2/CH_4 Ratio as Monitoring Parameters

First, Figure 5 shows the evolution of gas composition (CO_2/CH_4 ratio) together with the VFA composition and pH in the time between two digester feeds. These data refer to the digestion of SS=OFMSW when the reactor was operating in a pseudo–steady-state condition at an organic loading rate equal to 3.2kgTVS/(m³·day).[27] First, concerning the sensitiveness, the CO_2/CH_4 ratio appears to be a convenient monitoring parameter that is nearly as good as VFA or pH. Kroeker *et al.*[38] do not fully agree with what has been reported, but Capri and Marais conclude[39] that a digester can be monitored by only measuring

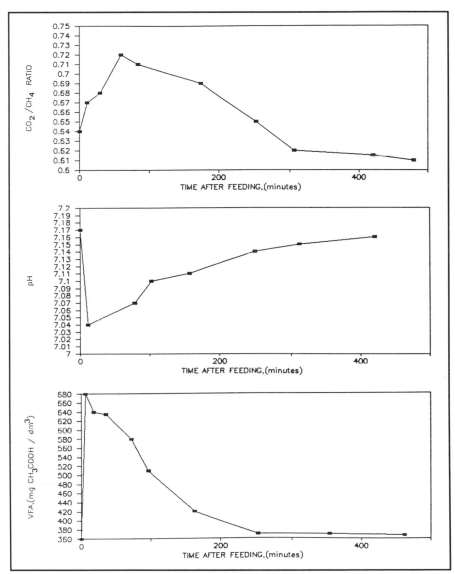

Figure 5. Evolution of gas composition (CO2/CH4 ratio), pH, and VFA after a feeding shock digesting SS-OFMSW.[27]

the pH and CO_2 partial pressure. This is a point in which there is not any general agreement. Possibly it depends on the system considered; surely, this specific topic requires more experimental evidence.

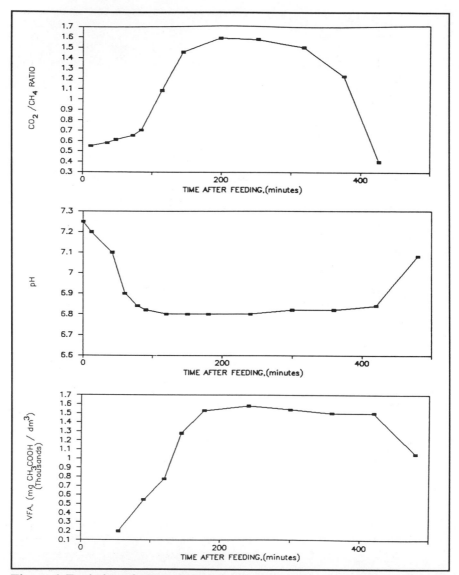

Figure 6. Evolution of gas composition (CO_2/CH_4 ratio), pH, and VFA after a feeding shock digesting wine stillage.[40]

However, it seems a good approach for the organic fraction of MSW digestion.

Second, the anaerobic digestion of wine stillage carried out at laboratory scale (anaerobic filters of six liters) by Moletta and Del-meyda[40] can be considered in order to try to generalize the approach. Figure 6 shows the evolution of the same parameters considered for the previous example after a feeding shock. The reactor (anaerobic filter) was loaded at $3.5kgCOD/(m^3 \cdot day)$ and was operating in mesophilic conditions ($35°C$).

The CO_2/CH_4 ratio increased at nearly the same rate as the VFA or pH. However, the authors found that the gas production rate was more sensitive than the composition ratio. Furthermore, although not reported, they measured the H_2 partial pressure and considered it a more sensitive stability monitoring parameter. Hydrogen is produced in very small quantities, however, it is very sensitive to digester disturbance and gives an early indication of failure. The problem is that this parameter requires an expensive and sophisticated technique that somehow limits the extension of its application.

Digester Stability Enhancement

The rapid fermentation of the putrescible fraction of the OFMSW can lead to process stability problems because of the susceptibility of methane bacteria to possible overloading. As a consequence, some authors[16,41] have recommended the addition of a chemical buffer to counter the acidity of the medium. Similar results can be achieved by using a fraction of the digester effluent supernatant to dilute the feeding wastes. This procedure was suggested by Le Roux and Koster[16,42] as a method of preventing digester failures and quantified at the University of Venice treating sourcesorted OFMSW in the mesophilic temperature range ($35°$ to $37°C$). Such an enhancement stability approach can be illustrated with the following experiment. This procedure appears to be the most appropriate from the biological point of view because the solution used to change the alkalinity is the same growth medium for the anaerobic consortia of microorganisms. The effluent used to dilute the reactor feeding was quantified according to the recycle ratio:

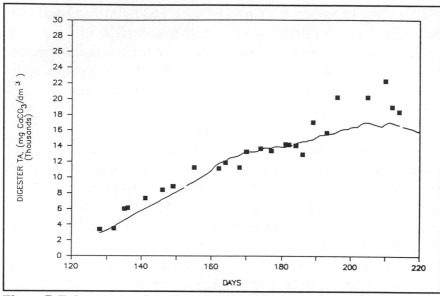

Figure 7. Enhancement of the digester stability by recirculation of reactor supernatant. (——) mathematical model; (...) experimental points

$$RR = \frac{\text{effluent supernatant}}{\text{effluent supernatant} + \text{OFMSW} + \text{water}} \tag{6}$$

This was maintained at the beginning of the experimental enhancement period between 0.87 to 0.72 for 35 days (see Figure 7 from Days 125 to 160), whereas in a second period for 60 days (from Days 161 to 220) it was between 0.6 to 0.44. During this time, the HRT was controlled at actual value, 15 to 18 days. Concurrently, the OLR increased from 1.2kg TVS/(m³·day) to 5.5kg TVS/(m³·day) (optimum value in accordance with the previous results.[27] The total alkalinity increased from approximately 2500 to approximately 20,000mg $CaCO_3/dm^3$ (see Figure 7), and the pH rose from values around 6.9 to values around 7.7 The biogas CO_2 content changed from 35 percent to 25 percent according to a profile similar to that of the pH. The digester reached a very stable operating condition after 40 days of optimization management. Gas production also increased to levels around $2m^3/(m^3 \cdot day)$, and in general, the conditions obtained were comparable with those of previous periods when they were the best for this substrate.[27] Experimental details of the the digester operative conditions and performance can be found elsewhere.[23]

Based on system management, the alkalinity increase was ascribed to the following factors: (1) the net balance of the feed alkalinity due to the addition of the supernatant fraction of the effluent, and (2) the improved biological environment inside the digester.

The enhanced biological medium was considered in order to explain the resulting reactor behavior because the first factor is not able to improve the reactor's alkalinity by itself as rapidly as can be seen in Figure 7. A balance of the factors affecting the reactor's alkalinity is represented (assuming the reactor to be completely mixed) by equation (7):

$$\frac{V \, d(TA)}{dt} = (Q-R) \times (TA_0) + (R) \times (TA) + TA_{env} - (Q) \times (TA) \quad (7)$$

where V is the digester volume, Q the diluted feed flow rate, R the recirculation flow rate, TA_0 the feed alkalinity (prior to dilution), and TA the digester alkalinity, equal to that of the stream leaving the reactor. TA_{env} is the alkalinity environmental term, which accounts for the physical-chemical and biological equilibrium factors. This term is difficult to quantify because of the complexity of the anaerobic digestion process of the substrate used. However, if the following assumptions are considered: TA_{env} is constant operating under stationary conditions; TA_{env} changes depend directly on the CH_4/CO_2 ratio and the pH value during the enhanced period; and the differential equation (7) can be integrated on the basis of one-day intervals to estimate the resulting alkalinity each day of the enhancement time, the profile of the increasing digester alkalinity can be illustrated by equation (8):

$$TA / V = [TA_0 (Q_i\text{-}R) + R\ TA_{i+1}] + [(TA_{env})_{ssc}\ (CH_4/CO_2)_{i+1}$$
$$(pH)_{i+1} / (CH_4/CO_2)_{ssc}\ (pH)_{ssc}] - [Q_i - TA_{i+1}] \quad (8)$$

where TA is the increasing alkalinity per day, the subscript "ssc" means steady-state conditions, and "i" is the day to which the measurements refer. A mean value for the terms $(TA_{env})_{ssc}$ can be calculated by equation (7) considering a steady-state period of the reactor; mean values for the $(CH_4/CO_2)_{ssc}$ ratio and $(pH)_{ssc}$ can be obtained similarly.

In agreement with the hypothesis put forward, the $[(CH_4/CO_2)_{i+1}$ $(pH)_{i+1}/(CH_4/CO_2)_{ssc}\ (pH)_{ssc}]$ ratio was inserted in equation (8), together with the balance elements, because it accounts for the stability status of the digester from both the physicochemical and biological point of view[22] during the enhancement management time.

By repeatedly applying equation (8), the increase of the digester alkalinity at intervals of one day was calculated, and the plot (solid line) is reported in Figure 7 together with the measured values. The theoretical and experimental data were found to agree closely. The discrepancy in the final part of the period was ascribed to variations of the analytical conditions.

Conclusions

The main conclusions to be drawn from the analysis made regarding future research and development in the field of the anaerobic biodegradation of solid waste are:

1. More work needs to be done to fully explain whether thermophilic conditions are applicable to all differently collected organic fractions of MSW with the same considerable advantages reported for MS-OFMSW pre composted. These results have to be compared with those of the two-phase anaerobic digestion process, which also needs further research work.

2. Source-sorted or separately collected OFMSW strategies have to be considered in the MSW final disposal to obtain the best energy-saving and environmental protection results.

3. Digester control and stability management have to be considered with a less empirical approach at full and demonstration scale levels.

These aims can be achieved by arranging a close cooperation between researchers and sector operators and transferring laboratory knowledge to the full-scale plants, where it is consequently verified in order to observe the scaling-up problems.

Notations

BO	Feed ultimate methane production rate
BO*	Digester content ultimate methane production rate
CSTR	Completely stirred tank reactor
f_B	Substrate biodegradability achieved
fTVS	Faction of TVS removed in the digester
GO	Feed ultimate biogas production rate
GO*	Digester content ultimate biogas production rate
GPR	Gas production rate
HRT	Hydraulic retention time
HS-OFMSW	Hand sorted organic fraction municipal solid waste
IS	Inert solids
k	First order kinetic constant
MSW	Municipal solid waste
MPR	Methane production rate
MS-OFMSWc	Organic fraction of municipal solid waste sorted by plant and precomposted
MS-OFMSWf	Organic fraction of municipal solid waste sorted by plant not precomposted
OFMSW	Organic fraction municipal solid waste
OLR	Organic loading rate
OLRr	Real organic loading rate
Q	Feed flow rate
R	Recycle flow rate
RR	Recycle ratio
SGPR	Specific gas production rate
SMPR	Specific methane production rate
SRT	Solid retention time
SC-OFMSW	Separately collected organic fraction of municipal solid waste
SS-OFMSW	Source sorted organic fraction of municipal solid waste

TA	Total alkalinity, end point: pH = 3.8
TA_0	Feed total alkalinity, end point: pH = 3.8
TA_{env}	Alkalinity generated inside the digester
TS	Total solids
TVS	Total volatile solids
TVSf	Feed total volatile solids content
TVSr	Reactor total volatile solids content
UASB	Upflow anaerobic sludge bed reactor
VFA	Volatile fatty acids
V	Reactor working volume
Subscripts:	
env	Environmental parameter
i	Day at which parameter is referred to
ssc	Steady state conditions

Acknowledgements

The authors acknowledge the "Instituto Trevigiano di Ricerca Scientifica del Comune di Treviso" for its auspices and support. Financial support from NaTO Grant No. 0178/87 is also gratefully acknowledged.

References

1. G. Vallini and A. Pera, *Biological Wastes* **28,** in press, (1989).
2. J. Mata and F. Cecchi, in *Proceedings of the First Workshop of the CNRE on Biogas Production Technologies* (Zaragoza, Spain), in press, (1989).
3. G. Cherubini, G. Adami, and G. Pasetto, in *Proceedings of SEP-Pollution - Rifiuti Solidi Urbani e Industriali* (Padua, Italy, 1988), pp. 425-431.
4. J.P. Peillex, personal comunication, 1988.
5. O. Begouen *et al.*, in *Fifth International Symposium on Anaerobic Digestion, Poster Papers*, A. Tilche, A. Rozzi, Eds. (Bologna, Italy, 1988), pp. 789-792.
6. I. Pipping and R. Valo, personal communication, 1988.
7. L. De Baere and W. Vestraete, *EEC Conference on Anaerobic and Carbohydrate Hydrolysis of Waste* (Luxembourg, 1984), pp. 195-208.
8. VALORGA, in *2nd Annual Int. Symp. On Ind. Resource Managem.*, February 17-20, Philadelphia, February 17-20 (1985).
9. L. De Baere, in *7th Symp. on Biotechn. for Fuels and Chemicals*, May 14-17 (Gatlinburg, TN , May 14-17, 1984).

10. L. De Baere and W. Vestraete, *Biocycle* **25**, 30 (1984).
11. M. Klein and H. Rump, in *Biomass for Energy and Industry, 4th E.C. Conference*, G. Grassi *et al.*, Eds. (Elsevier Applied Science, London, 1987), pp. 845-849.
12. G. Szikriszt *et al.*, in *Anaerobic Digestion 1988*, E.R. Hall and P.N. Hobson, Eds. (Pergamon Press, Oxford, 1988), pp. 375-382.
13. G. Hofenk *et al.*, EEC Contract Final Report ESE-E-R-040-NL, 1984, pp. 57.
14. A. Pauss, E.J. Nyns, and H. Naveau, in *EEC Conference on Anaerobic and Carbohydrate Hydrolysis of Waste* (Luxembourg, 1984).
15. B. Marty *et al.*, in *EEC Contractor Meeting Anaerobic Digestion*, Villeneuve D'Ascq [Lille], France, March 4-6 (1986).
16. N.W. Le Roux and D.S. Wakerley, *Conservation & Recycling* **2**, 163 (1978).
17. N.W. Le Roux, D.S. Wakerley, and M.N. Simpson, *Conservation & Recycling* **3**, 165 (1978).
18. M. Glauser, M. Aragno, and M. Gandolla, in *Bioenvironmental Systems, Vol. 3*, D.L. Wise, Ed. (CRC Press, Boca Raton, Florida, 1987), pp. 143-225.
19. F. Cecchi and J. Mata-Alvarez, in *Proc. Int. Conf. on Landfill Gas and Anaerobic Digestion of Solid Waste* (Chester, England, 1988), pp. 550-557.
20. P.G. Traverso and F. Cecchi, *Biomass.* **16**, 97 (1988).
21. F. Cecchi *et al.*, *Biological Wastes*, submitted.
22. F. Cecchi *et al.*, *Ingegneria Sanitaria* **35**, 339 (1987).
23. F. Cecchi *et al.*, *J. Chem. Technol. & Biotechnol.*, submitted.
24. F. Cecchi *et al.*, in *Rifiuti Urbani ed Industriali. Trattamento e smaltimento sviluppi normativi e tecnologici*, A. Frigerio, Ed. (Cl.Esse I, Milano, Italy, 1989), pp. 130-142.
25. F. Cecchi *et al.*, *Bio-Cycle* **30**, 68 (1989).
26. J. Mata-Alvarez and F. Cecchi, International Research Workshop on Biotechnology and Biodegradation (Vale De Lobos, Portugal, June 19-23, 1989).
27. F. Cecchi, P.G. Traverso, and P. Cescon, *Sci. Total Environ.* **56**, 183 (1986).
28. F. Cecchi *et al.*, *Environ. Technol. Letters* **9**, 391 (1988).
29. F. Cecchi *et al.*, in *Rifiuti Urbani Speciali Tossici e Nocivi*, A. Frigerio, Ed. (Cl. Esse. I, Milano, Italy, 1988), pp. 303-314.
30. F. Cecchi *et al.*, *Waste Management & Res.*, submitted.
31. F. Cecchi *et al.*, *Fifth EEC Conf. Biomass for Energy and Industry* (Lisbon, Portugal, October 9-13, 1989).
32. Y. Chen and A. Hashimoto, *Biotech. Bioeng. Symp.* **8**, 269 (1978).
33. F. Cecchi *et al.*, *Biomass*, in press, (1989).
34. F. Cecch *et al.*, *Biomass* **16**, 257 (1988).
35. F. Cecchi *et al.*, *Waste Manag. & Research*, submitted.
36. W.J. Wuicik and W.J. Jewell, *Biotech. Bioeng. Symp. Ser.* **10**, 43 (1980).
37. S.P. Graef and J.F. Andrews, *J. Water Pollut. Control Federation* **46**, 667 (1974).
38. E.J. Kroeker *et al.*, *J. Water Pollut. Control Federation* **51**, 718 (1979).
39. M.G. Capri and G.V.R. Marais, *Water Res.* **9**, 307 (1975).
40. R. Moletta and M.L. Delmeyda, in *Proc. 8th Int. Biotechnol.Symp.* (Paris, 1988), pp. 245.
41. M.G. Buivid *et al.*, *Resources & Conservation* **6**, 3 (1981).
42. I.W. Koster *et al.*, *ISWA Proceedings* **1**, 71 (1988).

Discussion

Salkinoja-Salonen: I would like to ask about the quality of the digested refuse after the operation. The landfills, as we all know, are a big problem because of the reactiveness of the waste inside the landfill. Is there an improvement of the landfill treatability of this waste after anaerobic digestion? For instance, does it leach less heavy metals from the noncompostable part of it. What is your experience?

Cecchi: I think that anaerobic digestion of the organic fraction of the municipal solid waste may be one step in the final disposal of this material. In fact, after digestion and composting, you can close the organic matter biological cycle by disposing of it on agricultural soil. Of course, if you dispose of this material in a landfill site, you can improve the environmental impact of the land-fill because the digested matter gives fewer leaching problems and so less reactiveness of the waste inside the landfill.Nevertheless, I think the aim of the approach illustrated is to closed biological cycles and not to improve the final landfill disposal. We have to compost the digested materials before they are used in agricultural soil, because there are some compounds in them that are phytotoxic to plants. Thus, you need an integration between composting and digestion technologies.

17

Kinetic Models Applied to the Anaerobic Biodegradation of Complex Organic Matter

correspondence

Joan Mata-Alvarez

*Department of Chemical
Engineering
University of Barcelona
C. Martii Franques 1
pat. 6-08028 Barcelona
Spain*

Franco Cecchi

*Department of
Environmental Science
University of Venice
Dorsoduro 2137
30123 Venezia
Italy*

Most relevant kinetic models applied to the biodegradation of complex waste are reviewed. Results obtained with the step diffusional model are compared with those obtained with the first order model. The latter model is simpler, but the step diffusional model better fits the experimental results because it is based on an approach that takes into account qualitative and quantitative chemical characteristics of the substrate.

The effects of external factors such as temperature and eventual changes of the quality of organic matter on the digestion performance are also examined. Increased of external temperature causes transformation to acetate of ethanol contained in the organic fraction of municipal solid waste fed to the digester. This transformation produces a clear effect on the process kinetics that are described by both the first order and the step diffusional model.

Introduction

Anaerobic digestion of substrates containing polymeric compounds is a very complex process. Several steps can be distinguished in this process. First, complex organic matter and polymers are hydrolyzed and fermented to fatty acids, carbon dioxide, and hydrogen. Then, fatty acids are converted by acetogenic bacteria to acetate.

Finally, methanogenic bacteria convert the hydrogen, carbon dioxide, and acetate to methane. This latter step is very important in order to maintain the low hydrogen concentrations thermodynamically necessary for the acetogenic bacteria. In order to ensure a stable digestion process, a proper balance between all these microbial populations must be maintained. Thus, the digester must be designed with careful consideration of parameters such as hydraulic retention time (HRT), organic loading rate (OLR), temperature, and pH.

Digester Design

Digester design is aimed mainly to calculate the required volume. Several factors directly affect the digester volume. First, the kinetics of the biodegradation process, which will be considered in detail in the text that follows. Second, temperature, which is directly related to the kinetics of the process. For instance, considering the anaerobic digestion process of the organic fraction of municipal solid waste (OFMSW), the process is faster when the digester is operated at thermophilic conditions than when it is operated at mesophilic conditions.[1] Some of our results (see preceding paper) seem to indicate a reduction of about 50 percent of the digester volume to treat the OFMSW selected by plant when the process is carried out at thermophilic conditions.

Another parameter affecting the digester volume is the organic loading rate. OLR is directly related to the concentration of the substrate (S_o):

$$OLR = S_o/HRT \tag{1}$$

On the other hand, the methane production (VMPR) per unit of digester volume is also directly related to the OLR:

$$VMPR = OLR \times SMPR \tag{2}$$

where SMPR is the specific methane production rate. If the HRT is constant, OLR will only depend on S_o, and SMPR can be considered relatively constant when the HRT is large enough (see preceding paper). As a consequence, VMPR will be proportional to S_o. This means that if the digester is fed with a larger S_o, the level of microorganisms concentration in the reactor will be higher, and more methane will be produced per day to work at the highest possible substrate concentration. The limits are imposed by the fluidity so as to avoid mass transfer and mixing problems. Inefficient mixing reduces the effective working volume and thus the process efficiency. Moreover, problems arising from the formation of a scum layer can result from poor mixing. A limit of the concentration within the reactor can be approximately 15 percent to 20 percent which places an upper limit on the feed concentration.[1,2]

Biomass concentration also affects the digester volume. A higher bacterial concentration increases the biodegradation rate. Several configurations are available to increase the microorganism concentration inside the digester. However, none of them is appropriate for the digestion of a high solids substrate. The traditional continuous stirred tank reactor (CSTR) offers the best possibility for successful application to complex, nonsoluble waste digestion. The following discussions are related to this configuration for the digester.

Kinetics of the Anaerobic Digestion of Complex Waste

Anaerobic digestion kinetics of complex organic waste is a very difficult topic. There are several steps involved that work at the same time and several microorganism species working together on a very complicated substrate. As a consequence, it is very difficult to develop an adequate kinetic model representing the degradation process, especially if non-steady–state conditions are present (overloads, starving periods, and so forth), even though these conditions are the most interesting from the industrial point of view. In fact, operating practice has shown that relying on steady-state assumptions could be dangerously misleading, given the inherently uncertain process dynamics and immeasurable variations of operating conditions.[3]

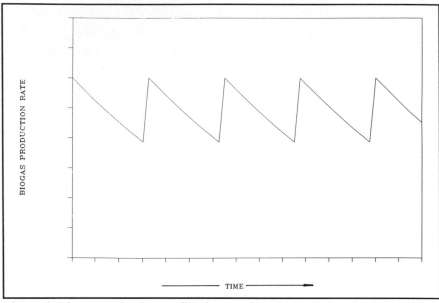

Figure 1. Biogas production profiles in a semicontinuously fed digester.

Several models present in the literature describe the anaerobic degradation process. They are useful to a limited extent, that is, for the same substrate at similar conditions and for predicting gas yield or solids reduction. Unfortunately, none of them is able to satisfactorily predict transition states, although some of them, using simplifications, have given good results in a limited range of situations.[4]

In a semicontinuous stirred tank digester, biogas production presents a profile that is a function of the feeding pattern. If substrate is fed at intervals of a given length p (min), the shape of organic matter concentration inside the digester will appear as in Figure 1. When a volume V_o of fresh substrate is fed at a concentration S_o, the same volume is withdrawn, with a concentration S_e. At this time substrate concentration in the digester can be computed in accordance with:

$$S_i = \frac{S_o V_o + S_e (V-V_o)}{V} \tag{3}$$

where S_i is the substrate concentration after feeding the digester of working volume V. The mean substrate flow rate is V_o/p (m³/min) and, as a consequence, the mean residence time will be:

$$HRT = p V/V_o \qquad (4)$$

During the period of time between one feed and the next one, substrate concentration S in the digester evolves in accordance with the kinetics of the fermentation process:

$$dS/dt = S(k,t) \qquad (5)$$

where k represents a vector containing the kinetic constants and t, the time. Limit conditions are, at $t = 0$, $S = S_i$, and at $t = p$, $S = S_e$.

As stated, several common kinetic models can be applied to mathematically describe the system. The most widespread considered here: models will be (1) First order, (2) Monod, (3) Inhibition model, (4) Diffusional, (5) Chen and Hashimoto (Contois), and (6) Step-diffusional, as proposed by the authors.

First Order Model

This model considers the microorganisms as "catalysts" and represents an overall mass transfer kinetic model for a "catalyzed" reaction. Although this is not a sophisticated model, it can provide a single and useful kinetic constant that will have applicability when dealing with complex systems such as that involved in the fermentation of refuse.[5,6]

The basic equation is:

$$dS/dt = -k S \qquad (6)$$

where k is the first order kinetic constant (time⁻¹) and S represents the biodegradable substrate concentration. Because this is a difficult parameter to be measured, another approach can be used. If B denotes the accumulated methane production for each unit of VS added, and B_o is the ultimate methane yield,[7] the concentration of biodegradable VS in the fermenter (S, mg/l) will be directly related to gas production in accordance with:

$$(B_o-B)/B_o - S/S_o \qquad (7)$$

Combinging equations (6) and (7), and integrating:

$$\frac{B_o - B}{B_o} = \exp(-kt) \qquad (8)$$

For a CSTR digester operating at steady state, a mass balance taking into account equation (6) yields:

$$S = S_o \frac{1}{1 + k \times (HRT)} \qquad (9)$$

If equation (7) is used, then:

$$B = B_o \frac{k \times (HRT)}{1 + k \times (HRT)} \qquad (10)$$

In this case, B represents the specific methane production rate for the given HRT.

Besides the application to describe the degradation of refuse mentioned before, the model has been used in the anaerobic digestion of cornstover[6] and pretreated straw.[8] Other studies using first order kinetics are those of Canovas-Diaz and Howell,[9] dealing with the anaerobic digestion of sugar in a biofilm reactor, those dealing with the anaerobic digestion of sewage sludge and pretreated straw,[10,11] and those dealing with the anaerobic digestion of brewery by-products.[12] Based on the first order model and taking into account that the remaining substrate is progressively less biodegradable, a modified approach was proposed by Singh et al.:[13]

$$\frac{dS}{dt} = - \frac{k\,S}{1+t} \qquad (11)$$

The model proved to be applicable to the anaerobic digestion of cattle waste. However, the justification of the model given before is strictly true if S is expressed as COD or VS concentration. If, on the contrary, S is expressed as biodegradable concentration using the approach given before (equation 8 or 10), the first order model is more appropriate.

Monod Model

This model is rigorously applicable to soluble substrates. Lawrence and McCarty[14] presented the basic equation:

$$\frac{dS}{dt} = - \frac{k\,S\,X}{K_s + S} \qquad (12)$$

which is normally used in combination with the growth rate equation:

$$\frac{dX}{dt} = Y\,\frac{dS}{dt} - k_d\,X \qquad (13)$$

Introducing μ, the specific growth rate:

$$\mu = \frac{dX/dt}{X} \qquad (14)$$

and neglecting the decay term in equation (13) yields:

$$\mu \; = \; \mu_{max} \; \frac{S}{K_s + S} \tag{15}$$

μ_{max}, the maximum specific growth rate is equal to k/Y. Equations in steady-state in a CSTR in the common case of a sterile feed ($X_o = 0$) are easily deduced. For substrate concentration, the corresponding equation is:

$$S \; = \; \frac{K_s}{\mu_{max}(HRT - 1} \tag{16}$$

Using equation (7) biodegradable concentration S can be expressed as a function of B:

$$B \; = \; B_o \; - \; \frac{B_o}{S_o} \; \frac{K_s}{\mu_{max}(HRT) - 1} \tag{17}$$

Lawrence[15] extended the application of Monod kinetics to municipal sewage sludge. This more complex waste made calculations somewhat more difficult, but assuming methanogenesis as the limiting step, the estimated constants gave reasonably good results. The Monod model has been applied to several wastes, as was pointed out by Chin,[16] and has been the basis of most anaerobic digestion models as, for example, the structured model developed by Bryers.[17]

Inhibition Model

The Monod equation does not account for inhibition, which may exist in the acidogenic phase.[18-21] Several mathematical models have been suggested to describe the effects of substrate inhibition.[22] The first equation, based on enzyme kinetics, was proposed for substrate inhibition by Haldane in 1930:

$$\mu = \mu_{max} \frac{1}{1 + K_i/S + S_i/K_i} \qquad (18)$$

where K_i is the inhibition constant and S_i the inhibition concentration. This model has been used for modeling the inhibition caused by the volatile fatty acids either ionized or not[23,24] and by phenol.[25] It also served to develop a dynamic model to predict volatile acid profiles, alkalinity, pH, gas flow rate, and gas composition.[26] Another inhibition expression was developed by Ierusalimsky:[20]

$$\mu = \mu_{max} \frac{S}{S + K_s} \frac{Ki}{S_i + K_i} \qquad (19)$$

This expression was used by Hendricks *et al.*[27] to study the inhibition of propionic acid and by Dinopoulou *et al.*[28] to study the acidogenic phase of the anaerobic digestion of a complex substrate based on beef extract.

When the inhibition is caused by the substrate, Haldane kinetics gives the following equation for substrate concentration in a CSTR digester:

$$S = \frac{-K_s + (K_s^2 - 4(1-(HRT)/X)K')^{1/2}}{2(1 - (HRT)/Y)} \qquad (20)$$

where K' is the inhibition constant.

Diffusional Model

The combination of the Monod rate equation together with mass transfer limitation equations can lead to the following overall rate equation:[29]

$$dS/dt = -k\, S^{0.5} \qquad (21)$$

where k is an apparent kinetic constant $[(g\ C/m^3)^{0.5}]$. In a CSTR digester this kinetic model yields the following equation for the substrate concentration leaving the reactor:

$$S = S_o + k(HRT)/2 - [(S_o + k(HRT)/2)^2 - S_o^2]^{1/2} \qquad (22)$$

Chen and Hashimoto Model

The Chen and Hashimoto model is an application of that of Contois to anaerobic digestion processes.[7,30] The Contois model is an expanded form of the Monod model that takes into account that mass transfer limitations may cause the specific growth rate to vary with population density. Although it is normally applied directly to gas production in terms of methane produced per kilogram of volatile solids added, its basic equation is:

$$\mu = \mu_m \ \frac{S/S_o}{K + (1-K)S/S_o} \qquad (23)$$

where μ is the specific growth rate (time^{-1}). If microorganism decay can be neglected, the combination of this latter equation with equations (13) and (14) gives:

$$\frac{dS}{dt} = -\mu_k \ \frac{S/S_o}{K + (1-K)S/S_o} \qquad (24)$$

where μ_k is $\mu_m X/Y$, which remains constant if X does. As mentioned before, this is approximately the case in a semicontinuously operated digester.

For a CSTR digester, a microorganism and a substrate mass balance leads to the following equation for methane produced per kilogram of TVS added:

$$B = B_0 \left(1 - \frac{K}{(HRT)\mu_m - 1 - K}\right) \qquad (25)$$

This equation can be used to estimate the constants of the model.

Chen and Hashimoto tested this model with sewage sludge data from O'Rourke,[31] municipal refuse data from Pfeffer,[5] and animal manure data from several authors, including their own.[7] Many other authors have used this model. See, for instance, Samson and LeDuy,[32] who studied the anaerobic digestion of algal biomass, or Lema *et al.*,[33] who modelized the biomethanization of landfill leachates.

Step Diffusional Model

This model has been proposed recently by the authors to take into account the different pathways of gas production rate between one feed and the subsequent one (see Figure 2), the complex scheme of carbon flow and interactions in the methanogenic syntrophic association,[34] and the characteristics of the compounds present in the substrate.[35]

The model was developed to represent mathematically the degradation rate OFMSW. Table 1 presents the main compound groups present in the source-selected OFMSW (SS-OFMSW) and mechanically selected (MS-OFMSW),on the basis of total volatile solids (TVS) fed to digester. Data to build this table comes from the values of volatile fatty acids (VFA) contained in the substrate,[36] data shown in Table 2 (see Materials and Methods), and the following estimates of insoluble compounds: cellulose (32 percent TVS basis), hemicellulose (15 percent TVS basis), and lignin (15 percent TVS basis).[37] Accordingly to Ghosh and Henry,[38] these compounds, in mesophilic conditions, are removed up to 32, 86, and 0 percent, respectively. Thus, more than half of the TVS of the MS-OFMSW are not biodegradable. The percentage of compounds of groups A (methanol and VFA having less than three carbon atoms) and B (ethanol and

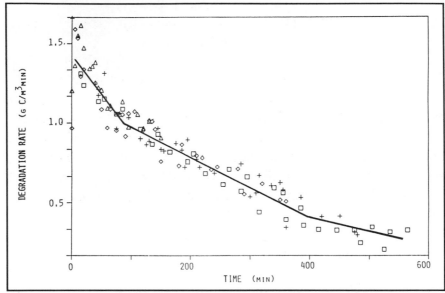

Figure 2. Anaerobic digestion of complex waste. Observed biogas production profiles between one feed and the subsequent one.

VFA having more than three carbon atoms) can vary, depending on the external temperature, as is later discussed.

The degradation rate of each group of compounds is related to a respective single straight line, which follows the pattern of the experimental points shown in Figure 2. These lines are described by the following three basic equations:

$$dS/dt = v_0 - 4a\, t/2 \tag{26}$$
$$dS/dt = v_1 - 4b\, t/2 \quad (t < t_1) \tag{27}$$
$$dS/dt = v_2 - 4c\, t/2 \quad (t_1 < t < t_2) \tag{28}$$

where v_0, v_1, v_2 and 4a, 4b, and 4c are the model constants. A further development of these equations is given in reference 35. It is clear that the model proposed has a strong diffusional character. The digester has a considerable amount of nonsoluble solids, which can act as a support for microorganisms. This is especially true for the methanogenic flora, so that diffusion of acetate seems to be the limiting step

Table 1
Organic Matter Distribution
Percentage Values of the Different Main Groups of Compounds of the OF* of
Source Selected and Mechanically Selected Municipal Solid Wastes (MSW)

	Compound Group	SS-OFMSW %TVS	MS-OFMSW %TVS
Acetate and compounds directly utilized by methanogenic bacteria (AcH, MeOH)	A	4.9	1.8
VFA $\geq C_3$ and EtOH	B	3.7	1.1
Free organic matter	C	21.6	8.1
Complex organic matter	D	44.5	36.8
Not biodegradable organic matter	E	25.3	52.2
Total organic matter		100.0	100.0

*OF=Organic fraction.

Table 2
Characteristics of Different Substrates Used to Perform the Kinetic Study

	TS g/kg	TVS g/kg	TCOD g/kg	TC %TS	N %TS	P %TS	STS %TS	SVS %TVS
PS	41.3	30.2	39.0	39.9	2.3	0.4	—	4.0
SS	53.1	24.4	40.0	25.0	2.6	0.2	2.6	1.5
SS-OFMSW	200.0	176.0	218.0	48.0	3.2	0.4	32.8	28.6
MS-OFMSW	208.2	106.7	121.4	17.9	1.8	—	21.7	11.8
SC-OFMSW	163.0	143.0	192.0	45.0	2.2	0.3	66.0	64.0

Experiments Using SS, Alone or Mixed With SC-OFMSW, Were Performed in Digester of Terni (2.2m³). Rest of Substrates Were Used in Treviso Digester (3m³).

(represented by the slope 4a). Subsequent steps might be regulated by the diffusion of extracellular enzymes to the nonsoluble compounds. In this sense, it would be possible to assume that the reactor has some of the characteristics of a carrier digester.

Materials and Methods

Experimental device. The experiments described in this paper were performed in two pilot plants situated in Treviso and Terni (Italy). They were equipped with stirred tank digesters of 3 and 2.2°m³ working volume, respectively, and were operated in the mesophilic temperature range ($35 \pm 0.5°C$).

The pilot plant in Treviso was used to treat SS-OFMSW and, after modifying the feeding system, to treat OFMSW coming from an industrial recycling plant located in S. Giorgio di Nogaro (MS-OFMSW). A complete description of the Treviso plant has been given in our preceding paper in this volume and in references 36 and 39 for the OFMSW-SS and in reference 40 for the MS-OFMSW.

The pilot plant in Terni was used to treat a mixture of sewage sludge and an OFMSW coming from a separated collection (OFMSW-SC) (fruit and vegetable market, restaurants, and so forth) so as to simulate a source-selected OFMSW. A description of this plant can be found in reference.[41]

Substrate. The characteristics of the different substrates fed to the digesters are summarized in Table 2. In all cases, the biomass was diluted before being stored in the feedstock tank. Digesters were fed several times a day (normally twice) according to the desired organic loading rate (OLR). Hydraulic retention time (HRT) was also variable, although it usually was approximately 15 days.

Analysis. A complete set of analyses was performed to monitor the process. References for them can be found in the literature already cited, although they normally followed guidelines from reference 42.

Kinetic model fitting. Digester substrate degradation rates have been estimated from the values of gas production. Biogas production rate was monitored after feeding in all the conditions tested. As a first step, data were corrected for pressure and water content and reduced to a common temperature basis using the following equation:[43]

$$\frac{GP \text{ at } T}{GP \text{ at } 35} = Z^{(T-35)} \tag{13}$$

where Z is a constant and GP represents the gas production at a given temperature. A mean value of 1.051 for Z has been found, after considering all the representative values.[35]

To facilitate the manipulation of data, biogas production rate is referred to as Total Carbon (TC) /min, and the concentrations of the substrates are expressed as TC.

Simple linearization techniques were applied to fit rate data. Kinetic model fitting was performed for each set of data corresponding to a given OLR. Another overall set of data comprising all the former data was also considered. These sets of data, concerning the TC consumption rate and TC concentration, represent mean values, because they have been obtained after averaging a significative number of experimental data.

Application of the Kinetic Models to the Anaerobic Digestion of the OF of MSW and Primary and Secondary Sludges

First order and step diffusional models were used to fit experimental data coming from a number of complex organic wastes. The following substrates were studied: organic fraction of municipal solid waste, source-sorted OFMSW-SS; organic fraction of municipal solid waste, mechanically sorted MS-OFMSW; primary sludge (PS); secondary sludge (SS); mixture, 20 percent SS, 80 percent organic fraction of municipal solid waste, separately collected, (SC-OFMSW); mixture, 50 percent SS, 50 percent SC-OFMSW.

Figure 3 shows a set of gas production profiles corresponding to each type of substrate studied. These results are the basis to perform the fitting to the kinetic models selected. Table 3 shows the estimated constants for both models, step diffusional and first order. As can be seen, constants v_0 and 4a have only been estimated for SS-OFMSW and SC-OFMSW, that is, for substrates containing compounds directly utilized by methanogenic bacteria (acetates, methanol, and so forth). Constants 4c and v_2 have been estimated in all the considered cases, as all the substrates contained cellulosic components. For these latter constants, there is some variability as a consequence of the

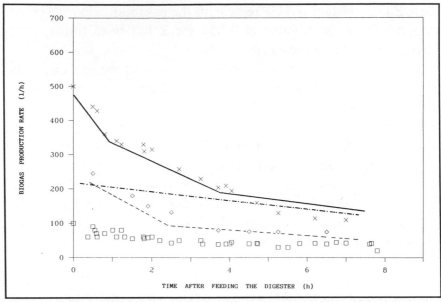

Figure 3. Observed biogas production profiles between one feed and the subsequent one, during the anaerobic digestion of the following substrates: organic fraction of municipal solid waste (source sorted) (OFMSW-SS)——— ; organic fraction of municipal solid waste (mechanically sorted) (OFMSW-MS) - - - - ; primary sludge (PS)- - - -; secondary sludge (SS) □ ; mixture of 20 percent SS and 80 percent organic fraction of municipal solid waste, separately collected (SC-OFMSW) X; mixture of 50 percent SS and 50 percent (SC-OFMSW) ◊.

experimental error, which is accentuated at low gas production rates. In general there is a good agreement among all the estimated values.

On the other hand, first order estimate exhibits a wide range of values, depending on the biodegradability of the individual substrate considered. Thus for SS, k is as low as 0.2 d^{-1}, whereas for SS-OFMSW, k is 3 d^{-1}. Table 4 shows first order constants on high solid substrates that have appeared in the literature. As can be seen, the values are comparable with those shown in Table 3. In particular, k for MSW refers to nonselected municipal solid waste so that it contains paper, plastics, and so forth, considerably reducing the constant value.

In accordance with the results reported in reference 35, values of constants 4a, 4b, and 4c are of the same order of magnitude as constant k of the diffusional model, which argues in favor of the diffusional character of the model.

Table 3
Estimated Kinetic Constants of the Step Diffusional and First Order Models Using Different Substrates

	SS-OFMSW	MS-OFMSW	PRIMARY* SS	SC-OFMSW SS 80% - 20%	SC-OFMSW SS 50% - 50%	SS* 100%
Step Diffusional						
v_0	1.43	—	—	1.67	—	—
4a	0.0100			0.0091		
v_1	1.15	—	0.71	1.22	0.89	—
4b	0.0030	0.0032	0.0025	0.0030		
v_2	0.75	0.64	0.32	0.80	0.45	0.25
4c	0.0010	0.0013	0.0003	0.0012	0.0007	0.0005
First Order						
k	3.00	0.30	1.11	2.20	1.50	0.28

*More experimental error involved.

Table 4
Other First Order Kinetic Constants of Complex Substrates Appearing in the Literature

Value of k (d^{-1})	Substrate	Reference
0.011	Straw methanization	(45)
0.017	Straw hydrolysis	(46)
0.15	Biological sludge hydrolysys	(11)
0.06	Pretreated straw	(8)
0.10	Brewery by-product rich in protein	(12)
0.15	MSW	(5)

A further check of the results was performed in terms of the analytical values of substrate composition, available for the SS-OFMSW. Values for the maximum degradation rate of the different steps v_0, v_1, v_2, and v_3 together with the corresponding slopes 4a, 4b, and 4c give rise to the values of t_1, t_2, and t_3.

Three zones named Z1, Z2, and Z3 can be considered. Z1

Table 5

Type of compounds	Analytic Value	Kinetic Estimation	Zone (see Figure 4)
A	28	19	Z1
B+C	145	137	Z2
D	255	265	Z3

Comparison of Analytical Values and Those Estimated From the Kinetic Relationships are Presented Corresponding to the Different Groups of Compounds Shown in Table 1. Values are Expressed as g C/m^3.

corresponds to the biogas production controlled by the methanogenic-acetogenic step. Its area gives an estimation of the contents of compounds directly convertible to methane (compounds of group A, see Table 1). Z2 corresponds to the acidogenic-acetogenic step control; its area is an estimation of the compounds named B and C in Table 1 (free organic matter; sugars; VFA, except acetic acid, ethanol, and so forth). Finally, Z3 represents an estimation of the nonsoluble compounds (group D), the solubilization of which represents the limiting step to the biogas production.

Analytical values in Table 5, and estimations from the kinetic relationships presented in Figure 4 are quite comparable.

Compared with the other models, the proposed one fits better to experimental data because of the step approach. As a consequence of taking several steps, more constants are involved, but the model is still simple enough for practical purposes. In fact, its complexity is a function of the substrate complexity, so that if it is applied to a substrate containing only cellulosic material, only one step has to be considered. Hence, the maximal substrate utilization rate is not always achieved for the acidic and soluble compounds.

Effects of External Temperature on the Anaerobic Digestion of Municipal Solid Waste

The reactor treating OFMSW was run under stationary conditions during what was approximately one year to study the

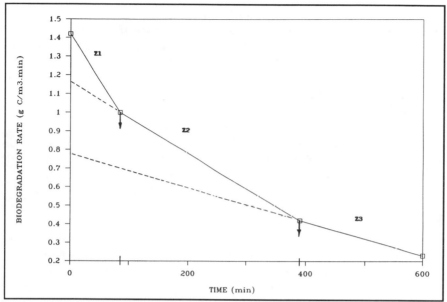

Figure 4. Estimation of the different groups of compounds presented in Table 5, from the kinetic relationships. Table 7 shows comparison with analytical values.

effect of the external temperature on digester performance. Table 6 illustrates the main operating parameters that were observed during that time.

Figure 5 shows the temperature evolution during a year in Treviso, where the experimental station is located. As can be seen, there is an ascending trend till August. After that month, temperature begins to decrease approaching a straight line. Experimental data from February to August were chosen so that the complete range of external temperatures could be considered. Mean temperatures of each month were selected to study their effect on substrate composition and process performance. Variables related to substrate composition were also averaged on a monthly basis.

Effects on Substrate Composition

The results showed that temperature produces a clear effect on VFA and ethanol content of the substrate.[44] However, their trends with

Table 6

Process Parameters (Mean Values) and Performance of Digester Feed and Reactor Characteristics During Six Month Steady-State Conditions of Pilot Plant Treating SS-OFMSW

Feed flow rate (dm^3/day)	60
Number of feed per day	2
Hydraulic/solids retention time (HRT/SRT) (day)	50
Organic loading rate (OLR) [kg TVS/(m^3/day)]	1.6
Gas production rate (GP) (m^3/day)	6.1
Specific gas production (SGP) (m^3/kgTVS fed)	0.9
Specific gas production (SGP*)(m^3/kgTVS fd.TVS r)	0.016
TVS removal (%)	81.9
CH_4 percentage (%)	60.1

	Feed		Reactor	
	Mean	**Range**	**Mean**	**Range**
TS (kg/m^3)	121.1	(103.1–139.4)	31.0	(23.8–37.0)
TVS (kg/m^3)	111.3	(94.6–127.1)	19.4	(14.1–24.8)
pH			7.1	(6.3– 7.4)
VFA and Alcohols (mg/l)				
Methanol	139	(107 – 189)	49	(7 – 290)
Ethanol	3283	(7107 – 1178)	257	(9 – 1749)
Acetic acid	5933	(2137 – 10756)	1560	(488 – 3583)
Propionic acid	422	(38 – 987)	552	(312 –5761)
Butyric acid	102	(24 – 286)	122	(21 – 249)
i-Butyric acid	100	(19 – 145)	552	(61 – 915)
Valeric acid	8	(2 – 37)	87	(81 – 152)
i-Valeric acid	11	(4 – 26)	637	(402 – 1101)
Lactic acid	—		—	

temperature are opposite: alcohol presence diminishes as temperature increases, whereas the VFA content increases. In fact, the amount of ethanol plus the acetic acid remains fairly constant during all the period. This behavior has been explained by the fact that bacteria responsible for the fermentation of ethanol to acetate are not very active at winter temperatures.[44] During summer, ethanol is fermented to acetate.

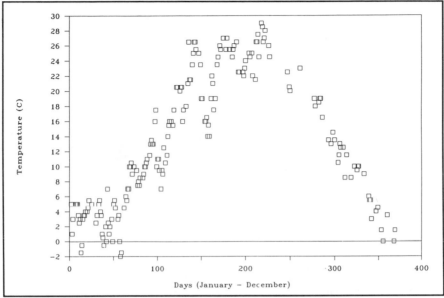

Figure 5. Temperature evolution during the year. The selected period was six months (February to August) to study the whole range of temperatures.

Effects on Reactor Performance

As the reactor temperature was kept constant at $35 \pm 2°C$, any effects on reactor performance were due to feed composition variations, that is, variations in the amount of acetate and ethanol.

As expected, due to the high value of the hydraulic and solids retention time, the final reactor behavior in terms of specific gas production rate did not vary too much. Thus, the reactor VFA concentration before any feeding was always the same, that is, it did not depend on the acids content of the feed. However, reactor performance was affected in terms of the biodegradation kinetics.[44]

As mentioned earlier, the quality of the feed can influence the gas production rate pattern and the kinetic behavior. Therefore, individual gas production profiles have been examined during all the period, to evaluate the quantitative effect on substrate utilization kinetics. Two representative examples of the gas production pattern between one feed and the subsequent one in winter and summer temperatures are shown in Figure 6.

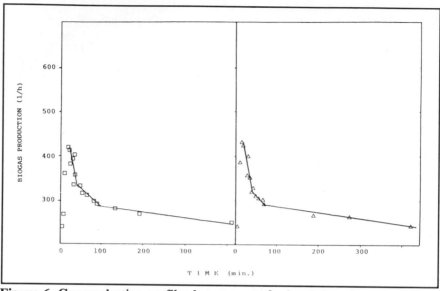

Figure 6. Gas production profiles between one feed and the subsequent one at 27°C and 9°C mean external temperature.

A first order model is quite appropriate to demonstrate the effect of temperature on kinetics. Figure 7 shows the whole first order Kinetic constants estimated. As can be seen, the constant increases as does the external temperature. This seems possible due to the feed quality change. The presence of a larger amount of easily degradable acetic acid accelerates the overall degradation process. One more observation comes from Figure 7, the evident existence of two ranges of kinetic constant values depending on temperature. In the first range, from 8 to 17°C, the kinetic constant averages 0.002min,$^{-1}$ whereas from 17 to 28°C, the value is more than two times higher.

The step diffusional model can also explain these profiles. During summer temperatures, the larger quantity of acetate makes the step regulated by methanogenesis (slope 4a) larger than the same step at winter temperatures. However, the constants involved are the same in both cases. Table 7 delineates the averaged estimated constants that were measured in both summer and winter external temperatures.

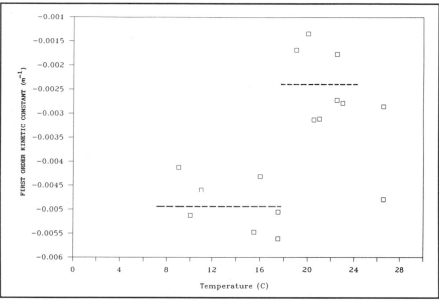

Figure 7. First order kinetic constant evolution with temperature. There are two levels of values corresponding to the temperature ranges 8-17°C and 18-28°C.

Conclusions

Several known kinetic models applied to the anaerobic digestion process of complex waste have been described. Among them, two have been selected to mathematically describe the biodegradation of some complex wastes, mainly the organic fraction of municipal solid waste and sewage sludges. A first order model fits reasonably well; its main advantage is its simplicity. However, to better represent the degradation rate process of complex wastes, the step diffusional model, which takes into account the different steps of the anaerobic process, has been used. This model emphasizes the characteristics of diffusional limitations, because they are likely to take place when treating wastes with a high content in suspended solids.

An appreciable seasonal influence on the process performance was observed during the digestion of the source-sorted organic fraction of MSW when the summer temperature was higher than 18°C. Thus, a double first order kinetic constant of substrate utilization was

Table 7
Constants of the Step Diffusional Model Obtained at 27°C and 9°C, Mean External Temperature Treating OFMSW-SS

	Summer	Winter
v_0	1.42	1.31
v_1	1.12	1.01
v_2	0.83	0.78
4a	0.0121	0.0111
4b	0.0030	0.0028
4c	0.0010	0.0009

observed and attributed to the changes in the quality of the feed, in particular to the transformation of the ethanol in the feed to acetate. On the other hand, using the step diffusional model, a different pattern of biogas production was observed, but the kinetic constants were approximately the same in all the cases.

Finally it should be noted that the step diffusional model does not solve the problem of general applicability to transition states mentioned earlier. However, it gives better results than the others, not only because the observed lack of fit is smaller but also because it is based on a new approach that takes into account substrate composition. Although this model is more complex, that is, more constants are involved, conceptually it is simple enough to be easily applied. Using information from the analytical values, makes the model more general and flexible, because it can be adapted and fitted to a particular substrate. In this sense it represents an effort to go further in the interpretation of rate data from the degradation of complex materials. However, more experimental work needs to be done to better appraise the new model presented, particularly with different substrates.

Acknowledgments

The authors acknowledge the "Instituto Trevigiano di Ricerca Scientifica del Comune di Treviso" for its auspices and support.

Financial support from NATO Grant No. 0178/87 is also gratefully acknowledged.

Notations

k	Kinetic constant (day^{-1}, first order model; [g C/m^3]$^{0.5}$, diffusional model; m^3/g VSS.d, Monod model)
K	Chen and Hashimoto, kinetic constant (dimensionless)
K$_I$	Inhibition constant (g C/m^3)
K$_s$	Saturation constant (g C/m^3)
n	Feeding times per day
p	Times between one feed and the subsequent one (min)
S	Substrate concentration in digester (g C/m^3)
S$_e$	Substrate concentration in digester just before feeding (g C/m^3)
S$_I$	Substrate concentration in digester after feeding (g C/m^3)
S$_o$	Substrate concentration (g C/m^3)
t	Time (day)
μ	Specific microorganism growth rate (day^{-1})
μ$_k$	Kinetic constant used in this study. It is equal to μ$_m$ X/Y (g C/m^3·d)
μ$_m$	Maximum specific microorganism growth rate (day^{-1})
V	Digester volume (m^3)
V$_0$	Volume fed to digester per time (m^3)
v$_0$	Maximum degradation rate for methanogenesis (g C/m^3·min)
v$_1$	Maximum degradation rate for acidogenesis (g C/m^3·min)
v$_2$	Maximum degradation rate for hydrolysis (g C/m^3·min)
X	Microorganisms concentration (g^{VSS}/m^3)
Y	Yield coefficient (g VSS/g C)
Z	Constant relating gas production at different temperatures (dimensionless)
4a	Kinetic constant representing proportionality constant between degradation rate and time for the methanogenic step (g C/m^3·min^2)
4b	Kinetic constant representing proportionality constant between degradation rate and time for the acidogenic step (g C/m^3·min^2)

4c	Kinetic constant representing proportionality constant between degradation rate and time for the hydrolytic step (g $C/m^3{\cdot}min^2$)

Abbreviations

CSTR	Continuous stirred tank reactor
GP	Gas production
HRT	Hydraulic retention time (day)
MS-OFMSW	Organic fraction municipal solid waste mechanically selected
MSW	Municipal solid waste
OLR	Organic loading rate (kgTVS/m^3·day)
OF	Organic fraction
OFMSW	Organic fraction municipal solid waste
PS	Primary sludge
SMPR	Specific methane production rate (m^{3}CH$_4$/kgTVS added)
SS	Sewage sludge
SS-OFMSW	Organic fraction municipal solid waste source selected
SC-OFMSW	Organic fraction municipal solid waste separately collected
TVS	Total volatile solids
TVSr	Total volatile solids in reactor
VFA	Volatile fatty acids
VMPR	Volumetric methane production rate (m^{3}CH$_4$/m^3·day)

References

1. F. Cecchi *et al.*, *Biomass* **16**, 241 (1988).
2. E.C. Clausen and J.L. Gaddy, in *International Biosystems Vol. III. Chapter 2*, D.L. Wise, Ed. (CRC Press, Boca Raton, Florida, 1989), pp. 15-39.
3. S. Marsili-Libelli, *Biotechnology Vol. 38*, A. Fiechter, Ed. (Springer-Verlag, Berlin-Heilderberg, 1989) pp. 90-146.
4. R.S. Billington, *J. Agric. Eng. Res.* **39** (2), 71 (1988).
5. J.T. Pfeffer, *Biotechnol. Bioeng.* **16**, 771 (1974).
6. J.L. Gaddy, Annual Progress Report to SERI, Document SERI/TR-9802011 (1981).
7. Y. Chen and A. Hashimoto, *Biotechnol. Bioeng. Symp.* **8**, 269 (1978).
8. R.A. Baccay and A.G. Hashimoto, *Biotechnol. Bioeng.* **17**, 885 (1984).
9. M. Canovas-Diaz and J.A. Howell, *Biotechol. Bioeng.* **32** (3), 348 (1988).
10. S.G. Pavlostathis and J.M. Gossett, *Biotechnol. Bioeng.* **27** (3), 345 (1985).
11. S.G. Pavlostathis and J.M. Gossett, *Biotechnol. Bioeng.* **28** (10), 1519 (1986).
12. J.D. Keenan and I. Kormi, *Biotechnol. Bioeng.* **19** (6), 867 (1977).
13. R. Singh, M.K. Jain, and P. Tauro, *Water Res.* **17** (3), 349 (1983).
14. A.W. Lawrence and P.L. McCarty, *J. Water Pollut. Contr. Fed.* **41**, R1 (1969).

15. A.W. Lawrence, *Advan. Chem. Ser.* **105**, 163 (1971).
16. K.K. Chin, *Water Res.* **15**, 199 (1981).
17. J.D. Bryers, *Biotechnol. Bioeng.* **28**, 638.(1985).
18. R.J. Zoetemeyer *et al., Water Res.* **16**, 633 (1982).
19. Dela Torre *et al., Second Symposium on Bioconversion and Biochemical Engineering, Volume 2*, T.K. Ghose, Ed. (New Delhi, India, 1980), pp. 113-131.
20. N.D. Ierusalimsky, *Microbial Physiology and Continuous Culture: Third International Symposium*, E.O. Powell *et al.*, Eds. (1967) pp. 23-33.
21. D. Hill and C.L. Barth, *Water Pollut. Control Fed.* **49**, 2129 (1977)
22. V.H. Edwards, *Biotechnol. Bioeng.* **12**, 679 (1970).
23. R. Moletta, D. Verrier, and G. Albagnac, *Water Res.* **20**, 427 (1986).
24. S. Marsili-Libelli and M. Nardini, *Environ. Technol. Lett.* **6**, 602 (1985).
25. M.T. Suidan *et al., J. of Environ. Eng.* **114**, 6, 1359 (1988).
26. J.F. Andrews and S.P. Graef, in *Anaerobic Biological Treatment, Advances in Chemistry Series, Vol. 105* , R.F. Gould, Ed. (1981), pp. 126-162.
27. B. Hendricks, R.A. Korus, and R.C. Heimsch, *Biotechnol. Bioeng. Symp.* **15**, 241 (1985).
28. G. Dinopoulou, R.M. Sterritt, and J.N. Lester, *Biotechnol. Bioeng.* **31** (9), 969 (1988).
29. M.T. Suidan, B.E. Ritmann, and V.K. Traeguer, *Water Res.* **21**, 481 (1987).
30. D.E. Contois, *J. General Microbiol.* **21**, 40 (1959).
31. J.T. O'Rourke, Ph.D. Dissertation, Standford University, 1968.
32. R. Samson and A. Leduy, *Biotechnol Bioeng.* **28** (7), 1014 (1986)
33. J.M. Lema, E. Ibañez, and J. Canals, *Environ. Technol. Lett.* **8** (11), 555 (1987).
34. M. Glauser, M. Aragno, and M. Gandolla, *Bioenvironmental Systems, Vol. III*, Donald Wise, Ed.(CRC Press, Boca Raton, Florida, 1987) pp. 143-225.
35. F. Cecchi *et al., Biomass*, submitted. (1988)
36. F. Cecchi and P.G. Traverso, *Chim. Ind.—Quad. Ing. Chim. Ital.* **22**, 9 (1986).
37. H.J. Gijzen *et al., Biological Wastes* **22**, 81 (1987).
38. S. Ghosh and M.P. Henry, *Biomass* **6**, 257 (1985).
39. P.G. Traverso and F. Cecchi, *Biomass* **16**, 97 (1988).
40. F. Cecchi *et al.*, submitted.
41. F. Cecchi *et al., Env. Techn. Letters* **9**, 391 (1988).
42. *Standard Methods for the Examination of Water and Wastewater, 16ᵗʰ Edition*, (American Public Health Association, American Water Works Association, Water Pollution Control Federation, 1985), pp. 1193.
43. Metcalf and Eddy (McGraw-Hill, Inc., New York, 1985).
44. F. Cecchi *et al.*, submitted.
45. J. Mata-Alvarez and J. Gonzalez, *International Biosystems, Chapter 3*, D.L. Wise, Ed. (CRC Press, Boca Raton, Florida, 1989), pp. 41-64.
46. P. Llabres-Luengo and J. Mata-Alvarez, *Biological Wastes* **23**, 25 (1988).

Discussion

Omenn: Concerning the 25 percent to 50 percent nonbiodegradable fractions depending on the method of sorting: How does the toxicity of those fractions compare with the many different toxicities of the organic fractions that are biodegradable? Is there any general way to describe the relative toxicity of different fractions of municipal solid waste?

Mata-Alvarez: Normally toxicity comes from the presence of heavy metals in the municipal solid waste. When we deal with the organic fraction of municipal solid wastes separated at source, that is properly selected by you at home, we have practically no heavy metals because of this previous separation made. In a mechanical plant sometimes there is the presence of heavy metals in the final organic fraction of municipal solid waste, which can be a problem. As far as for the question of the presence of toxicants in biodegradable or nonbiodegradable components, we have no data because we have not analyzed the metals on these fractions.

Visscher: Can you say something about the feasibility of this system, especially costs in comparison with incineration and landfill.

Mata-Alvarez: I think that this system when applied in a mechanical plant can be more economical than the classical approach of aerobic composting because composting time can be reduced. Besides, this process generates a significant quantity of gas that can be burned to produce energy for the whole plant. The present treatment is not for producing energy, and it has costs like any other treatment plant, but it has certain economical advantages. As far as for the approach of selecting municipal solid waste at home, this is more for the future, because it needs a training of the people, but it could have many advantages with regards to the application of the digested material on the land because it can be converted into a compost free of toxicants. Compared with other techniques, landfilling sometimes can be less expensive, but it is not a solution in many instances, especially in populated areas, nor is it a preferred long-term solution. Incineration, if performed in a proper way, is much more expensive.

Cecchi: I think the approach presented here is difficult to quantify in terms of economical aspects because we have to consider all of the technologies involved in the municipal solid wastes final disposal. It is awkward to speak about the economics of the anaerobic step because it can be part of an integrated plant. So far there are a few plants planned in Europe that are taking into account this strategy. The plant at Bergamo is a famous example in Italy. In this town there are four anaerobic digesters (2000 cubic meters each) under construction in the same area where the water treatment plant is located together with a new incinerator. So an economical analysis needs to consider all these facilities.

Omenn: In my home city, Seattle, Washington, 40 percent of municipal wastes are now sorted at the source. Trucks with multiple compartments come around weekly, and many citizens participate (voluntarily). The problem now for the city is that the value of the recyclable materials has gone down as the large supply exceeds the demand from firms that pay to use it to recycle. Now the city must bear an increasing cost to subsidize the recycling operation.

Experience with Field Applications: Successes and Failures

18

Cleanup of Old Industrial Sites

correspondence
Mirja Salkinoja-Salonen
Peter Middeldorp
Maria Briglia
University of Helsinki
Department of General
Microbiology
Mannerheimintie 172
00300 Helsinki, Finland

Risto Valo
DN-Bioprocessing Ltd.
Läkkisepänkuja 7
00680 Helsinki, Finland

Max Häggblom
New York University
Medical Center
Department of Microbiology,
550 First Avenue
New York, NY 10016

Adam McBain
University of Strathclyde
Department of Applied
Microbiology
Glasgow United Kingdom

The authors discuss the general problems of using microbes to remediate chemically contaminated soils. Laboratory experiments and field experience are described for one category of chemically contaminated soils (wood-preserving sites), where bioremediation under field conditions appeared possible. Chlorophenol degrading actinomycetes were shown to actively bioremediate the contaminated soils. Immobilized inoculant was found superior to liquid inoculum. Bioremediation was feasible for a wide range of concentrations (one to 9000mg/kg) of chlorophenol. At older sites, a part the chlorophenol was sometimes inaccessible to biodegradation by an unknown mechanism. Chlorophenol-degrading inoculants remained viable in soil a very long time so reinoculation was rarely needed. A gram-positive inoculant (*Rhodococcus*) was superior to a gram-negative inoculant (*Flavobacterium*) in survival and degradation capacity. Transforming reactions such as biomethylation of chlorophenol and its downstream metabolic intermediates were in some soils enhanced by external soil amendments. The response was unpredictable. Therefore testing for mineralization in the laboratory is recommended for each soil before using soil amendments at field scale.

Biodegradability and Soil Pollution

Man's industrial activity involves the release of a huge spectrum and quantity of different organic chemicals into the environment. Biodegradation of practically all intentionally produced organic chemicals has been assayed. Biodegradation data from the worldwide literature have been assembled in data banks. The data recently became available as well on compact diskettes for personal computers.[1]

A search through the available biodegradability literature shows that the most usual test for biodegradability has been and still is the disappearance test: if the chemical of input was not found or its amount had become less, it was assumed that it had become biodegraded.

This loose interpretation of biodegradation has given a false feeling of safety. The finding that natural soil microbes converted the widely used chemical cleaning solvents tri- and tetrachloroethylene into the leukemia-causing agent vinyl chloride[2,3] has shocked scientists, authorities, and the general public. In addition, chemicals designed for use on land, for instance, the agricultural pesticides simazine and atrazine (N-ethyl- and isopropyl 6-chloro-S-triazines, respectively), have caused extensive pollution of both surface water and ground water. Clearly, environmental biodegradability and the laboratory biodegradability are two different things.

The days when soil was considered a safe storage for used up chemicals, or soil filtration a method to turn polluted surface water into safe artificial groundwater are past, never to return. Every industrialized country has thousands of chemically contaminated areas that need to be restored to prevent catastrophes like widespread pollution of groundwater or health hazards to people living in the vicinity.

In this paper, we discuss general problems involved in the use of biological methods to remediate contaminated soils and, more specifically, our experience in the cleanup of abandoned wood-preserving sites.

Table 1

The Reasons for the Persistence of an Organic Chemical in Soil

Condition
1. Incompatibility with microbial growth: too dry, hot, or cold; oxygen unsuitable; aerobic vs. anaerobic growth.
2. Insufficient nutrients for degrader to grow; degraders compete unsuccessfully for nutrients, oxygen or space.
3. Chemical compound unavailable for the microbes; for instance, those present as large particles or droplets, are encapsulated by a barrier (plastic, clay, or other impermeable matter).
4. Degraders compete unsuccessfully with biotransforming microbes for substrate; biotransformation masks degradation.
5. Easily degradable carbon is available and causes catabolic repression of the degrading enzymes.
6. Concentration of the chemical is below the threshold value of the degradation (environmental Km value).
7. Metabolic products of the chemical are toxic and poison the degraders.
8. Biophysical factors (redox potential, acidity, temperature, metals required as cofactors that are absent, and so forth) are unfavorable for the degrading enzymes (important when extracellular enzymes should attack large or water-insoluble molecules).
9. There are toxic chemicals around that inhibit some metabolic step in the degradation.
10. There are no microbes present with the biochemical capacity of degrading the compound in question.

Results and Discussion

What determines whether or not a chemical will degrade in the soil? At least ten possible reasons can be brought up for the persistence of an organic chemical in soil (Table 1). Condition 1 (Table 1) is the easiest to meet. One only needs to know the oxygen demand of and the temperature requirement for the desired degradation process. These factors are easily measured with the soil in question in the laboratory.

But if adjusting Condition 1 does not start degradation, it is not easy to guess what is the correct way to proceed. Adding nutrients (fertilizer) is popular in the conditioning of oil-contaminated land. This is a logical approach, because hydrocarbons contain no nitrogen or phosphorus. Huntjens *et al.*[4] found that mineralization of 3500ppm of oil in soil ($20\mu g$ CO_2-C /h) was only slightly enhanced by 40ppm phosphorus and was even suppressed by nitrogen compounds (200 or 400ppm N from ammonium nitrate). "Oil content" (as measured by infrared absorbance) is often seen to decrease faster after fertilizing. The disappearance of more "oil" than was mineralized to carbon dioxide indicates that other products may accumulate. Few controlled studies, where a complete materials balance has been made, have been reported.

Gas chromatographic analysis of old oil contaminated sites and areas where wood preservation has been performed with creosote always shows a hill of unresolved complex material (UCM). This material is extractable into organic solvents but cannot be resolved by the usual derivatization methods into single peaks. We found the UCM to contain more nitrogen than does crude oil or creosote, probably covalently bound. Maybe nitrogen fertilization favors bio-transformation into UCM (see Condition 4, Table 1), which would explain its retarding effect on mineralization.

Oil has been around for millions of years, so it is not surprising that oil-degrading bacteria are widespread in nature. Many hydrocarbon-degrading bacteria and yeasts have been isolated and characterized. The biochemistry and genetics of hydrocarbon degradation has been studied in great detail.[5] However, successful soil bioremediation enhanced by externally added degrader microbes has yet to be described. All the land farming of oily soils and waste oil has so far relied on indigenous degraders.

Most aromatic halogen compounds are alien to the biosphere were taken into massive production without adequate knowledge of their biodegradability. This has led to global pollution, for example, by the polychlorinated biphenyls (PCBs) (see chapter by D. Bedard in this volume), chlorobenzenes, and chlorophenols.

Till recently, pentachlorophenol was the pesticide used more than any other, approximately 25 million kg/year in the wood and textile industry and in agriculture.[6,7] We studied 15 former and present wood-preserving sites and found chlorophenol in high concentrations in soil (up to 10,000mg/kg) at every site.[8-10] We also observed that the concentration did not noticeably decrease when measured at the same sites for three subsequent years, even though chlorophenol use had been discontinued[8-10] on the site. Similar observations were reported also from other countries.[11] Sweden was the first country to ban chlorophenols (1978), and many countries have since followed. However, the pollution persists.

Use of Microbes to Clean Contaminated Soil

Do microbial inoculants help to remediate soil? Seeing the great number of reports on the biodegradation of the various chemicals that have caused serious pollution of soil, and have threatened surface water and groundwater, it is actually surprising that there are so few reports on attempts of using microbes for soil cleanup. The likely explanation is that there were few successes to report. It is known from the research on agricultural inoculants that it has been difficult to establish, for instance, efficient di-nitrogen–fixing *Rhizobium* and vesicular-arbuscular mycorrhiza into their intended host plants under field conditions, even though short-term successes were achieved with presterilized or fumigated soils under greenhouse conditions.[12]

Aerobic chlorophenol degradation has been observed in soil water, bioreactors, and mixed bacterial cultures.[13-24] The number of degraders varied in Finnish soils from none to more than 10 million per gram of fresh soil.[25] Several aerobic bacteria that degrade poly-chlorophenols have been described.[26-37] Many of these strains degrade several different polychlorophenols, but poorly or not mono- or di-chlorophenols.[38,39] The biochemistry and genetics of chlorophenol degradation are beginning to be understood and have recently been reviewed.[38,39]

We report here on the results of work on bioremediation of chlorophenol-contaminated soil. We found that it was possible to initiate chlorophenol degradation in soil by introducing degrading organisms. In cases where sufficient indigenous degraders were already present, bioremediation was possible also in the absence of added organisms.

Figure 1 demonstrates the onset of chlorophenol degradation in soil by added degrader organisms. To monitor for mineralization, U-^{14}C–labeled pentachlorophenol (PCP) was added to natural soil containing 600 mg of pentachlorophenol per kg of soil. It is seen that 80mg (Figure 1A, sandy soil) to 150mg (Figure 1B, peaty soil) of the chlorophenol were mineralized to carbon dioxide per kg of soil per month after degrading bacteria (*Rhodococcus chlorophenolicus* PCP-1[26,27]) were added. When no degraders were added, there was no significant mineralization of pentachlorophenol.

Whereas the results in Figure 1 were from laboratory pilots (^{14}C-substrate could not be used in-field), Table 2 shows the results of a field site: 50m^3 of soil, bioremediated at a former landfill site at Heinola, southern Finland. This soil had been stored in windrows on that landfill since 1981, with no significant change in its chlorophenol content. Table 2 shows that biological treatment during the first four months decreased the chlorophenol content by 83 percent, and a"background" chlorophenol level was reached in three years' time.

Competition Between Biodegradation and other Reactions of Chlorophenols in Soil

Figure 1 shows what happened when both degrading and biomethylating bacteria, competing for the same substrate, pentachlorophenol, were added: *R. rhodochrous*, methylates chlorophenols into the corresponding anisols,[40] which are unavailable for biodegradation by *R. chlorophenolicus*.[41,42] Figure 1 shows that the methylators, although added in an amount equal to the degraders (10 million active cells/gm fresh soil), did not suppress mineralization.

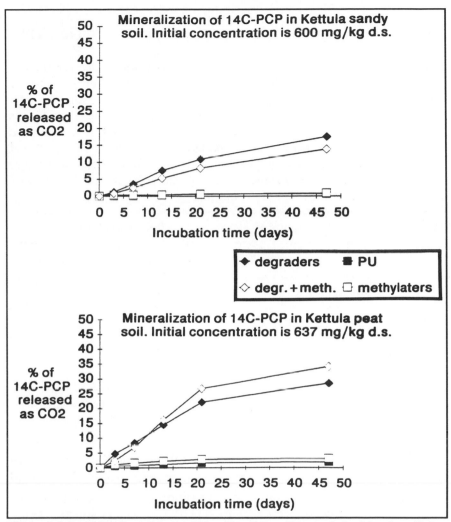

Figure 1. Mineralization of pentachlorophenol in soil amended with mineralizing and/or biomethylating bacterial cultures. Two soils containing 600mg of pentachlorophenol per kilogram were spiked with 50,000cpm/50gm of U-^{14}C–labeled pentachlorophenol and monitored for ^{14}C–carbon dioxide evolution. Soil A was sandy: volatile solids contents, 2.5 percent (w/w); pH 5.1 (aq); soil B was peaty: volatile solids contents, 33 percent; pH, 6.0 (aq). The response as evolution of ^{14}C–labeled carbon dioxide occurred (monitored as in References 13, 22) is shown on the figures for the soil inoculated in different ways either with *Rhodococcus chlorophenolicus* PCP-1, a chlorophenol degrader, or with *R. rhodochrous* DSM 43241, a chlorophenol methylator,[42,43] or with both, each with 10 million active cells per gram of soil.

Table 2
Bioremediation of Chlorophenol Contaminated Soil in Field

$50m^3$ of gravel soil: pH (in water), 6.0; volatile solids 31 percent (wood residues); water-soluble nitrogen content, 0.08 percent; total nitrogen, 0.19 percent; nutrients soluble in 1M ammonium acetate as follows: P, 160mg/kg; K, 390mg/kg; Mg, 330mg/kg. Total aerobic bacteria were counted on standard plate count agar as previously described[49] and chlorophenol-mineralizing bacteria were monitored with ^{14}C-carbon dioxide formation from ^{14}C-pentachlorophenol by the MPN-method.[50] Chlorophenols were assayed by gas chromatography mass spectrometry after acetone extraction using internal and external standards as described.[8,40,51] Extraction efficiency was 80 percent to 100 percent.

| Date | Sum of Contents of Penta-, Tetra-, Tri-, and Dichlorophenols | | ——— Bacterial Count ——— | |
			Total heterotrophs	Pentachlorophenol Mineralizing
	mg/kg	%	——— millions /g soil ———	
1.6.1984	212	100	80	5
5.10.1984	38	17		
10.10.1985	16	7	70	5
Oct. 1987*	0.3	0.1	77	3

*The contribution of the different chlorophenols was as follows: pentachlorophenol, 0.042mg/kg; 2,3,4,6-tetrachlorophenol, 0.216mg/kg; 2,4,6-trichlorophenol; 0.0034mg/kg.

We had observed methylators to compete successfully for substrate against degraders when studied in an axenic system.[42,43] We had also seen that competitiveness of three randomly chosen methylator strains, *R. rhodochrous* (DSM 43241), *Rhodococcus* sp. Pl (IMET 7412), and Anll7 (IMET 7497), was strongly enhanced if carbohydrate was added to the mixed culture.[41,42]

Biomethylation is an undesirable reaction from the environmental viewpoint. We found that some biomethylating strains not only biomethylated chlorophenols, but also the catechols arising from the biodegradation of mono- and dichlorophenols[38,39] and the chlorinated *p*-hydroquinones arising as the first metabolites from polychlorinated phenols,[28,29,39,41,44,45] into the corresponding chloromethoxyphenols and chloro-dimethoxybenzenes. These compounds appear nonbiodegradable other than under anaerobic conditions.[39,46] Another undesirable property of the methyl derivatives is the probability to bioaccumulate because of the higher log Kow values. We measured the Kow values of all tri- and tetrachlorophenols, methoxy-chlorophenols, and dimethoxy-chlorobenzenes, and found an increase of 0.4 to 0.6 units for each hydroxyl group replaced by a methoxyl, which resulted in a shift from approximately 4.0-4.8 to 4.4-5.7 (results not shown).

Table 3 shows the results of an experiment designed to measure the formation of anisols in soils contaminated with pentachlorophenol during bioremediation with *R. chlorophenolicus* PCP-1. The results show that the addition of a huge methylator inoculum (250 million cells/gm of soil) had little effect on the amount of anisols found: 3.5mg/kg in the absence and 4.0mg/kg in the presence of the added methylator inoculum. It thus seems that the indigenous methylating microbes were not complemented by externally added ones. On the contrary, added degrader inoculum (a high inoculum was used because of the high level of pollution in the soil) very significantly initiated degradation of pentachlorophenol in soil. Degradation was in this case not hindered by the presence of methylating organisms. Because biomethylating capacity was common with *Rhodococcus* and many other bacteria,[39] methylating activity is likely to be indigenously present in soils.

We obtained similar results with some soils when biodegradable wastes such as distillery and/or wood-debarking waste were added to 1 percent of soil dry weight. With other soils, the methylation reaction was enhanced by externally added carbon source, reflecting the results obtained in axenic systems (results not shown). The behavior of the soils was unpredictable; therefore, laboratory studies are necessary with each soil before starting fieldwork.

Physical and Biological Accessibility of the Pollutant in Soil

With very old, contaminated sawmill sites, we frequently observed that the resident chlorophenol contaminant was less acces-

Table 3
Degradation and Methylation of Pentachlorophenol in Soil

A sandy soil (pH in KCl, 4.6; volatile solids, 2.4 percent) and a peaty soil (pH in KCl, 4.7; volatile solids, 33 percent) were inoculated with 100 million active *Rhodococcus chlorophenolicus* cells per gram and/or with a similar number of *R. rhodochrous* cells, both immobilized to polyurethane. Glucose and yeast extract were added when indicated to 2.5g/kg each. Moisture was adjusted to 60 percent of water-holding capacity. Soil was enclosed in sealed polyethylene bags to avoid evaporation of water or volatile metabolites of the chlorophenols. Analysis was as described,[8,31,40,51] with an extraction efficiency of 80 percent to 100 percent. Initial pentachlorophenol in the peat soil was 1860mg/kg and in the sand 685mg/kg.

Soil type	Inoculated with	Carbohydrate added	Pentachlorophenol contents on Day 30		Pentachloroanisol contents on Day 30
	*	†	mg/kg	% degr.	mg/kg
Peat	–	–	–	1900	0	3.5
Peat	+	–	–	1460	20	1.4
Peat	–	+	–	1800	0	4.0
Peat	+	+	–	1370	25	1.6
Peat	+	–	+	1340	32	0.5
Peat	+	+	+	1140	37	0.6
Sand	–	–	–	670	0	0
Sand	+	–	–	580	13	0.12
Sand	–	+	–	680	0	0.32
Sand	+	+	–	590	11	0.16
Sand	+	–	+	490	26	0.18
Sand	+	+	+	600	11	0.16

* -Inoculated with Degrader
† -Inoculated with Methylator

sible to biodegradation than the same chlorophenol compound more recently added to soil. Figure 2 shows biodegradation of pentachlorophenol in the soils from two old sawmill sites. Both soils had been under bioremediation treatment in the field for 2 years. The original chlorophenol contents of Toras-soil (300m³) was 9000mg/kg and of Lappeenranta (500m³) was 500mg/kg, meaning that on Day 0 (see

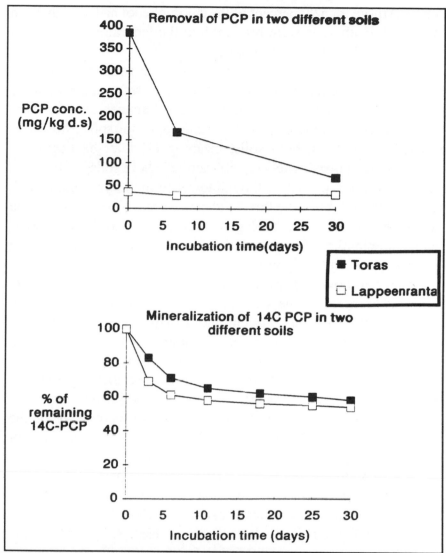

Figure 2. Pentachlorophenol degradation in soil at two old bioremediation sites. Toras soil was peaty, pH 5.7 (aq.), and contained an average of 9000mg of chlorophenols when bioremediation operation was started in 1986. Lappeenranta soil was gravel, pH 6.8 (aq.), and had contained 500mg of chlorophenols when bioremediation was started in 1987. In 1988, when the concentration of pentachlorophenol was as indicated on Day 0 samples of the field-scale windrows were taken into the laboratory and spiked with 1000 Bq of U-^{14}C–labeled pentachlorophenol (39,000GBq/mmol). The concentration of pentachlorophenol and the evolution of ^{14}C-carbon dioxide was monitored for 30 days, and results are as shown.

Figure 2) more than 90 percent of the chlorophenol had already been consumed. Both soils were brought into the laboratory and spiked with U-^{14}C–labeled pentachlorophenol.

Figure 2 shows that pentachlorophenol was consumed from the Toras soil during the 30 days of observation from approximately 400mg/kg to approximately 100mg/kg, but in Lappeenranta soil there was no change. The added ^{14}C-pentachlorophenol spike, however, behaved similarly in both soils, meaning (1) that the degrading bacteria were approximately equally active in both soils, and (2) that the concentration of PCP, although lower in the Lappeenranta soil, was sufficiently above the threshold concentration below which the bioreaction slows down ("biodegradation Km"). Also, Table 2 shows that biodegradation of chlorophenol in soil could continue to a very low concentration (<< 1ppm).

Figure 3 shows the results of an experiment where the apparent biodegradation Km value was sought. Clean, uncontaminated soil was spiked with various concentrations of pentachlorophenol and subsequently inoculated with the degrading microbes. The figure shows that pentachlorophenol was mineralized quite efficiently down to concentrations of 0.08μM or 21μg/kg (wet weight). The reaction velocity slowed a little when the initial pentachlorophenol concentration was below 53μg/kg (0.2μM). The specific activity of of the 14C–labeled pentachlorophenol available (25.6 mCi/gm) did not allow testing for concentrations below 0.08μM.

The experiment that Figure 3 represents was performed in soil-water slurry (>100 percent of water holding capacity) because it is impossible to mix the minute quantities of added chlorophenol homogeneously into the soil if too little liquid is used. As a result, toxic inhibition was observed at 0.5mg of chlorophenol per kilogram (0.02mM) and higher. This is because *Rhodococcus* are very sensitive towards chlorophenol toxicity at high water content. At low moisture content, biodegradation proceeded succesfully even at huge concentrations (9000mg/kg). Sensitivity was also partially due to the fact that in this experiment a liquid inoculum was used (instead of immobilized) to distinguish between the biological and physical barriers.

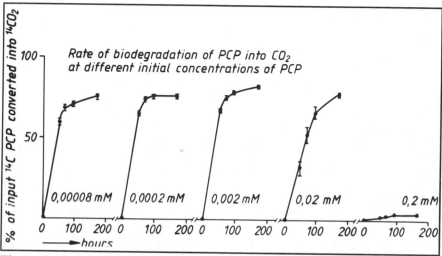

Figure 3. Biodegradability of pentachlorophenol at varying concentrations. Five-gram aliquots of agricultural soil (Seveso 1976, Italy, stored dry on laboratory bench for 3 years) in 45ml of water were spiked with varying amounts (shown in figure) of nonlabeled pentachlorophenol and 1000Bq of U-^{14}C–labeled pentachlorophenol (0.9GBq/gm) and 100 million pentachlorophenol degrader cells each (experiment in triplicate). Evolution of ^{14}C–labeled carbon dioxide is shown (monitored as described in References 13 and 22).

So the reason for the inaccessibility of the "old" chlorophenol for biodegradation in Lappeenranta soil is unclear. We found that the inaccessibility correlated with unavailability of chlorophenol to non-polar solvents (diethyl ether, hexane), although good extraction (recovery >90 percent) was obtained by our usual method , extraction with hydrophilic solvents (acetone extraction of wet soil, reference.[8]

We found unavailability also with other chemicals, notably with the polychlorinated dibenzo-*p*-dioxins and -furans, which also occurred in these soils[8] as impurities in the technical chlorophenol used at the sawmills. We noticed that unavailability was a time-connected development occurring more rapidly with the dioxins than with the chlorophenols. Figure 4 shows how physical inaccessibility "developed" in two months for 2,3,7,8-tetrachlorodibenzo-*p*-dioxin (TCDD) mixed into soil. The figure shows that while on Days 0 and 30, 80 percent or more of the added dioxin was extractable from the soil into

Figure 4. Extractability of
^{14}C–labeled 2, 3, 7, 8-
tetrachlorodibenzo-*p*-di-
oxin (TCDD) from soil in
course of time. 2.5ug
(11,200cpm) of 2,3,7,8-
TCDD were added to 5-
gram aliquots (water
added to 80 percent w/w)
of the same agricultural
soil as described in Figure
3 and analyzed for ben-
zene-soluble ^{14}-C after
varying times of incuba-
tion in closed vessels
(50ml) at room tempera-
ture. To monitor for the
efficiency of extraction, 1,
2, 3, 4-tetrachlorodibenzo-
p-dioxin was added (10μg/
flask) as internal standard
immediately prior to ex-
traction. 14C-2, 3, 7, 8-
TCDD recoveries shown
were corrected for extraction recovery obtained by
GLC for 1,2,3,4-TCDD

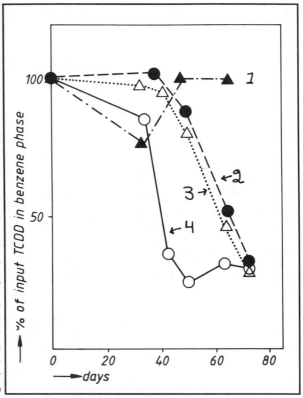

(>90 percent at all times). 1, uninoculated 2, with liquid inoculum of 100 million
pentachlorophenol degrading cells plus phosphate buffer and ammonium salts;[13] 3
as described in 2 but with no nutrient salts; 4, with inoculum of bark-immobilized
pentachlorophenol degrading cells (same amount of cells as in 2 and 3).

nonpolar solvent in an ultrasonic bath, the extraction efficiency
subsequently dropped to approximately 30 percent.

The following observations indicate that no real biodegradation
occurred: (1) there was no stoichiometric volatile or water-soluble
metabolite detected from ^{14}C-labeled 2,3,7,8-TCDD; (2) on repeated
extractions using hydrophilic solvent (acetone-water) in ultrasonic
bath, close to 100 percent of the dioxin was recovered.

We do not have a documented explanation for this phenomen,
but we thought it is useful to report, because this kind of phenomena
easily could be interpreted as biodegradation if no radiolabeled

substrate can be used. This phenomenon may be connected to some biological factor, as we did not observe it (or much less severely) in sterile, uninoculated controls. We suggest a mechanism by which the lipid-soluble chemical is first trapped by microbial cells, and the microbes then slowly invade the micropores of the clay or other soil materials. Hydrophobic solvents are unlikely to penetrate the soil micropores, which are polar in nature.

Our temporary conclusion is that biological and physical barriers (see condition 3, Table 1) may halt biodegradation of the compounds studied here more likely than concentration thresholds (see condition 6, Table 1).

Establishment and Survival of Chlorophenol Degrading Bacteria in Soil

The previously described results (Figures 1-3, Tables 2,3) demonstrate that *Rhodococcus chlorophenolicus*, when inoculated into natural, nonsterile soil, was able to biodegrade chlorophenol in that soil. The *Rhodococcus* inoculum was introduced as a polyurethane-immobilized culture. In this way, the inoculum established itself in soil stably. Figure 5 shows the pentachlorophenol-mineralizing activities of nonimmobilized and various immobilized inoculae. It shows that although liquid inoculum was ineffective (Figure 5B, No. 5 and 6), degradation was very much enhanced when the same quantity of inoculum was blended with bark chips (Figure 5A, No. 2; Figure 5B, Nos. 3 and 7).

Polystyrene anion exchange resin or crushed unglazed pottery did not similarly stimulate the activity. We later found that polyurethane[47] was even more effective, and we have subsequently used it.

To see if another chlorophenol degrader would behave similarly to *R. chlorophenolicus* in soil bioreclamation, laboratory experiments analogous to those described in Figure 1 were performed with a gram-negative chlorophenol-degrader *Flavobacterium* sp.[48] donated by R. L. Crawford. We found that the *Flavobacterium* inoculum vanished

Figure 5. Pentachlorophenol mineralizing activity of inoculants added as liquid or immobilized culture into soil. Five-gram portions of agricultural soil in 20ml of water, 0.2mM in pentachlorophenol, in bottles of 100ml, were spiked with 22,000cpm (**A**) or 13,700cpm (**B**) of U-^{14}C-pentachlorophenol (0.9GBq/gm). Chlorophenol mineralization was monitored for by ^{14}C-carbon dioxide evolution as described.[13,22] **A.** To flask 1, heat-inactivated in

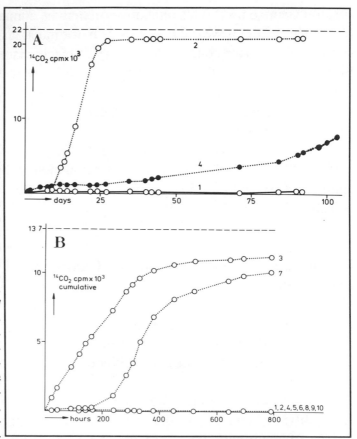

oculum was added; to flask 2, an inoculum absorbed onto bark chips (*Pinus sylvestris*); and to flask 4, a liquid inoculum. **B.** Flasks 1, 4, 5, 6, and 7 were inoculated with pentachlorophenol mineralizing liquid culture. Crushed unglazed pottery (1gm) was added to 4, polystyrene anion exchange resin particles (1gm) to 8 and sterilized bark chips (1gm) to 2 and 7. Flask 3 was inoculated with the same culture as 1, 4, 5, 6, and 7, but culture was absorbed to bark chips (1gm) before introducing it into the flask. Flasks 2, 8, 9, and 10 were uninoculated controls, 8 with polystyrene resin (1gm), 2 and 9 with bark chips and crushed unglazed pottery, respectively.

from the soil two weeks after inoculation, and there was also no decrease in soil contents of pentachlorophenol. The *Flavobacterium* sp. was in liquid culture, under conditions previously described,[34] and comparably active to *R. chlorophenolicus* PCP-1. It thus seems that some other biological property other than just the capacity of the organism to degrade is important. We do not know what the properties are that help to maintain survival in soil. This is clearly an area that needs further research before bioremediation can become a reliable large-scale practice for the conditioning of contaminated soils.

Acknowledgments

This work was financially supported by the Maj and Tor Nessling Foundation (M.B & MSS), Center for Technology Development TEKES, Finland, (MSS, PM & RV); The Carnegie Trust for the Universities of Scotland and the Bellahouston bequest fund (AMcB), US EPA grant No. 68-03-2936 IERL, Cincinnati, OH (MSS), and The Ministry of Education, Scholarship Office Italy (MB). M.H. is a holder of a Helsinki University Young Scientist's Fellowship. The authors would like to thank Riitta Boeck for expert laboratory assistance, Erkki Äijö for instrument maintenance, dr R. Huetter for the gift of ^{14}-C–labeled 2,3,7,8-TCDD, and P. Paasivuo and S. Räisänen for the gifts of unlabeled 1,2,3,4- and 2,3,7,8-labeled TCDD, respectively.

References

1. Environmental Fate Database (CHEMFATE), Numerica Online Services.
2. T. Vogel and P.L. McCarty, *Appl. Environ. Microbiol.* **49**, 1080 (1985).
3. R.D. Kleopfer *et al.*, *Environ. Sci. Technol.* **19** (3), 277 (1985).
4. J.L.M. Huntjens, H. de Potter, and J. Barendrecht, *Contaminated Soil*, J.W. Assink and W.J. van den Brink, Eds. (Martinus Nijhof Publishers, Dordrecht, 1986), pp.121-124.
5. J.A. Shapiro *et al.*, in *Genetic Control of Environmental Pollutants*, G.S. Omenn and A. Hollaender, Eds. (Plenum Press, New York, 1984), pp. 229-238.
6. J.T. Wilson and C.W. Ward. *Developm. Ind. Microbiol. Vol. 27* (Elsevier and the Society for Industrial Microbiology, 1987) pp. 109-116.
7. R.C. Dougherty, in *Pentachlorophenol, Chemistry, Pharmacology, and Environmental Toxicology*, K.R. Rao, Ed. (Plenum Press, New York, 1978) pp. 351-361.
8. V. Kitunen, R. Valo and M. Salkinoja-Salonen, *Environ. Sci. Technol.* **21**, 96 (1987).
9. M.S. Salkinoja-Salonen *et al.*, in *Current Perspectives in Microbial Ecology*, M.J. Klug and C.A. Reddy, Eds. (American Society for Microbiology, Washington, D.C., 1984), pp. 668-678.
10. R. Valo *et al.*, *Chemosphere* **13**, 835 (1984).

11. Discussion Document Pentachlorophenol. (Agriculture Canada Food Production and Inspection Branch Canada, 1987), pp. 87-02.
12. Proceedings of the Society of Chemical Industry Symposium, "Microbial Inoculants in Agriculture," 14 February 1989, London.
13. J.H.A. Apajalahti and M.S. Salkinoja-Salonen, *Microbiol Ecology* 10, 359 (1984).
14. E.J. Brown *et al., Appl. Environ. Microbiol.* 52, 92 (1986).
15. J.E. Etzel and E.J. Kirsch, *Dev. Ind. Microbiol* 16, 287 (1974).
16. E.J.Kirsch and J.E. Etzel, *J. Water Poll. Contr. Fed.* 45, 359 (1973).
17. G.M Klecka and W.J. Maier, *Appl. Environ. Microbiol.* 49, 46 (1985).
18. D. Liu, K. Thomson, and K.L.E. Kaiser, *Bull. Environ. Contam. Toxicol.* 29, 130 (1982).
19. L.P. Moos *et al., Water Res.* 17, 1575.
20. J.J. Pignatello *et al., Appl. Environ. Microbiol.* 46, 1024 (1983).
21. J.J. Pignatello *et al., Can. J. Microbiol.* 32, 38 (1986).
22. M.S. Salkinoja-Salonen and J. Apajalahti, EPA Industrial Environmental Research Laboratory Report on Project 68-03-2936, Cincinnati, Ohio (1982).
23. R.Valo, J. Apajalahti, and M.S. Salkinoja-Salonen, *Appl. Microbiol. Biotechnol.* 21, 313 (1985).
24. I. Watanabe, *Soil Biol. Biochem.* 10, 71 (1978).
25. R. Valo and M. Salkinoja-Salonen, *Appl. Microbiol. Biotechnol.* 25, 68 (1986).
26 J.H.A. Apajalahti and M.S. Salkinoja-Salonen, *Appl. Microbiol. Biotechnol.* 25, 62 (1986).
27. J.H.A. Apajalahti, P. Kgrphnoja, and M. Salkinoja-Salonen, *Intern. J. Syst. Bacteriol.* 36, 246 (1986).
28. J.P. Chu and E.J. Kirsch, *Appl. Microbiol.* 23, 1033 (1972).
29. J.P. Chu and E.J. Kirsch, *Dev. Ind. Microbiol.* 14, 264 (1973).
30. R.U. Edgedill and R.K. Finn, *Eur. J. Appl. Biotechnol* 16, 179 (1982).
31. M.M. Higgblom, L. Nohynek, and M. Salkinoja-Salonen, *Appl. Environ. Microbiol.* 54, 3043 (1988).
32. J.S. Karns *et al., Appl. Environ. Microbiol.* 26, 1176 (1983).
33. E.A. Reiner, J. Chu, and E.J. Kirsch, in *Pentachlorophenol, Chemistry, Pharmacology, and Environmental Toxicology*, K. R. Rao, Ed. (Plenum Press, New York, 1978), pp. 67-81.
34. D.L. Saber and R.L. Crawford, *Appl. Environ. Microbiol.* 50, 1512 (1985).
35. G.J. Stanlake and R.K. Finn, *Appl. Environ. Microbiol.* 44, 1421 (1982).
36. T. Suzuki, *J. Environ. Sci. Health* B12, 113 (1977).
37. I. Watanabe, *Soil Sci. Plant Nutr.* 19, 109 (1973).
38. W. Reineke and H.-J. Knackmuss, *Ann. Rev. Microbiol.* 42, 263 (1988).
39. M. Häggblom, *J. Basic Microbiol.*, in press.
40. M.M. Häggblom, J.H.A. Apajalahti, and M.S. Salkinoja-Salonen, *Appl. Environ. Microbiol.* 54, 683 (1988).
41. M.M. Häggblom, J.H.A. Apajalahti, and M.S. Salkinoja-Salonen, *Appl. Environ. Microbiol.* 54, 1818 (1988).
42. M.M. Häggblom, D. Janke, and M.S. Salkinoja-Salonen, *Microbial Ecol.* in press.
43. M.M. Häggblom *et al., Arch. Microbiol.*, in press.
44. M. Salkinoja-Salonen *et al.*, in Water Research Pollution Report 6: "Behaviour of Organic Micropollutants in Biological Wastewater Treatment" (CEC EUR 11356, 1987), pp. 75-80.

45. J.H.A. Apajalahti and M.S. Salkinoja-Salonen, *J. Bacteriol.* **169**, 675 (1987).
46. A.H. Neilson, A.-S. Allard, and M. Rereberger, in *The Handbook of Environmental Chemistry, Vol.2, Part C, Reactions and Processes*, O. Huizinger, Ed. (Springer, Berlin Heidelberg, New York, 1985), pp. 29-86
47. I. Pascik and H.-J. Henzler, *Anaerobic Digestion*, 1988 Proceedings Fifth International Symposium on Anaerobic Digestion, Bologna, Italy, May 22-26, 1988), pp. 491-497.
48. R.L. Crawford and W.W. Mohn, *Enzyme Microbiol. Technol.* **7**, 617 (1985).
49. *Standard Methods for the Examination of Water and Waste Water, 16th Ed* (American Public Health Association, New York, NY, 1985).
50. *Manual of Methods for General Microbiology* (American Society for Microbiology, Washington, D.C., 1981).
51. M. Häggblom, J. Apajalahti, and M. Salkinoja-Salonen, *Appl. Microbiol. Biotechnol.* **24**, 397.

Discussion

Kamely: When you did the first oil experiment, you said you added nutrients and when you measured, the concentration of oil went down. Did you measure at that first experiment what the breakdown products were?

Salkinoja-Salonen: The product that we recorded here is the ^{14}C labeled carbon dioxide, which means that it is really mineralized. We have shown in laboratory work that you can get 90 percent mineralization of the carbon to carbon dioxide, whereas 10 percent goes into biomass. I think it is essentially a complete mineralization reaction.

Kamely: That was done under laboratory conditions. Do you have any idea what happens if you carry out the same experiment in the environment?

Salkinoja-Salonen: Yes, we have quite a lot of ideas. The other experiment that I showed was done under field conditions without the radioactive compound. Here you see approximately the speed by which it is biodegradable. We have looked into the mass spectra of all these soils, and the only chlorinated compound that we find is the anisol. Sometimes, you find quite a bit of anisol. For example, we have found four percent of the resident organic chlorine as anisol, but in that case there were no degraders added. When we add degraders, we always find less, but we find it.

Kamely: So there are other processes going on that you cannot account for at this time?

Salkinoja-Salonen: Yes, if you are unlucky.

Kamely: When you do that in the field, how reproducible are the results of one experiment to the other if you carry them in the field under the same conditions? Do you get a lot of variability from one experiment to another?

Salkinoja-Salonen: Every field experiment has been different. We take soil into the laboratory and work with it until we find out the best moisture, analyzer, and amendment to get the maximal mineralization rate. We do it that way. We have not found any simple recipe; to apply every soil is individual.

Buswell: The experiments show the increased mineralization when you add immobilized bacteria as opposed to, say, just a liquid culture. Is that due to an increased metabolic conversion by the immobilized bacteria, or is it the fact that the organisms survive better in the soil because they are immobilized?

Salkinoja-Salonen: It is the latter.

Janssen: You mentioned that one cause of persistence could be that concentrations are below the threshold level enzymes. Enzyme kinetics is assumed to follow Michaelis-Menten. Alexander has shown there are different substrates in different systems, and that first-order kinetics are followed for the mineralization of very low concentrations of substrates. Is there any experimental evidence for the existence of threshold concentrations. If there is a situation in which this occurs, would the proper explanation be that there is only enough energy for survival and not enough energy for growth of microbial cultures?

Salkinoja-Salonen: I think you may well be right. The reason why we began to think about whether there was something like a threshold concentration is that sometimes the biodegradation could stop in this case at approximately 14 milligrams. We thought maybe this is too low to biodegrade. However, later we could treat other soils in which we could go down to below one milligram. So I do not think there is a real threshold.

Janssen: Of course, you say this is a soil system in which all the factors like availability of the compounds could also play a role.

Salkinoja-Salonen: I think that is the most important.

Eveleigh: Should we isolate the bacteria out of the entire population as a percentage of total bacteria, then characterize it for survivability and put it back into the system?

Salkinoja-Salonen: We put PCB degraders, almost 10^8 organisms in different windows to see how they survive under different conditions. You can try all kinds of amendments. After three months you still have approximately 10^7 organisms. This is a standard plate-count but faces an unknown substrate. It is a challenge for the geneticists here to engineer degrader organisms for survival.

Eveleigh: The problem as I see it is being able to get survival. Surely that should be addressed in the isolation procedure. Do not give the challenge away to the geneticists and say we do not know how it survives. Try and work it out.

19

Bacterial Transformation of Polychlorinated Biphenyls

Donna L. Bedard

*GE Corporate Research and Development
Schenectady,
New York*

Aerobic bacteria are proving versatile and effective agents for biodegrading polychlorinated biphenyls (PCBs). Four natural isolates have been shown to degrade many tetra- and pentachlorobiphenyls and some hexachlorobiphenyls. The enzymes responsible for PCB metabolism in these organisms fall into two genetically distinct classes that differ markedly in congener reactivity preferences. Because the reactivities complement each other, treating Aroclor 1242 with a mixture of two bacteria representing each class of enzymes has been particularly effective. *In situ* bioremediation of Aroclor® 1242 (Monsanto, St. Louis, MO) has been demonstrated.

Extensive reductive dechlorination of PCBs in anerobic sediments of lakes, rivers, and harbors has been documented. Laboratory experiments have demonstrated that this dechlorination proceeds by step-wise removal of *meta* and *para* chlorines and results in the accumulation of mono– to trichlorobiphenyls that are easily degraded by aerobic bacteria. It appears that natural microbial populations already have the capacity to biodegrade most if not all of the PCBs that contaminate the environment. Research aimed at stimulating the activity of these organisms should make it possible to accelerate biodegradation of PCB contaminants

Introduction

Polychlorinated biphenyls (PCBs) have attracted concern because of their persistence, their bioaccumulation, and their possible health effects. PCBs were used worldwide for a wide range of applications for more than 50 years. Major uses included transformer oil, capacitor dielectric fluid, heat transfer fluid, fire retardants, and plasticizers. The properties that made PCBs useful industrial chemicals; thermal and chemical stability, resistance to chemical corrosion, and general inertness, have contributed to their widespread persistence in nature near the sites of their production, use, storage, or disposal. Because of their hydrophobic nature, PCBs have accumulated primarily in soils and aquatic sediments where they adsorb strongly to organic matter.

PCBs are a family of compounds (congeners) consisting of a biphenyl nucleus carrying one to 10 chlorines; hence, there are 209 possible PCB congeners that differ in the number and position of the chlorines. Because the commercial PCBs (Aroclors) commonly contain more than 60 to 80 congeners, they pose a particulary difficult challenge as candidates for bioremediation.

Bacterial Oxidation of PCBs

There have been numerous reports of bacteria that are capable of degrading PCBs. The literature prior to 1982 has been thoroughly reviewed,[1] but there have been a number of reports of bacteria with exceptional ability to degrade PCBs since that date, and several reports of novel dioxygenase attack on PCBs. Four strains of bacteria are particularly noteworthy for their ability to degrade a broad spectrum of PCBs: *Acinetobacter* sp. P6,[2] *Corynebacterium* sp. MB1[3,4] *Alcaligenes eutrophus* H850,[3-5] and *Pseudomonas* sp. LB400.[6]

Acinetobacter sp. P6 was extensively characterized by Furukawa and co-workers.[1,2] When grown on biphenyl or 4-chlorobiphenyl (4-CB), *Acinetobacter* sp. P6 can oxidize a broad range of PCB congeners, including many tetrachlorobiphenyls and some penta- and

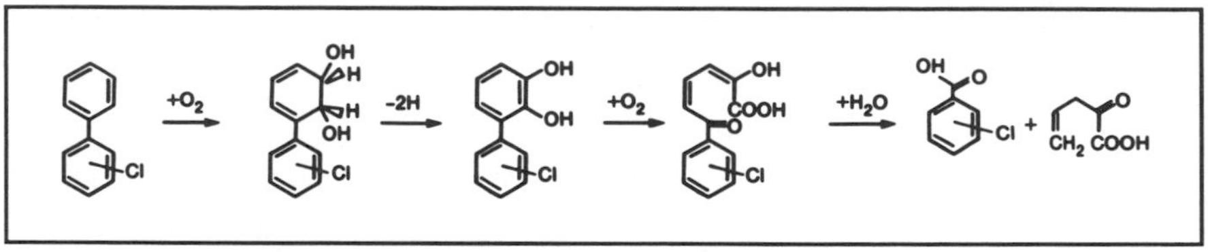

Figure 1. Pathway for the degradation of PCBs.

hexachlorobiphenyls.[7] *Corynebacterium* sp. MB1 was isolated as a contaminant from a culture of *Acinetobacter* sp. P6. Although never compared side by side, the two strains appear to have very similar PCB-degradative competence. Both oxidize PCBs via dioxygenase attack at carbon positions 2,3 followed by dehydrogenation, *meta* ring-fission between carbons 1 and 2, and cleavage to generate chlorobenzoic acid and a five carbon fragment (Figure 1). Both can oxidize some dichlorophenyl rings, most notably those with chlorine substituents at carbon positions 2,3 and 3,4, but neither strain has been shown capable of oxidizing a trichlorophenyl ring.

A. *eutrophus* H850 and *Pseudomonas* sp. LB400 were isolated at different times and from different locations, yet they have remarkably similar congener specificity. Both strains have a superior ability to degrade PCBs via attack on 2-, 2,4-, 2,5-, 2,3,6- and 2,4,5-chlorophenyl rings, all of which are common substituents in the commercial PCB mixtures (Aroclors). Because of this, they degrade many tetra- and pentachlorobiphenyls and some hexachlorobiphenyls. These strains also metabolize biphenyl and PCBs via a 2,3-dioxygenase pathway (see Figure 1), but in addition they metabolize PCBs containing a 2,5-chlorophenyl ring via 3,4-dioxygenase attack (Figure 2, A).[8,4] It appears that the 3,4-dihydrodiol cannot be dehydrogenated or further metabolized in these microorganisms except by a second 3,4-dioxygenase attack to generate a *bis*-diol.[8]

Both A. *eutrophus* H850 and *Pseudomonas* sp. LB400 can oxidize 2,4,5,2',4',5'-CB to a single-ring product, 2',4',5'-trichloroacetophenone,[4,6,8] but the route of degradation of this congener has not been understood as it has no unchlorinated 2,3- or 3,4- position available for dioxygenase attack. However, we have recently obtained evidence that the 2,3-dioxygenase in these organisms can

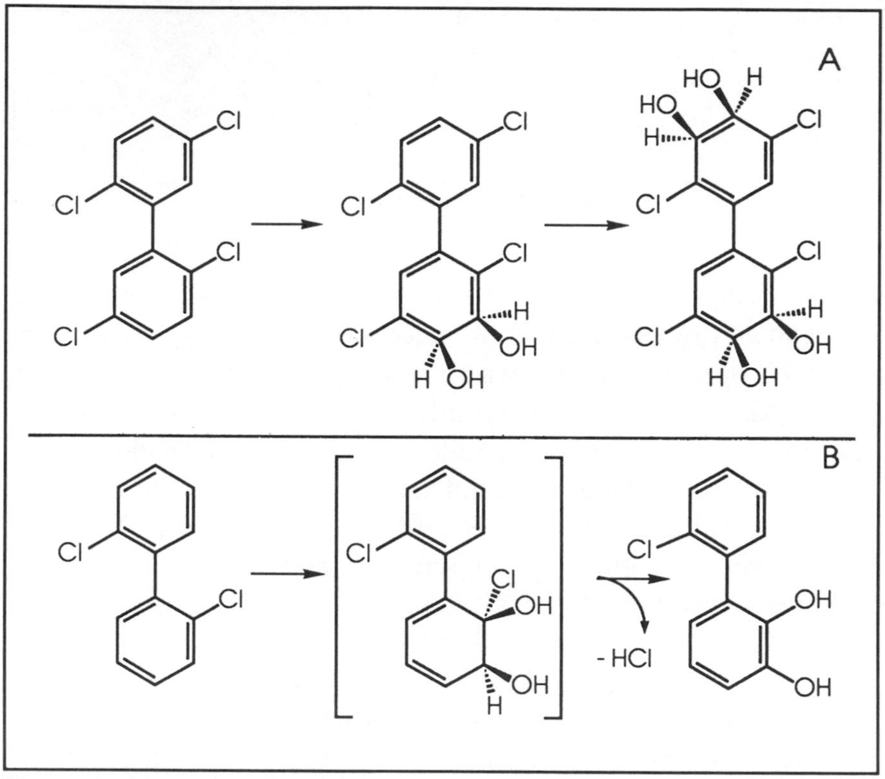

Figure 2. Alternative dioxygenase attacks on PCBs that occur in *Alcaligenes eutrophus* H850 and *Pseudomonas* sp. LB400: **(A)** 3,4 dioxygenase attack; **(B)** 2,3-dioxygenase attack at an *ortho*-chlorinated carbon.

attack at an *ortho*-chlorinated carbon and may even exhibit a preference for attack at a chlorinated position in PCB congeners containing chlorines at carbon positions 2,2'.[9] Figure 2, panel B illustrates the proposed reaction. Instead of a dihydrodiol, an unstable intermediate would form that would spontaneously lose a chloride ion to form a dihydroxy-chlorobiphenyl. The dihydroxy-chlorobiphenyl could then be further metabolized via the biphenyl 2,3-dioxygenase pathway. Dioxygenase attack at the *ortho*-chlorine of the 2,5-chlorophenyl ring of 2,5,2',5'-CB would result in loss of the *ortho*-chlorine and would generate 2,5,3'-trichloro-5',6'-dihydroxybiphenyl, the same intermediate that would result from conventional 2,3-dioxygenase attack on the 3-chlorophenyl ring of 2,5,3'-CB. In other words, once the 2-

chlorine of a 2,5-chlorophenyl ring is removed, the ring would be metabolized exactly like a 3-chlorophenyl ring. Because the oxidation of a 3-chlorophenyl ring of a PCB generates chloroacetophenones,[4,10] this would explain the production of chloroacetophenones from the metabolism of PCBs containing a 2,5-chlorophenyl ring. Presumably 2,4,5,2',4',5'-CB could be metabolized in much the same way.

It is not yet clear whether a single PCB–biphenyl dioxygenase with relaxed specificity is responsible for all three types of dioxygenase attacks that have been observed in *A. eutrophus* H850 and *Pseudomonas* sp. LB400. It is clear, however, that there are at least two classes of PCB/biphenyl dioxygenases that differ markedly in congener reactivity preferences. The type of dioxygenase found in *Acinetobacter* sp. P6 and *Corynebacterium* sp. MB1 is particularly well suited to the degradation of the more planar PCB congeners such as 4,4'-CB and 3,3'-CB and to congeners with a single *ortho*-chlorine, such as 2,4,5,4'-CB. The class of dioxygenase typified by *A. eutrophus* H850 and *Pseudomonas* sp. LB400 preferentially degrades congeners containing an *ortho*-chlorine on each ring (2,2') and congeners containing a 2-, 2,4-, 2,5-, 2,3,6-, or 2,4,5-chlorophenyl ring, but has a limited ability to degrade congeners containing 4-chlorophenyl rings. This is clearly illustrated by the fact that the latter two strains cannot degrade 2,4,5,4'-CB but can degrade 2,4,5,2',4',5'-CB. The PCB congener reactivity preferences of these two dioxygenase classes complement each other so well that treatment of Aroclor 1242 with both *Corynebacterium* sp. MB1 and *Pseudomonas* sp. LB400 resulted in total degradation of almost all congeners in the Aroclor.[11]

Aroclor 1254 is a more difficult substrate because it is more highly chlorinated, but substantial degradation of this Aroclor by several bacteria has now been demonstrated in the laboratory. Most PCB degradation assays have been conducted with resting-cell suspensions because this permits the correlation of degradation activity to cell number and therefore provides a means of more direct comparisons between strains. However, because the bacteria probably gain little or no energy from the metabolism of the more highly chlorinated congeners, the metabolism of PCBs would not be optimal under resting-cell conditions unless nutrients and cofactors were replenished. Recently, a direct comparison was made of the ability of two bacterial strains, *Acinetobacter* sp. P6 and *Arthrobacter* sp. B1B, to oxidize Aroclor 1254 as resting cell suspensions and as cells actively growing on biphenyl.[7] The authors found that for both bacterial strains, growing cells were superior to resting cells in terms of the total amount of PCB degraded, the extent of depletion of specific congeners, and the diversity of congeners that were degraded. Resting cells of *Acinetobacter* sp. P6 degraded 17 percent of Aroclor 1254 (10ppm) and the components of 19 of the 40 capillary gas-chromatographic peaks of Aroclor 1254. Cells of the same strain growing on biphenyl degraded 32 percent of the Aroclor and the components of six additional peaks.[7] The congeners that were degraded by growing cells included 2,5,2',5'-CB and several other congeners containing a 2,5-chlorophenyl ring. These are congeners against which this strain has been reported to have only weak activity.[2] At this point, only resting cell data are available for *A. eutrophus* H850. However, even under these conditions H850 degraded the components of 21 of 44 capillary peaks to effect a degradation of 35 percent of Aroclor 1254.[5] Because the congeners that were selectively degraded by *Acinetobacter* sp. P6 and *A. eutrophus* H850 differed, treatment of Aroclor 1254 with both strains should result in even better degradation.

Genetics of PCB Degrading Bacteria

Until recently little was known about the genes that encode the enzymes responsible for PCB degradation, but the genes encoding the entire PCB degradation pathway have now been cloned from *Pseudomonas* sp. LB400, *A. eutrophus* H850, and *P. putida* OU83,[12-14] and the genes for part of the pathway have been cloned for several other *Pseudomonas* strains.[15,16] The recombinant *Escherichia coli* containing the insert from *Pseudomonas* sp. LB400 has been shown to degrade Aroclor 1242 nearly as well as the donor strain, but unlike *Pseudomonas* sp. LB400, the recombinant did not require growth on biphenyl to achieve high levels of degradative activity.[12] In addition,

DNA-DNA hybridization experiments comparing the genes for PCB degradation from *Pseudomonas* sp. LB400 with those of seven other PCB-degrading strains showed that these genes are closely related in *Pseudomonas* sp. LB400 and *A. eutrophus* H850 but that they are genetically distinct from the other six strains.[17] The six strains included *Corynebacterium* sp. MB1 and four other species with PCB congener selectivity preferences similar to albeit narrower than that of *Corynebacterium* sp. MB1. These results confirm the existence of at least two distinct classes of genes encoding PCB degradation.[17] In the region of DNA encoding PCB metabolism, *A. eutrophus* H850 and *Pseudomonas* sp. LB400 showed a strong conservation of restriction sites, yet no other sequence similarities were detected in the two genomes. The authors inferred that these genes must have been acquired through some form of DNA transfer and that the genes for PCB degradation can be spread within bacterial populations in the environment.[17] However, in these two strains the PCB degradation pathway does not appear to be plasmid-encoded.[17]

Degradation of PCBs in Soil

There is little evidence for PCB degradation in soil in nature, yet bacteria capable of degrading PCBs are easily isolated from PCB-contaminated soils by enrichment with biphenyl. The natural substrate for the biphenyl–PCB-degradative enzymes has not been identified, but at present it appears that biphenyl or a monochlorobiphenyl is required as a growth substrate in order to achieve maximum activity of the enzymes involved in PCB degradation. Our laboratory studies have shown that *A. eutrophus* H850, *Pseudomonas* sp. LB400, and *Corynebacterium* sp. MB1 all have reduced PCB-degrading activity when grown on carbon sources such as glucose, succinate, glutamate, histidine, or Luria broth rather than biphenyl. The PCB congeners that persist in soil generally have three or more chlorines and will not support the growth of any of the PCB-degrading bacterial strains described in the literature. This is a major obstacle to PCB degradation *in situ*. Because the PCB congeners that are present at spill sites will not support growth, we know of no way to enrich or sustain a PCB-degrading population unless biphenyl is added.

Some work has been done on the degradation of PCBs in soil. Two papers describe laboratory experiments investigating the conditions under which Aroclor 1242 (100ppm) in soil could be degraded.[18,19] In these experiments it was found that no significant degradation occurred unless biphenyl was added (3.3mg/kg). The addition of biphenyl alone (without bacterial inoculum) resulted in approximately 60 percent degradation of the PCB in 49 days. When a single inoculum of *Acinetobacter* sp. P6 was also added, 70 percent of the PCB was degraded, including a higher proportion of tetrachlorobiphenyl. Some congeners such as 2,5,2',5'-CB were refractory.

Plating assays were conducted to determine the growth kinetics of the bacterial population in the soil capable of using biphenyl as a carbon source. After the addition of biphenyl, the population increased rapidly for 10 to 15 days, then declined exponentially when the biphenyl was exhausted.[19] This suggests that sustained degradation of PCBs would require repeated applications of biphenyl or some other substrate that would sustain the activity of the PCB-degrading population. It was also established that 72.5 percent of the degraded PCB was mineralized to carbon dioxide, carbonate, and bicarbonate. This result indicates that microorganisms indigenous to the soil were capable of mineralizing the by-products of PCB degradation: chlorobenzoic acids and chlorinated organic acids.

The experiments just described were conducted with clean soil that was treated with PCBs in the laboratory. However, actual spills are often contaminated with other organic pollutants such as oil. If the PCBs are sequestered in dispersed oils or waxes, their bioavailability may be quite limited. In addition, the nature of the soil (sand, clay, organic content) affects the sorption of the PCBs and hence their bioavailability.

Recently, a series of laboratory experiments was conducted using PCB-contaminated soil obtained from a drag strip in South Glenns Falls, New York.[11,20] The PCB was partially evaporated (depleted in di- and trichlorobiphenyls) Aroclor 1242 at a concentration of 525ppm. Initial studies were conducted under optimal conditions to determine if the PCB could be degraded: 0.4g of soil was incubated with 2ml of *Pseudomonas* sp. LB400 (1 O.D.$_{615nm}$, 30°C, 250rpm for 3 days). Under these conditions, 50 percent of the PCBs were degraded. However, percolation experiments of the same soil dosed three times per week with *Pseudomonas* sp. LB400 showed a much lower rate of degradation. In undisturbed soil, 50 percent of the PCB in the top centimeter was degraded in 15 weeks, but only 10 percent of the PCBs below a depth of one centimeter was degraded. When thoroughly mixed after each application of bacteria, 35 percent degradation at all depths was achieved in 23 weeks.

Following these laboratory studies, a field test was conducted in a site at the drag strip in South Glenns Falls from June to late October, 1987.[20] *Pseudomonas* sp. LB400 was again applied three times a week. Half of the 3m x 3m test plot was left undisturbed and half was rototilled weekly. At the end of the 19-week test, 25 percent degradation had occurred in the top centimeter, but significantly less degradation occurred below the surface. In the half that was mixed, 19 percent of the PCB was degraded throughout the 15cm depth. Undoubtedly, cell viability, temperature conditions, and moisture control all affected the outcome of the field test, but the oil and other organic pollutants in the soil were probably also a major factor.

Organic pollutants appeared to be the major obstacle to biodegradation of Aroclor 1242 in an industrial sludge from a settling tank that we investigated.[21] The sludge was composed of oily coarse sand containing about 500ppm of Aroclor 1242 with small amounts of Aroclors 1221, 1016, and 1254. Additional organic compounds present in the sludge included trichlorobenzenes, di(2-ethylhexyl) phthalate (DEHP), mineral oil, kerosene, and No. 2 fuel oil. The PCBs in the sludge were completely refractory to degradation by high cell densities of either *Pseudomonas* sp. LB400 or *A. eutrophus* H850. When subsequent experiments ruled out water-soluble inhibitory agents as the source of the problem, we suspected the other organic pollutants in the sludge. The most prominent of these was DEHP, which we estimated was present at approximately a 150:1 ratio relative to the PCB (w:w). DEHP is an oily substance that is extensively used as a plasticizer. Aroclor 1242 has a very low solubility in

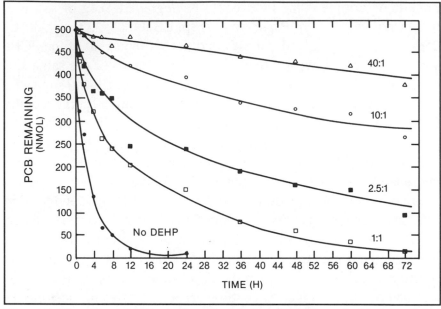

Figure 3. The effect of di(2-ethylhexyl) phthalate (DEHP) on the biodegradation of 2,4'-CB by *Alcaligenes eutrophus* H850. The 2,4'-CB was incubated with resting cells of *A. eutrophus* H850 in the presence of various amounts of DEHP. The ratios on the graph refer to the molar ratio of DEHP to PCB.

water (288ppb) but is readily soluble in oil. In fact, the octanol:water partition coefficient for Aroclor 1242 is 196,500.[22] The partitioning of PCB into an oil phase such as DEHP would be expected to depress its availability for biodegradation.

In a resting-cell assay[23] we compared the biodegradation of Aroclor 1242 (10ppm) by *A. eutrophus* H850 in the presence and absence of a 150-fold excess of DEHP. The sample without DEHP was 78 percent degraded in 72 hours, but no degradation of the PCB was detected in the presence of DEHP. A second experiment examined the effect of DEHP on the biodegradation of 2,4'-CB. The results are shown in Figure 3. In the absence of DEHP, the PCB was nearly 50 percent degraded in two hours, but when DEHP was added at the same molar concentration as the PCB, it took six hours to degrade half the PCB. With a 10-fold molar excess of DEHP, the PCB was still not 50 percent degraded at 72 hours, and with a 40-fold molar excess, less than 25 percent of the PCB was degraded in 72 hours.

It is apparent from these experiments that DEHP, even at low concentrations, had a strong negative effect on PCB degradation. We have established that *A. eutrophus* H850 can grow in the presence of 10 percent DEHP, so the observed effect on PCB biodegradation cannot be attributed to toxicity. Other possible explanations are (1) the DEHP might compete with PCB for, or otherwise affect, the PCB-degrading enzymes, or (2) the DEHP might sequester the PCB and make it unavailable for degradation. We favor the latter possibility.

Reductive Dechlorination of PCBs in Anaerobic Sediments

In 1984 Brown *et al.*[24] reported that extensive dechlorination of PCBs had occurred in the anaerobic sediments of the Hudson River south of Hudson Falls, New York. Existing usage records indicate that this PCB was originally almost entirely Aroclor 1242 that was released from a capacitor manufacturing plant between 1952 and 1971. Aroclor 1242 is primarily composed of tri- and tetrachlorobiphenyls (see Figure 4) and contains only 0.7 percent 2-chlorobiphenyl and 11.5 percent dichlorobiphenyl, but the PCB extracted from the anaerobic river sediments was composed of 10 to 43 percent 2-chlorobiphenyl and 21 to 50 percent dichlorobiphenyls. Capillary gas chromatography showed particularly prominent peaks of lower congeners with *ortho*-chlorines: 2-, 2,2'-, 2,6-, 2,3'-, 2,3-, 2,4-, 2,6, 2'-, 2,6,3'-, and 2,6,4'-CB.[24-26] The authors concluded that anaerobic microorganisms were selectively removing chlorines from the *meta* and *para* positions of the more highly chlorinated PCB congeners, and this resulted in the accumulation of *ortho*-chlorinated mono-, di-, and trichlorobiphenyls. Furthermore, because several distinct dechlorination patterns were seen, the authors concluded that several different populations of microorganisms were involved.

Extensive dechlorination of Aroclor 1260 (primarily hexa- and heptachlorobiphenyls) was seen in the anaerobic sediments of Silver Lake (Pittsfield, Massachusetts), which is located next to a transformer manufacturing plant. The PCB extracted from the sediments showed a 90 to 98 percent loss of the hexa- and heptachlorobiphenyl

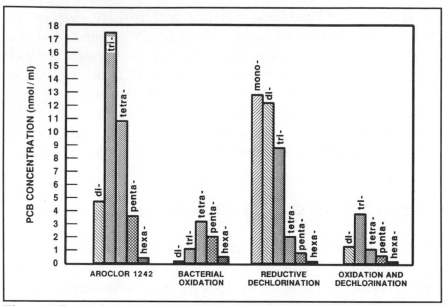

Figure 4. Comparison of the effect of bacterial oxidation, reductive dechlorination, or both on Aroclor 1260. The data were taken from Figure 1 and Table 1 in Bedard and co-workers[5] and were compiled by Vogel, Nies, and Anid.[32] Bacterial oxidation: resting-cells of *Alcaligenes eutrophus* H850 were incubated with 10ppm of Aroclor 1242 at 30°C for 48 hours. Reductive dechlorination: environmentally dechlorinated Aroclor 1242 was extracted from Hudson River sediment. Oxidation and dechlorination: environmentally dechlorinated Aroclor 1260 from Hudson River sediment was incubated with resting-cells of *A. eutrophus* H850 as previously described.

peaks of Aroclor 1260 and the appearance of large amounts of tri- and tetrachlorobiphenyls. (These homologs account for less than one percent of the total PCB in Aroclor 1260, but they account for 57 to 82 percent of the total PCB in the altered Aroclor extracted from the sediments.[25,26] Evidence for dechlorination of PCBs in anaerobic sediments at several other spill sites was also found. These included freshwater sediments from Waukegan Harbor, Illinois; the Hoosic River (North Adams, Massachusetts); the Sheboygan River (Sheboygan, Wisconsin); and sediments from two marine sites: the Acushnet Estuary (New Bedford, Massachusetts), and Escambia Bay (Pensacola, Florida).[25-27]

Experiments in several laboratories have now confirmed that reductive dechlorination of PCBs occurs in PCB-contaminated sediments cultured under anaerobic conditions.[28-32] Quensen, Tiedje, and Boyd[28] transferred anaerobic microorganisms from a PCB-contaminated Hudson River sediment sample that showed evidence of extensive dechlorination to an autoclaved PCB-free sediment that had been amended with 700ppm of Aroclor 1242 in the laboratory. After 16 weeks' incubation in a minimal medium under methanogenic conditions, 53 percent of the total chlorine was removed. Furthermore, 2-CB, a congener not present in Aroclor 1242, represented 63 percent of the total PCB at the end of the incubation, and 2,2'- and 2,6-CB increased from 1 percent to 14 percent. The observed dechlorination pattern was very similar to environmental dechlorination pattern C, one of the three dechlorination patterns most commonly seen in the region of the Hudson River from which the inoculum was obtained.[25,26]

In more recent experiments[29] conducted under similar conditions (again with Hudson River sediment), extensive dechlorination of Aroclors 1242 and 1248 (500ppm on the basis of dry sediment weight) was seen in only eight weeks. By 12 weeks, most tetra- and pentachlorobiphenyls were 80 to 90 percent depleted and *ortho*-substituted mono- and dichlorobiphenyls had accumulated. Dechlorination of Aroclors 1254 and 1260 was also observed but at much slower rates. When the same sediments were incubated with biphenyl, 2-CB, 2,2'-CB, or 2,6-CB, no dechlorination or degradation was observed, indicating that these compounds are terminal dechlorination products for the methanogenic consortia. Two of the more toxic PCB congeners, 3,4,3',4'- and 2,3,4,3',4'-CB were individually added to sediment incubations with Aroclor 1242. Both were completely removed by dechlorination.

Two other laboratories have also observed dechlorination of Aroclors 1242[31,32] and 1260[31] in laboratory experiments with Hudson River sediment incubated under methanogenic conditions. In these experiments, several distinct dechlorination patterns were observed under slightly different culture conditions. Taken in various combinations, these dechlorination patterns account for the environmental dechlorination patterns previously reported for Hudson River sedi-

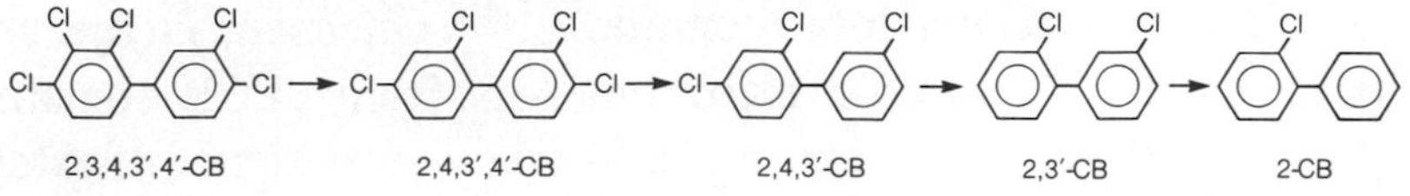

Figure 5. Reductive dechlorination of 2,3,4,3',4'-CB as proposed and later confirmed in the laboratory.

ments[25,26,33] and suggest that the Hudson River sediments contain several different populations of anaerobes that are able to dechlorinate PCBs.

Dechlorination of Aroclor 1242 in Silver Lake sediment has now been observed in the laboratory, but at slower rates than in Hudson River sediment.[29,31]

Dechlorination studies with single congeners have also been initiated. These studies have confirmed that the dechlorination of 2,3,4,3',4'-CB (one of the more toxic congeners) occurs by stepwise removal of all the *meta*- and *para*-chlorines, resulting in the formation of 2-CB, a congener that is easily metabolized by aerobic bacteria and by many higher organisms, including man. Several different sequences of dechlorination of this congener have been seen depending on the incubation conditions, particularly the carbon source and the reduction potential of the medium.[30] The sequence most often seen in Hudson River sediment (Figure 5) is in fact the pattern of dechlorination predicted for this congener based on analysis of the dechlorinated PCBs in Hudson River sediments.[34] The major intermediates are 2,4,3',4'-, 2,4,3'-,and 2,3'-CB

Biodegradation of PCBs in Anaerobic Sediments

Rhee and co-workers[35] have recently reported evidence for the biodegradation of endogenous PCBs (in untreated anaerobic sediments from the Hudson River) incubated in the laboratory under an N_2 atmosphere for seven months.[35] Statistically significant decreases on the order of 33 to 63 percent were observed in congeners ranging from mono- to tetrachlorobiphenyls. Notably, the PCBs in the sediment used in this experiment were already extensively dechlorinated. Sixty-one percent of the PCB was composed of only three congeners: 2-, 2,2'- and 2,6-CB. These congeners have been repeatedly described as terminal dechlorination products in the Hudson River sediments.[24-26,28,29] In the untreated sediment, 2-CB was decreased by 63 percent and 2,2'-CB by 49 percent over the course of the experiment. Amending the sediment with biphenyl had little effect on the degradation of the mono- and dichlorobiphenyls but significantly enhanced the biodegradation of the more highly chlorinated congeners.

No biodegradation products have been identified from the experiments just described.[35] Clearly, this needs to be done. There are various reports of the anaerobic degradation of other halogenated compounds, but in all cases the biodegradation occurred only after complete dehalogenation.[36-39] Although the authors found no evidence of dechlorination, it is possible that 2-CB, 2,2'-CB, and other congeners in these sediments were completely dechlorinated to biphenyl prior to biodegradation. Regardless of the mechanism, these results suggest that the bacterial population indigenous to the Hudson River sediments has the ability to mineralize PCBs.

It should be noted that all reported observations of reductive dechlorination of PCBs occurred with methanogenic consortia. In contrast, the anaerobic incubations that resulted in biodegradation were not methanogenic, although the reduction potential was very low (-210 to -310mv as indicated by a platinum electrode versus a silver/silver chloride electrode).

Discussion

Research over the past decade has demonstrated that aerobic bacteria are versatile and effective agents for biodegradation of PCBs. Four strains of bacteria representing four different species have been shown to oxidize many tetra- and pentachlorobiphenyls and some hexachlorobiphenyls. It has been shown that at least two genetically distinct classes of PCB-degradative enzymes exist and that the PCB congener reactivity preferences for these two classes complement each other. Thus, treatment of Aroclor 1242 with a mixture composed of one organism of each class degrades nearly all of the components of the Aroclor. Laboratory experiments have demonstrated that both *Acinetobacter* sp. P6 and *A. eutrophus* H850 can each degrade approximately one third of the total PCB in Aroclor 1254. Because the congener selectivity patterns of these two strains complement each other, it is to be expected that a mixture of the two organisms would be even more effective.

There are at least four primary factors limiting the degradation of PCBs in soil:

1. Degree of chlorination of the PCB. Generally, PCBs with five or more chlorines are more refractory than the lower congeners, yet recent studies on the biodegradation of Aroclor 1254 show considerable promise.[5,7] Genetic engineering may permit the development of recombinant organisms with increased degradative capabilities.

2. Solubility and bioavailability of the PCB. In order to be degraded, the PCBs must come in contact with the cells. This problem can be minimized under incubation conditions that involve rapidly mixing or shaking the contaminated soil with cell suspensions under controlled conditions (essentially a small bioreactor). Mixing may also be effective for *in situ* treatment. The presence of oil or other organic pollutants may increase the problem of availability due to partitioning of the PCB into the organic phase. This could be alleviated through identification of effective bacterial strains for degradation of these contaminants.

3. Inability of the PCB-degrading bacteria to use PCBs (except monochlorobiphenyls) as growth substrates. This means that the PCB-degraders have no selective advantage over other soil bacteria. Furthermore, high levels of PCB-degradative activity have not been achieved unless the cells are grown on biphenyl. In fact, the best activity has been found when cells are actively growing on biphenyl. There are two ways that this problem might be overcome. First, biphenyl or another suitable carbon source might be added to the contaminated soil. Research would be required to identify alternative growth substrates. Second, genetic engineering might be used to combine the pathways for PCB biodegradation and chlorobenzoic acid degradation in a single organism in order to develop recombinant strains capable of mineralizing PCBs.

4. Temperature and moisture conditions. In situ treatment of PCBs will require developing ways of preventing wide variations in temperature and moisture. Some organisms may be more tolerant than others of such fluctuations and might be good candidates for the basis of new strains developed through genetic engineering.

The prospects for PCB removal in aquatic sediments are excellent. It appears that anaerobic dechlorination of PCBs in both freshwater and marine sediments is widespread. Furthermore, it appears that several populations of microorganisms may be involved. Like the aerobic PCB-degrading bacteria, these populations exhibit different congener selectivity patterns.

Reductive dechlorination of PCBs in anaerobic sediments has now been confirmed in three different laboratories. Efforts are needed to determine the optimal culture conditions for dechlorination (carbon source, mineral requirements, temperature) and the conditions under which the organisms responsible can be enriched and possibly isolated. Ideally, the dechlorinating organisms should be isolated and characterized. At a minimum, conditions must be established for maintaining stable dechlorinating consortia, preferably on a defined medium in the absence of sediment.

There is a need to monitor the progress of dechlorination in sediments where it is known to be occurring (such as the Hudson River) in order to identify the limitations of the dechlorinating system that is operative in the sediment. Because different populations exhibit distinct congener selectivity patterns, it may be possible to inoculate sediment with a second population of PCB-dechlorinating bacteria that will aid the activity of the endogenous population.

In addition, efforts are needed to analyze other aquatic sediments for evidence of reductive dechlorination of PCBs. If evidence of dechlorination is not found or if it is not occurring rapidly enough, laboratory experiments should be done to determine if there are conditions under which reductive dechlorination of PCBs can be stimulated in the sediment. This may require the addition of an essential nutrient (carbon source, phosphate, nitrogen source, trace metals) or may require inoculation with dechlorinating microorganisms from another sediment.

At the time of this writing no evidence has been found for dechlorination of the *ortho*-chlorinated congeners that accumulate as a result of the removal of *meta*- and *para*-chlorines from more highly chlorinated congeners. These congeners (2-, 2,2'-, 2,6-, 2,6,2'-CB) can all be degraded by naturally occurring aerobic bacteria that were originally isolated from the same sediments in which the dechlorination occurred.[3,5] Therefore, it should be possible to develop conditions to promote aerobic degradation of these congeners by introducing oxygen. The benefit of such a sequential anaerobic-aerobic treatment is apparent from Figure 4. Further efforts in this area are already in progress.[32] Alternatively, anaerobic populations that can completely dechlorinate or biodegrade the *ortho*-chlorinated lower congeners may already exist in the sediments. Rhee and co-workers[35] observed significant depletion of these congeners in unamended Hudson River sediment incubated in the laboratory. Further experiments are needed to clarify the mechanism of the depletion of these congeners.

In summary, it appears that natural microbial populations already have the capacity to biodegrade most if not all of the PCBs that contaminate the environment. Through research directed at understanding the growth requirements of these populations, it should be possible to accelerate biodegradation of the PCBs that persist as environmental contaminants.

References

1. K. Furukawa, in *Biodegradation and Detoxification of Environmental Pollutants*, A.M. Chakrabarty, Ed., (CRC Press, Inc., Boca Raton, FL, 1982), pp.35-37.

2. K. Furukawa, N. Tomizuka, and A. Kamibayashi, *Appl.Environ. Microbiol.* **38**, 301, (1979).
3. D.L. Bedard *et al.*, *Appl. Environ. Microbiol.* **51**, 761 (1986).
4. D.L. Bedard *et al.*, *Appl. Environ. Microbiol.* **53**, 1103 (1987).
5. D.L. Bedard *et al.*, *Appl. Environ. Microbiol.* **53**, 1094 (1987).
6. L.H. Bopp, *J. Indust. Microbiol.* **1**, 23 (1987).
7. H.-P.E. Kohler, D. Kohler-Staub, and D.D. Focht, *Appl. Environ. Microbiol.* **54**, 1940 (1988).
8. L. Nadim *et al.*, in *Proceedings of the 13th Annual Research Symposium on Land Disposal, Remedial Action, Incineration, and Treatment of Hazardous Waste, EPA/600/ 2-86/090*, (U.S. Environmental Protection Agency, Cincinnati, OH, 1987), pp. 395-402.
9. D.L. Bedard, in *Research and Development Program for the Destruction of PCBs, Eighth Progress Report* (General Electric Company Corporate Research and Development Center, Schenectady, NY, 1989), pp. 15-23.
10. D.L. Bedard, M.L. Haberl, and R.J. May, in *Research and Development Program for the Destruction of PCBs, Sixth Progress Report* (General Electric Corporate Research and Development Center, Schenectady, NY, 1987), pp. 9-16.
11. R. Unterman *et al.*, in *Reducing Risks from Environmental Chemicals Through Biotechnology*, G.S. Omen *et al.*, Eds. (Plenum Press, New York , 1988) pp. 253-269.
12. F.J. Mondello, *J. Bacteriol.*, **171**, 1725 (1989).
13. F.J. Mondello and J.R. Yates, in *Proceedings of the Fifteenth Annual Research Symposium on Remedial Action, Treatment, and Disposal of Hazardous Waste*, in press.
14. A. Khan and S. Walia, *Appl. Environ. Microbiol.* **55**, 798 (1989).
15. K. Furukawa and T. Miyazaki, *J. Bacteriol.* **166**, 392 (1986).
16. K. Kimbara *et al.*, *J. Bacteriol.* **171**, 2740 (1989).
17. J.R. Yates and F.J. Mondello, *J. Bacteriol.* **171**, 1733 (1989).
18. W. Brunner, F.H. Sutherland, and D.D. Focht, *J. Environ. Qual.* **14**, 324 (1984).
19. D.D. Focht and W. Brunner, *Appl. Environ. Microbiol.* **50**, 1058 (1985).
20. R.D. Unterman *et al.*, in *Research and Development Program for the Destruction of PCBs, Seventh Progress Report* (General Electric Company Corporate Research and Development Center, Schenectady, NY, 1988), pp. 7-15.
21. D.L. Bedard and J.A. Bergeron, in *Research and Development Program for the Destruction of PCBs, Seventh Progress Report* (General Electric Company Corporate Research and Development Center, Schenectady, NY, 1988) pp. 17-21.
22. S.F.J. Chou and R.A. Griffen, in *PCBs and the Environment, Chapter 5*, J.S. Waid, Ed. (CRC Press Inc., Boca Raton, FL, 1986).
23. D.L. Bedard *et al.*, *Appl. Environ. Microbiol.* **51**, 761 (1986).
24. J.F. Brown, Jr., *et al.*, *Northeast. Environ. Sci.* **3**, 167 (1984).
25. J.F. Brown, Jr., *et al.*, *Science* **236**, 709 (1987).
26. J.F. Brown *et al.*, *Environ. Toxicol. Chem.* **6**, 579 (1987).
27. J.F. Brown *et al.*, in *Research and Development Program for the Destruction of PCBs, Seventh Progress Report* (General Electric Company Corporate Research and Development Center, Schenectady, NY, 1988), pp. 61-72.
28. J.F. Quensen, III, J.M. Tiedje, and S.A. Boyd, *Science* **242**, 752 (1988).
29. J.M. Tiedje, S.A. Boyd, and J.F. Quensen, in *Research and Development Program for the Destruction of PCBs, Eighth Progress Report* (General Electric Company Corporate Research and Development Center, Schenectady, New York, 1989), pp. 37-47.
30. D.A. Abramowicz, M.J. Brennan, and H. Van Dort, in *Research and Development*

Program for the Destruction of PCBs, Eighth Progress Report (General Electric Company Corporate Research and Development Center, Schenectady, NY, 1989), pp. 49-59.

31. D.A. Abramowicz, H.M. Van Dort, and M.J. Brennan, in *Research and Development Program for the Destruction of PCBs, Eighth Progress Report* (General Electric Company Corporate Research and Development Center, Schenectady, NY, 1989), pp .61-70.

32. T.M. Vogel, L. Nies, and P.J. Anid, in *Research and Development Program for the Destruction of PCBs, Eighth Progress Report* (General Electric Company Corporate Research and Development Center, Schenectady, NY, 1989), pp .71-80.

33. J.F. Brown *et al.*, in *Research and Development Program for the Destruction of PCBs, Eighth Progress Report* (General Electric Company Corporate Research and Development Center, Schenectady, NY, 1989), pp. 85-90.

34. J.F. Brown, Jr., personal communication.

35. G.Y. Rhee *et al.*, *Water Res.*, in press.

36. S.A. Boyd *et al.*, *Appl. Environ. Microbiol.* **46**, 50 (1983).

37. S.A. Boyd and D.R. Shelton, *Appl. Environ. Microbiol.* **47**, 272 (1984).

38. A. Horowitz, J.M. Suflita, and J.M. Tiedje, *Appl. Environ. Microbiol.* **45**, 1459 (1983).

39. J.M. Suflita, J.A. Robinson, and J.M. Tiedje, *Appl. Environ. Microbiol.* **45**, 1466 (1983).

Discussion

Kamely: Have you studied the fate of the biphenyl-degrading bacteria? What happens to them when they finish degrading the biphenyl? Do they die off or can you recover them anytime you add biphenyl again?

Bedard: That experiment has not been done. That was Brunner and Focht's work. They did not report on trying to revive the bacteria.

Kamely: Has anybody tried to add nutrient or fertilizers or enhancers with these PCB-degrading bacteria to see if they can enhance the rate of degradation?

Bedard: No, they have not. One point that I did not make is that the PCB-degraders will not degrade PCBs optimally unless they are grown on biphenyl. That is, the cells are not fully "turned-on" unless they are grown on biphenyl. Biphenyl is the only substrate that we know that can induce maximal PCB-degradation activity. Focht and Brunner found the same thing. When they inoculated the soil with bacteria and did not add biphenyl, they got minimal degradation of PCBs.

Ribbons: I was very interested in the dihydroxylation you showed of the 2,5,2',5'-tetrachlorobiphenyl molecule. You described it as a 3,4-dihydroxylation. That is very important for chemists. I would suggest to you that, in fact, it is still just a 2,3-dihydroxylation with respect to the chlorines as opposed to the other aromatic ring, and so it really looks like the toluene system with a great big substituent at the bottom.

Bedard: Yes, it could be thought of that way, but it is a novel position of attack on the PCB.

20

Biotechnology in Hazardous Waste Management in The Netherlands

K. Visscher
J. Brinkman
E.R. Soczó

*Laboratory for Waste and
Emission Research (LAE)
National Institute of Public
Health and Environmental
Protection (RIVM)
P.O. Box 1
3720 BA Bilthoven
The Netherlands*

Application of biological processes in controlling environmental problems has increased decidedly over the past decade. A characteristic and important aspect of biological processes is that pollutants are degraded into products that are part of naturally occurring cycles.

Generation of more fundamental knowledge on microbiological degradation offers the possibility of broadening the field of application, especially for degrading not easily biodegradable pollutants. This creates the opportunity for developing biological methods for treating of hazardous and toxic wastes.

Research in the Netherlands has so far resulted in important applications including treatment processes for industrial wastewater, processes for cleaning contaminated soil, and polluted air purification. However, more research is necessary in order to apply present and future microbiological knowledge to specific environmental problems. The Dutch Government supports this type of environmentally and often economically relevant research.

This article looks at technological aspects of developments in biotreatment of hazardous wastes, and techniques relating to several fields of application.

Introduction

In recent years biotechnology has made considerable progress, and with growing knowledge of the relevant microbiological processes, it can now be stated that the possibilities for using biotechnology in dealing with environmental problems have increased dramatically, especially in the field of solid waste and wastewater treatment.

In comparison with physicochemical techniques, biotechnological methods have the advantage that use is made of microbiological mineralization processes by which substances foreign to the environment (xenobiotics) are converted to inorganic end products that are part of natural recycling processes. The fact that microbiological processes can offer a solution for these problems cannot be considered to be a recent development. The knowledge of wastewater treatment by microorganisms has been available for the last one hundred years. The production of compost from different sorts of waste has long been the usual method of processing this type of waste. In these applications use is made of mineralization processes that are part of natural recycling processes.

The processes just mentioned are applied in the first place to prevent the uncontrolled release of large quantities of oxygen-binding substances into the environment.

From fundamental microbiology it is known that a great number of xenobiotics can be biologically degraded. Theoretically, this opens the possibility of using biotechnological methods to remove the environmental bottlenecks concerning these substances. Research has started in certain areas of study, and in some cases it has already led to concrete applications. Although certain fundamental microbiological research still has to be carried out, the emphasis is now put on the development of new technologies in order to apply present and future microbiological knowledge to specific environmental problems. This type of environmentally and often economically relevant research is stimulated within the context of the Dutch Research and Development Programme for Environmental Biotechnology. This program is financially supported by the Ministry of Housing, Physical Planning and Environment and by the Ministry of Economic Affairs.

For the setting up and the execution of the program, a Working Party on Environmental Biotechnology has been installed. The actions of this Working Party are coordinated by the RIVM/LAE.[11]

An overview will be given of the developments, stimulated by this program, in the field of processing hazardous waste. The overview will be divided into the most important fields of application, namely the purification of polluted air, the cleaning of soil, and wastewater treatment. Before discussing these items, attention will be paid to more general technological aspects with respect to these applications.

Technological Aspects

Certain technological aspects are important for a further development of processes for the treatment of hazardous waste.

Concentration of microorganisms. By a high concentration of active biomass, the size of the reactor can be reduced. This is an essential condition in order to achieve successful technological developments. Because of a high concentration of microorganisms, there is an additional benefit in the fact that the conversion of toxic components can be speeded up to such a degree that the concentration of these components in the reactor can be kept below the toxification limit of the microorganisms. There are various methods to achieve and maintain such a high concentration of microorganisms. These methods are related to the immobilization of microorganisms on carrier material, the use of membrane reactors, or the separation of microorganisms from the treated wastestream and for return to the reactor. The method to be applied is dependent on the medium that contains the pollution. For example, in the case of a biological filter for air cleaning, immobilization can be achieved relatively easily by fixing the organisms on the solid carrier. Concerning application in wastewater treatment, particularly in cleaning polluted soil, still much effort has to be directed to developing suitable methods.

Mixing and mass transfer. A good mixing for intensive contact between microorganisms, polluting elements, nutrients, and other products is necessary for an effective degradation. The biodegradation can be impeded when the polluted elements are not easily accessible to the microorganisms. This can occur when the pollution is present in low concentrations between other organic components or when the pollution has been strongly adsorbed. It is also possible that no transportation medium (such as water) is available or can be used in order to bring nutrients and polluted elements into intensive contact with the microorganisms.

The problems just described involve technical points that in principle can be solved. In particular, use can be made of the know-how about existing technologies already used in process industry and in processing of chemical waste and wastewater. However, a considerable amount of technological research still has to be carried out in order to develop optimal processes both technologically and economically.

Emission of intermediate products. Compounds that are not soluble in water can be converted by microorganisms into intermediate products that are soluble. In addition, volatile compounds can be formed which, for example, will escape in aerated systems. In these cases, there is a danger that the environmental problem is partly replaced. On the other hand, it may be necessary to remove toxic intermediate products from the system in order not to impede the degradation process.

These factors are closely related and can have a strong effect on each other. With the further development of these technological processes, it will be necessary to keep all these aspects in view.

Purification of Polluted Air

In recent decades biofiltration systems have been developed to clean air by means of microbiological degradation processes. With biofiltration the polluted air is led through a filter (Figure 1) that mainly consists of a natural packing material such as compost.

In this packing material a wide variety of microorganisms can be

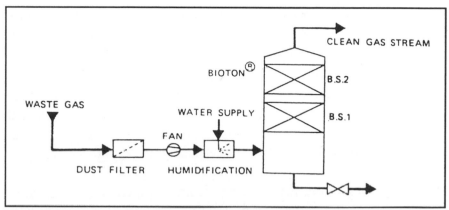

Figure 1. Flow sheet of a two-step biofilter: BS 1 and BS 2 are biological sections in which different microbial populations can be maintained.[5]

found that have the potential of degrading a large number of organic compounds. In The Netherlands, the application of biofiltration started in 1978 when biofilters were used at sewage treatment plants to process polluted air that caused obnoxious odor problems. The surface load of these systems was relatively low (20-100 m³ /m³•h).

In the last few years, the field of application was also extended to industry for the removal of smells and the biogradation of chemicals like alcohols, esters, ketones, and so forth.[2]

This extension of application field was made possible by developments of technical and microbiological research that led to biofiltration systems in which a high conversion rate could be combined with high gas flows and low drops in pressure. The packing material has been very much improved in recent years; aging of the filter packing can be retarded which assures an extended period (years) of relatively high biological activity. The pressure drop of the filter bed can also be decreased considerably, and gas velocities of approximately 400mh⁻¹ and elimination capacities of 100 to 200g organic carbon m⁻³ packing material h⁻¹ for easily biodegradable compounds can be obtained. Costs are in the range of 0.25 to 1.25 U.S. dollars per 1000m³ waste gas to be treated.[5]

In addition, the elimination of xenobiotic compounds retains more attention. For example, the Laboratory for Physical Technology of the Technical University of Eindhoven has studied the degradation of a mixture of ethyl acetate, butyl acetate and toluene in the process air from a lacquer factory. It revealed that the first three mentioned components could be degraded without many problems. Degradation of toluene, however, was not started until the carrier material had been inoculated with bacteria isolated from soil samples from an area near a gas station. To maintain optimal degradation conditions for all four compounds involved, it proved necessary to operate a two-step process.

When degrading the polluted air from a pharmaceutical company containing the compounds acetone, ethanol, isopropanol, and methylenechloride, similar results could be observed. During semitechnical research, it turned out that the component acetone could be almost completely degraded in the first step; the same occurred for ethanol and isopropanol in the second step.

The degradation of methylene chloride, however, was not achieved. When a third step involved inoculation with a culture of *Hypomicrobium* sp. the fourth component was degraded with relative high speed. This research has led to the installation of a full-scale plant.

The experiments just presented also have shown that the accumulation of degradation products in biofilters can cause problems. Accumulation of chlorides was shown to lead at the end to a complete stop of the methylene chloride degradation. This makes a regeneration of the filter necessary. Another problem appeared to be the generally low rates of microbiological elimination of recalcitrant xenobiotics.

Because of the difficulties just mentioned in using biofilters for degradation of xenobiotics, research is now directed to the application of trickling filters. In a trickling filter, the gas flow is moving cocurrently or countercurrently with a water phase through a bed of inert packing material with an attached biolayer. First results on laboratory scale with gas flow rates up to $500 mh^{-1}$ show elimination capacities of up to $200 g/m^3$ reactor hours for dichloromethane and $80 g/m^3$ reactor hours for dichlorethane. Degrees of conversion were achieved up to 70 percent for both substances.[15]

Soil Cleaning Techniques

In January 1983, the Interim Soil Clean-up Act was put into force in The Netherlands. It is expected that by 1997, under this act, approximately 2000 contaminated sites will have been cleaned up. Up to now approximately 3500 contaminated sites have been investigated; however, only in the case of 800 sites has a comprehensive investigation been carried out. Nearly 400 contaminated sites have now been cleaned up. The total expenditure for the investigation and the cleanup was subsidized by the government at a cost of approximately 1.5 billion guilders.

For the enforcement of this act, the development of adequate investigation and cleanup methods was very important.

The initial emphasis has been on the development of thermal and extraction techniques. Since 1984, however, there has also been a strongly increased interest in the development of alternatives such as biological treatment techniques.[6]

The aim of the biological soil treatment is to create favorable environmental conditions in the soil for improvement of the microbiological activity and consequently the enhancement of the biodegradation of the contaminants. Favorable conditions for the microbes mean roughly sufficient oxygen and nutrients supply, a pH ~7, and temperature between 25 and 30°C. The moisture content and a good soil structure are also very important for biological activity.[4]

At present three kinds of biological treatment can be distinguished: landfarming, *in situ* biorestoration, and bioreactors. The landfarming method and *in situ* biorestoration are operational; however, the latter will be improved and tested in the near future. The bioreactors are still in the developmental stage.

Landfarming. In the case of the most simple landfarming method (used by De Ruiter), the contaminated soil is spread out over a sand layer with a drainage system to a depth of approximately 40cm. Prior to this, the soil is protected by means of a plastic layer [approximately 0.5mm polyvinyl chloride (PVC)]. Landfarming is also carried out under so-called conditioned circumstances. This means that during the cleanup process, a better control of parameters such as oxygen,

Table 1
A Few Clean-up Results From Full-scale Landfarming[16]

Company	Type of Soil	Contamination Type	Initial concentration mg/kg dm	Final concentration mg/kg dm
De Ruiter	Clayish Sand	Heavy Oil	3,000- 8,000	1,000
	Loamy sand	Heavy Oil	5,000-20,000	1,000
Mourik	Clayish sand	Kerosene	1,000-10,000	500
	Clayish Sand	Aromatics	100	3
Heidemij	Clayish Sand	Mineral oil	12,000	500

water contents, and temperature is achieved. In the case of the system of Mourik, forced aeration is used for the enhancement of the oxygen supply. The landfarming plots are usually covered, and the air is cleaned by means of a compost filter. By letting in hot air, the soil temperature can be increased. In the case of the so-called Cum Bac system of Heidemij, the temperature of the soil is raised by the "greenhouse" effect. Forced aeration and heating make it possible to increase the depth of the layer of the soil to be cleaned to approximately 100 to 150cm, while a quicker breakdown of substances is also achieved. Some treatment results are summarized in Table 1. It can be concluded that good results have been achieved with the treatment of contaminated sand and clayish or loamy sands. Experience has shown that this technique is in general suitable for the removal of different types of oil and aromatic hydrocarbons. After one "growing season," the final oil concentrations reached are in most cases between 400 and 1000mg/kg dry matter.

A high level of decontamination (90 to 99 percent) can be obtained in the case of lower PCAs. However, a much lower degradation level can be reached (in a longer period) in the case of higher PCAs.

The cleanup costs of landfarming are in the range of 25 to 40 U.S. dollars per ton of soil.[16]

In situ biorestoration. In situ biorestoration is based on the stimulation of the natural degradation processes in the soil itself. The groundwater is used as a medium for addition of oxygen, nutrients, and eventually detergents and organisms to stimulate biodegradation of the contaminants. The water is infiltrated via drains, trenches, or wells.[16] The pumped-up water containing the dissolved degradation products and a part of the contaminants is treated above the ground and usually recycled. Before starting the biorestoration, the floating layer must be removed. To prevent the contamination from spreading, isolation by means of hydrological or civil-engineering intervention strategies is required.[16]

In situ biorestoration of petrol polluted sandy soil is being investigated at the RIVM (National Institute of Public Health and Environmental Protection) in cooperation with the Netherlands Organization for Applied Scientific Research (TNO). In six columns, process parameters such as nutrient addition (nitrogen, phosphorus), oxygen source (nitrate, peroxide, or air), and substrate addition (acetate) are varied. Biodegradation occurred in the columns where oxygen sources had been added or recirculation of the purified groundwater took place. In these columns 35 to 80 percent of the gasoline turned out to be degraded. With the addition of nutrients and hydrogen peroxide, a reduction from 2900 to 6400mg gasoline per 1kg soil (depending on depth) to 10 to 600mg gasoline per 1kg soil after six months could be observed.[1] However, removal by leaching, especially of volatile aromatics, also turned out to be important. A full-scale experiment at a petrol station where the subsoil has been contaminated with 30,000 liters of gasoline from a leaking tank will start soon. The groundwater that is extracted is recycled after purification by air stripping and biofiltration of the contaminated air.[1] Peroxide will be used as oxygen source. In the last two years, a few cleanup projects were successfully completed. The method can be used for sandy soils contaminated by oil compounds and aromatics.

Bioreactors. Research into the development of bioreactors has only started during the last three years. Generally, it can be stated that development of bioreactors offers the possibility to shorten treatment time of polluted soil from one or two seasons (landfarming, *in situ* biorestoration) to less then two weeks because of the better process control and availability of contaminants for the microorganisms. Furthermore, bioreactors can be of importance for the biological treatment of soil contaminated with substances of low biodegradability (such as halogenated hydrocarbons) and for soils that are generally difficult to treat (such as clay).

Researchers at The University of Groningen are working on the selection and characterization of microorganisms that can degrade halogenated hydrocarbons. Parallel to this research, TNO carries out pilot plant experiments on the mixing characteristics of soil in various types of reactors in order to identify the most suitable process conditions for different kinds of soil. The first results of this experiments are promising. For example, in sandy loam, the concentration of gasoline turned out to be reduced from 10g/kg dry matter to 1.5g/kg dry matter after eight days' retention time in a slurry reactor. Also, low PCAs turned out to be degraded from 99 to 100 percent. On the other hand, degradation of higher PCAs, such as benzopyrene and anthracene was only 30 to 80 percent. (TNO, personal communication).

In the future, research will be directed towards the improvement of the bioavailability of contaminants and the possibilities of inoculation of selected microorganisms.[16]

A completed project in this field is the research on the degradation of hexachlorocyclohexanes (HCH) that has been carried out by the RIN (Research Institute for Nature Conservation) in cooperation with LU-Wageningen (Agricultural University Wageningen). The LU has done laboratory research on the various degradative pathways under different conditions (aerobic, methanogenic, denitrifying) and on possible degradation products. On the basis of the laboratory results, it can be concluded that the degradation rate of α-HCH is fastest under aerobic conditions. Based on these results, the RIN did some experiments in containers with "wet" soil (approximately 20 percent water) and "slurry" (approximately 30 percent of water). In continuously aerated slurry conditions, a decrease of α-HCH from 300 to 40 to 60mg/kg dry matter could be observed. Neither during experiments previously mentioned nor under any other conditions was a reduction of β-HCH observed.[7]

Delft University of Technology is conducting research into the possibilities of microbiological degradation of various substances in a three-phase (air, liquid, solid) slurry reactor, the so-called Pachuca reactor. The design procedure of this slurry reactor entails three steps: study of the kinetics of the decontamination process, technological studies regarding construction and scaleup aspects, and total treatment process design.[4, 16]

Summarizing, it can be concluded that bioreactors seem to offer possibilities, particularly for the cleanup of soil with pollutants of low biodegradability. It is generally expected that the possibilities for using bioreactors can be extended to other wastestreams polluting the environment.

Purification of Wastewater

Since the enforcement in The Netherlands of the law on the pollution of surface water in 1970, the application of biological waste water treatment has increased enormously. Until 1980, effluent was treated almost exclusively in aerobic activated sludge systems. Subsequently the anaerobic technique proved a good alternative, especially in terms of saving both energy and costs. At present, the anaerobic technique is used in many branches of industry.

In the last decade, interest in the role and behavior of xenobiotics has increased. This has been partly stimulated by the growing possibilities of detection. It became possible to determine very low concentrations of many sorts of micropollutants. Automatically, the question arises as to whether pollution of the surface and groundwater with these xenobiotics could be prevented. At first, attention was almost exclusively drawn towards physicochemical detoxification methods for xenobiotics, especially filtration stages in activated carbon columns after an aerobic biological treatment. In the last few years, however, biotechnological methods have come into the picture. For example, experiments have been carried out at the Institute for Inland Water Management and Waste Water Treatment (DBW/RIZA) with the addition of activated carbon to an active sludge system by which

Table 2
Wastewater Composition of Chemische Industrie Rijnmond[14]

Wastewater Composition	
	(mg/l)
COD total	30.500
Formiate	5.800
Acetate	19.500
Propionate	100
Phenol	450
Formaldehyde	900
Benzene	200 – 400
Toluene	500 – 1000
pH	2 – 3

wastewater from a tank accommodation storage company was purified. During the experiments, shock loadings with aniline were simulated. It turned out that the addition of activated carbon substances to the active sludge had a stabilizing influence on the purification process.[9] To support this development, the RIVM has started a fundamental research project in which the biodegradation of cresol in chemostat cultures and gas lift reactors is being investigated.

Anaerobic wastewater treatment also offers possibilities for the biodegradation of xenobiotic compounds. Semitechnical and pilot research in an Upflow Anaerobic Sludge Bed (UASB) reactor of wastewater from the Chemical Industry Rijnmond (for composition, see Table 2) showed that toxic substances such as phenol and formaldehyde could be degraded from 99 to 100 percent. A full-scale UASB plant has been constructed based on this research.[14]

A recent development concerns the biotechnological cleaning of groundwater that derives from soil cleaning. The physical and chemical techniques that have been used so far have certain disadvantages such as frequently high costs and environmental objections (rest material, emissions). Research in The Netherlands has concentrated on the development of bioreactors for the removal of xenobiotic compounds, such as aromatics, PCAs, HCHs, and monochlorobenzene from groundwater.[3]

A project that has already led to application concerns the treatment of groundwater polluted with HCH, chlorobenzene, and benzene at a former pesticide production site. As a treatment system, two sand filters and three activated carbon filters were first planned. Pilot plant research was carried out with a trickling filter and a rotating biological contractor. The results were promising: 50 percent removal of HCH and 99 percent removal of benzene and monochlorobenzenes. Besides the activated carbon filters, two rotating biological contractors were then installed for groundwater pretreatment. The required activated carbon was reduced to less than 10 percent and biological pretreatment resulted in this situation in a cost reduction for groundwater treatment of 30 to 40 percent.[10]

Future Research

In general, results of research on the topics we have discussed have been promising so far. Further research is useful and will be supported by the Dutch government in the framework of the already mentioned research program on Environmental Biotechnology.[11]

Also, more attention will be paid to increase the fundamental know-how in the field. With the aforementioned developments, bottlenecks have been met that were previously difficult to solve because of a lack in fundamental know-how. Moreover, it is expected that stimulation of fundamental research will give more opportunities to develop desirable applications in the field. In this context, research projects will be initiated on such topics as:

1. Biodegradation of xenobiotics: relevant microorganisms, degradation pathways, molecular and genetic base of degradation, relevant environmental factors, modeling of biodegradation processes

2. Use of selected microorganisms in biological purification

systems: influence on microbial adaptation processes, way of inoculation, and maintenance of selected microorganisms.

3. Microbial leaching of heavy metals from solid waste: development of technical know-how.

4. Availability of contaminants for microorganisms in soil
systems: possibilities to increase biodegradation rate by increasing availability, production, and role of biological emulsifiers.

5. Immobilizations of microorganisms: attachment of microorganisms and stability of immobilized microbial systems.

On the other hand, projects for the development of proper
solutions for existing environmental problems still will be started up
in the framework of the mentioned research program. These projects
will usually be carried out in collaboration with various institutes and
universities. Engineering consultants and firms will also participate at
an early stage in those projects.

This cooperation between scientists, industrial researchers, and
governmental representatives has contributed to a great extent to the
rapid progress of the development of environmental biotechnology in
The Netherlands. The execution of the research program and other activities of the Working Party on Environmental Biotechnology has
proved to be a necessity for the fruitful communication between the
parties involved.

References

1. R. van den Berg, D.H. Eikelboom, and J.H.A.M. Verheul, *Second Interim-Report of the Second International Meeting of the NATO/CCMS Pilot Study* (RIVM, Bilthoven, The Netherlands, 1988).
2. A.H.M. van Bergen, Ed., *Biofiltratie. Eindrapport van de Werkgroep Biofilters* [Biofil-tration. Final Report of the Working Party on Biofiltration] (Publikatiereeks Lucht, nr. 72, Ministry of Housing Physical Planning and Environment, Leidschendam, The Neth-erlands, 1987).
3. DHV Consultancy, *Bioreactoren voor de reiniging van Grondwater. Onderzoeksvoor-stel Fase b.* [Bioreactors for the Purification of Groundwater. Research Proposal, Phase b] (Amersfoort, The Netherlands 1988).

4. R.H. Kleijntjes *et al.*, *Process Development for Biological Soil Decontamination in a Slurry Reactor* (Paper delivered at the 4th European Congress on Biotechnology, 1987).
5. S.P.P Ottengraf, *Trends in Biotechnology* **5**, 132 (1987).
6. E.R. Soczó, J.J.M. Staps, and K. Visscher, *Biotechnologische Bodemsanering. Rapportage van de Workshop 20 en 21 Maart 1986 te Bilthoven* [Biological Soil Clean-up Techniques. Report of the workshop in March 20-21, 1986, Bilthoven] (RIVM Report No. 851105002, National Institute of Public Health and Environmental Hygiene, Bilthoven, The Netherlands, August 1986).
7. E.R. Soczó, J.J.M. Staps, and K. Visscher, *Resources, Conservation and Recycling* **1**, 65 (1988).
8. E.R. Soczó and K. Visscher, *Resources and Conservation* **15**, 125 (1987).
9. L.V.M. Teurlinckx and R. Anthonijsz, *Biologische Zuivering van Industrieel Afvalwater met Poederkooldosering*, [Biological Treatment of Industrial Wastewater with Activated Carbon Addition], (Rijkswaterstaat, DBW/RIZA) Nota nr. 86-022, Lelystad, The Netherlands,1986).
10. L.G.C.M. Urlings, F. Spuij, and J.P. van der Hock, *Biological Treatment of Groundwater Polluted with HCH, Chlorobenzene and Benzene on a Former Pesticide Production Site in Bunschoten, The Netherlands* (Tauw Infra Consult B.V., Deventer, The Netherlands, 1988).
11. K. Visscher and W.H. Rulkens, Eds., *Onderzoeks- en Ontwikkelings- Programma Milieubiotechnologie*, [R&D Programme Environmental Biotechnology] (Publikatiereeks Milieubeheer Report nr. 29, Ministry of Housing, Physical Planning and Environment, Leidschendam, The Netherlands, 1985).
12. K. Visscher, *Biotechnologie in Nederland* **2**, 58 (1985).
13. S. Keuning and D.B. Janssen. *Microbiologische Afbraak van Zwarte en Prioritaire Stoffen voor het Milieubeleid* [Microbiological Degradation of High Priority Compounds in Environmental Policy], (Ministry of Housing, Physical Planning and Environment, Leidschendam, 1987).
14. Gist Brocades N.V., *Chemische Industrie Rijnmond B.V. Anaerobe Afval- waterzuivering Chemische Industrie Rijnmond B.V.* [Anaerobic Wastewater Treatment Chemical Industry Rijnmond B.V.].(Ministry of Housing, Physical Planning and Environment, Leidschendam, 1988).
15. S.P.P. Ottengraf, R. Diks, and C. van Lith, *Proceedings 2nd Netherlands Biotechnology Congress* (Netherlands Biotechnological Society, Zeist, 1988).
16. E.R. Soczó, *Review of Soil Treatment Techniques in The Netherlands,* Anlæg til behandling af forurenet grundvand, perkolat og jord, Hearing, December 1988, Industri og Handelsstyrelsen, Denmark)(Article in English), 1988.

21

Diversity of Toluene Degradation Following Long Term Exposure to BTEX *In Situ*

Jerome J. Kukor
*Department of Microbiology
and Immunology
University of Michigan
Medical School*

correspondence

Ronald H. Olsen
*Department of Microbiology
and Immunology
University of Michigan
Medical School
Ann Arbor, MI 48109-0620*

Aquifer remediation has been conducted for three years by a purge and treat system utilizing granular activated carbon (GAC) filtration of the groundwater at a gas production facility contaminated with aromatic petroleum hydrocarbons: benzene, toluene, ethylbenzene, and xylenes (BTEX). Analyses have been made of groundwater and GAC particles for presence and metabolic diversity of microorganisms capable of degrading BTEX under aerobic and denitrifying conditions. Seven bacterial isolates were selected for detailed investigation. Determination of growth substrate profiles and also oxygen consumption profiles for toluene-induced cells indicated that catabolic diversity was significantly broader than the induction specificity used by the microorganisms for degradation of aromatic hydrocarbons. *Pseudomonas pickettii* PKO1 was selected as a model organism for genetic analysis of BTEX catabolism by such microorganisms. A 27 kilobase *Bam*HI restriction endonuclease DNA fragment cloned from strain PKO1 and expressed in *P. aeruginosa* PAO1 allowed the latter strain to utilize benzene, toluene, phenol, and *m*-cresol under aerobic conditions and toluene and ethylbenzene under anaerobic, denitrifying conditions.

Introduction and Background

Groundwater is a major resource in the United States, where it provides approximately 40 percent of the water supply for domestic use, both rural and urban, including widespread use for irrigation.[1] Owing to its use for human consumption and to the increasing incidence of groundwater contamination by anthropogenic chemicals, there is mounting concern in the public, private, and scientific sectors about the threat of synthetic chemicals moving through the soil into aquifers and affecting the supply of acceptable quality water. In Michigan, the vast majority of households that derive their domestic water supply from groundwater utilize shallow wells that are readily affected by mobile groundwater contaminants. Also, nearly 2000 sites have been identified that will require cleanup because of hydrocarbon leaks and spills. Chemicals from industrial storage sites, from spills at production facilities, from leaking underground storage tanks, and leaking dump sites are commonly identified as sources of contaminants that reach groundwater. Waste solvents such as polychlorinated biphenyls, primarily of industrial origin, are capable of reaching groundwater more rapidly than many other synthetic chemicals. Thus, highly mobile chemicals can present a significant health hazard as common contaminants of the domestic water supply.

One currently used technology for remediation of groundwater contaminated with aromatic hydrocarbons is activated carbon adsorption (for a review of this process, see references).[2] Groundwater is pumped from a contaminant plume through columns of granular activated carbon (GAC), which are configured so that the effluent water contains a predetermined (usually micrograms per liter) level of the target contaminants. The carbon adsorption process is relatively nonspecific and has broad application for treatment of complex waste streams where the composition is not fully known. Major drawbacks to the use of GAC adsorption treatment processes are rapid exhaustion of the capacity of carbon for sorption of target compounds and the high costs of frequent regeneration or replacement of the carbon.

Activated carbon treatment units that receive an influent of groundwater from natural aquifers invariably come in contact with microorganisms and microbial products. The ability of activated carbon to adsorb substrate material, inorganic ions, and dissolved gases can result in the development of a complex microbial layer, sometimes referred to as a slime layer or biofilm, on the surface of GAC particles. There are operational disadvantages associated with the presence of a biofilm layer on carbon adsorbers due primarily to increased pressure drops through columns,[3] blockage of water passage, and adsorption interference.[4,5] Despite the disadvantages, it is clear from numerous studies[6-10] that microbial activity can increase the useful life of activated carbon columns for adsorption of recalcitrant or nondegradable compounds. The mechanism proposed for the extended life is that microorganisms in the biofilm utilize readily degradable compounds, leaving more adsorption sites on the carbon for recalcitrant compounds.

In 1984, groundwater beneath a gas plant facility in northern Michigan became contaminated with aromatic hydrocarbons, primarily benzene, toluene, and xylenes (BTX). The extent and distribution of BTX contamination in the shallow aquifer beneath the gas plant has been characterized by sampling soil and water quality from monitoring wells and soil borings.[11,12] The maximum BTX concentrations initially detected in groundwater at the site were 353μg/L benzene, 108μg/L toluene, and 5280μg/L xylenes. From a hydrogeological description of the site, the contaminant plume area was estimated to be 430 meters in length and 200 meters in width. Groundwater remediation efforts were begun at the site in late 1985. Four purge wells were installed along the center line of the contaminant plume, and groundwater pumped from each well was piped to two parallel GAC column trains that consisted of a series of three columns, each holding 6600kg of GAC. Effluent water was monitored for BTX concentrations to assure that the discharge limit of 1μg/L was achieved. The effluent water was then discharged to the groundwater through a subsurface drain field that was upgradient to the area of contamination. Assessment of the time-related variation of total soluble BTX mass in the groundwater beneath the gas plant site during the three years of treatment has indicated a general decline, to a current level of approximately 200μg/L total BTX.

The GAC column trains at the northern Michigan gas plant site have operated more or less continuously in an undisturbed manner for 3 years. Calculations based on the total mass of BTX removed from the contaminant plume relative to the expected breakthrough point for BTX that would have been predicted on the basis of equilibrium capacity for the GAC mass indicated that the carbon column trains at the site had far exceeded their nominal bed capacity for adsorption of BTX. The implication from this finding is that biodegradation is occurring in the GAC columns, in addition to adsorption of BTX into the GAC. In early 1989, we obtained GAC particles and groundwater from the carbon adsorption treatment column trains at the gas plant facility in northern Michigan. Our objectives were to analyze the microbial composition of the GAC slurry with respect to catabolic diversity for BTX utilization, under both aerobic and denitrifying conditions.

Selection Strategy for Isolation of Microorganisms

The selection strategy employed for isolation of bacteria from GAC particles and groundwater from the northern Michigan gas plant site is illustrated in Figure 1. Four parallel isolation procedures were used. The first isolation procedure involved dilution plating onto Vogel and Bonner's (VBG) glucose-citrate media[13] under aerobic conditions, followed by washing of the colonies that arose on VBG plates to MMO minimal medium[14] containing toluene as sole carbon source, with incubation under both aerobic and anaerobic, denitrifying conditions. The second isolation procedure involved direct dilution plating from GAC or groundwater samples onto MMO toluene media, with selection under both aerobic and anaerobic, denitrifying conditions. The third isolation procedure involved liquid enrichment in 100ml of VBG media under aerobic conditions, followed by plating from the liquid enrichment to MMO toluene media, with selection under aerobic and anaerobic, denitrifying conditions. The fourth isolation procedure involved liquid enrichment in 100ml of MMO toluene media under both aerobic and anaerobic, denitrifying condi-

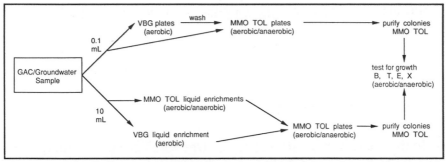

Figure 1. Selection strategy used for isolation of microorganisms from granular activated carbon (GAC) and groundwater samples. Abbreviations are as defined in text.

tions, followed by plating from the enrichment cultures onto solid MMO toluene media, under both aerobic and anaerobic, denitrifying conditions. Bacterial colonies obtained on MMO toluene plates from the four selection schemes were screened for differences in colony morphology, size, and pigmentation and were then purified repeatedly for production of discrete, isolated colonies on solid media. Purified bacterial isolates were tested for their ability to utilize various aromatic hydrocarbons as sole carbon source by inoculating plates containing the appropriate solid medium with a small patch of cells obtained from a single colony. Bacterial isolates were obtained by inoculating 0.1 ml of groundwater and associated GAC particles from the GAC columns onto solid media or by inoculating 10 ml of the GAC-groundwater slurry into liquid media.

Volatile, non-water-soluble, aromatic hydrocarbons were added to solid media as vapor by incubating plates in a sealed, glass desiccator jar that contained a 1-cm^2 piece of filter paper saturated with 50 to 100 μl of the hydrocarbon. For liquid cultures, 50 to 100μl of the non-water-soluble hydrocarbons were placed in a 0.5 x 5 cm glass test tube that was attached to a supporting glass rod, which was fixed to the lid of the culture vessel.

Anaerobic incubations were conducted in BBL GasPak jars (Becton Dickinson & Co., Cockeysville, MD), which contained a nitrogen-carbon dioxide-hydrogen atmosphere, with methylene blue impregnated strips as indicators of anoxic conditions. Media for anaerobic incubations contained potassium nitrate at a final concentration of 10mM.

The identity of selected bacterial strains obtained from the selection schemes just described was determined by utilization of API rapid NFT strips (Analytab Products, Plainview, NY).

For oxygen uptake experiments, cells were grown at 30° C with aeration overnight in 25ml of MMO media that contained 0.3 percent sodium lactate as the carbon source. One ml of the overnight culture was used to inoculate 50ml of fresh MMO medium that contained 0.3 percent sodium lactate plus the appropriate inducing aromatic carbon source. The cultures were incubated at 30°C with aeration until the cell density (A_{425}) reached 0.8 to 1.0. Cells were harvested by centrifugation at room temperature and were washed twice in 10ml of 50mM sodium-potassium phosphate buffer, pH 6.8. Washed cells were used immediately for oxygen uptake assays. Oxygen consumption was determined polarographically in a 3-ml stirred cell with a YSI 5300 apparatus (Yellow Springs Instruments, Yellow Springs, OH).

Catabolic Diversity of Microbial Isolates From GAC

The liquid enrichment and dilution-plate selection scheme described in the previous section yielded 43 bacterial isolates that differed from one another in morphological and physiological properties as well as their overall catabolic profiles for utilization of benzene, toluene, xylene, or ethylbenzene as growth substrates. From these 43 isolates, seven were selected for more intensive investigation. These seven isolates (Table 1) were *Pseudomonas fluorescens* 711, *P. fluorescens* K1-1, *Pseudomonas* sp K3-2, *P. putida* 713, *Acinetobacter calcoaceticus* 113, *P. pickettii* 311, and *P. cepacia* N27. In addition, we included in our detailed analyses *P. pickettii* PKO1, a strain recently isolated by us from sandy aquifer material in southeastern Michigan,[15] and *P. putida* PPO300.[16] This strain of *P. putida* is designated PPO300 in our laboratory and is identical to strain U of Dagley[17] and strain 144 of Stanier *et al.*[14] *Pseudomonas putida* PPO300 has previously been investigated for its ability to catabolize

Table 1
Growth Substrates for Typical Isolates from Granular Activated Carbon (GAC) Slurry

Isolate number/ (bacterial strain)		TOL	BZE	E-BZE	XYL
PKO1/(*P. pickettii*)	Ar	+	+	+	−
	An	+	+	+	−
711/(*P. fluorescens*)	Ar	+	−	+	−
	An	−	−	+	nd
K1-1/(*P. fluorescens*)	Ar	+	−	+	−
	An	−	−	−	−
K3-2/(*Pseudomonas* sp.)	Ar	+	+	+	−
	An	−	−	−	−
713/(*P. putida*)	Ar	+	+	+	−
	An	−	−	−	−
113/(*A. calcoaceticus*)	Ar	+	+	+	−
	An	−	−	−	−
311/(*P. pickettii*)	Ar	+	−	−	−
	An	+	−	−	−
PPO300/(*P. putida*)	Ar	+	+	−	−
	An	−	−	−	−
N27/(*P. cepacia*)	Ar	+	+	+	m,p
	An	+	+	+	nd
PpF1/(*P. putida*)	Ar	+	+	+	−
	An	−	−	−	−
PaW1/(*P. putida*)	Ar	+	−	−	m,p
	An	−	−	−	−
KR/(*A. xylosoxidans*)	Ar	+	+	+	−
	An	−	−	−	−
G4/(*P. cepacia*)	Ar	+	+	−	−
	An	+	+	+	nd

Abbreviations: TOL, toluene; BZE, benzene; E-BZE, ethyl benzene; XYL, xylene; Ar, growth under aerobic conditions; An, growth under anaerobic (denitrifying) conditions; *o*, ortho; *m*, meta; *p*, para; nd, not determined. Growth (+) was determined by the formation of discrete, isolated, opaque colonies on solid media.

phenol and cresols;[16,17] we have determined that this microorganism is capable of utilizing toluene as sole source of carbon for growth. Also included in Table 1 for the purpose of comparison are four strains, *P. putida* F1;[18-20] *P. putida* PaW1 (also designated strain mt-2); *Achromobacter xylosoxidans* KR, which was formerly designated *P. mendocina* KR (this strain was originally identified as *P. mendocina* KR,[24] but repeated testing in our laboratory indicates that it is an isolate of *A. xylosoxidans*); and *P. cepacia* G4,[21] for which detailed information is available concerning the pathways by which they metabolize toluene. The results in Table 1 show that there is considerable catabolic diversity among the isolates obtained from the groundwater-GAC slurries. In addition to the ability to utilize toluene as sole carbon source for growth under aerobic conditions, most of the isolates were also able to grow on benzene as well as ethylbenzene. The latter compound frequently occurs in hydrocarbon spills together with BTX. *Pseudomonas cepacia* N27 was the only isolate capable of growing on *m*- and *p*-xylene. None of the isolates could use *o*-xylene as sole carbon source for growth. There was much less overall catabolic diversity among the GAC isolates for degradation of aromatic hydrocarbons under denitrifying conditions. Several of the isolates were able to grow on a single aromatic substrate when nitrate was present in the media, as exemplified by *P. fluorescens* 711 or *P. pickettii* 311. However, *P. cepacia* N27 was a noteworthy exception to the overall pattern, being able to grow on toluene, benzene, and ethylbenzene. In this respect it resembles *P. cepacia* G4.

The four reference strains included in Table 1, *P. putida* F1, *P. putida* PaW1, *A. xylosoxidans* KR, and *P. cepacia* G4, each metabolize toluene by a different oxygen-dependent pathway. As illustrated in Figure 2, the pathway utilized by *P. putida* PaW1 involves sequential oxidation of the methyl group with catechol as the substrate for *meta* ring cleavage. This is the well-characterized pathway encoded by the TOL plasmid pWW0.[22,23] *P. putida* F1, which has been extensively investigated by Gibson and co-workers,[18-20] incorporates two atoms of oxygen directly into the aromatic nucleus to produce a *cis*-dihydrodiol, which is then dehydrogenated to produce 3-methyl catechol, the substrate for *meta* ring cleavage. Toluene is metabolized

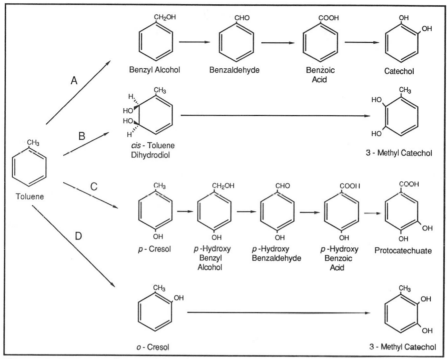

Figure 2. Pathways for aerobic microbial degradation of toluene: A, pathway that occurs in *P. putida* PaW1; B, pathway that occurs in *P. putida* F1; C, pathway that occurs in *A. xylosoxidans* KR (formerly *P. mendocina* KR); D, pathway that occurs in *P. cepacia* G4.

by *A. xylosoxidans* KR via an initial hydroxylation, producing *p*-cresol, followed by sequential oxidation of the methyl group to *p*-hydroxybenzoate.[24] *p*-Hydroxybenzoate is hydroxylated to protocatechuate, which is metabolized by an *ortho* cleavage pathway that is analogous to the well-studied *ortho* fission pathway for catabolism of *p*-hydroxybenzoate known for other pseudomonads.[25] The most recently described route for oxidative degradation of toluene is that found in *P. cepacia* G4.[21] In this strain, a nonspecific monooxygenase hydroxylates toluene to *o*-cresol. The same enzyme continues hydroxylation to produce 3-methyl catechol, which is the substrate for meta ring fission. Each of the four pathways for metabolism of toluene as previously described contains distinctive intermediates that are indicative of the pathway. As shown in Table 2, toluene grown cells

Table 2
Oxygen Uptake for Toluene Grown Cells

Bacterial isolate	Pathway	TOL	p-CRE	4HBZL	3MCAT	CAT	o-CRE
PaW1	A	+++	+/–	+/–	+/–	+++	nd
PpF1	B	++	+/–	+/–	+++	++	nd
KR	C	+	+++	+++	+/–	+	nd
G4	D	+	+/–	–	++	++	+++
PKO1	B	++	+/–	+/–	+++	++	–
711	(C,D)	+++	+	+	+++	++	+
K1-1	(C,D)	+++	+	+	+++	++	+
K3-2	B	+	+/–	+	++	+/–	nd
713	B	+++	+	+/–	+++	+	+/–
311	B	++	–	–	++	+/–	–
PPO300	D	+	–	+	+	+	++

Symbols represent μM oxygen consumed per min per cell suspension normalized to a density (A_{425}) of 1.0; – = 0.00; +/– = 0.00-0.02; + = 0.02-0.05; ++ = 0.05-0.10; +++ = >0.10. Abbreviations: TOL, toluene; p-CRE, p-cresol; 4HBZL, 4-hydroxybenzyl alcohol; 3MCAT, 3-methyl catechol; CAT, catechol; o-CRE, o-cresol; nd, not determined.

of *P. putida* F1 exhibit significant oxygen consumption when given 3-methyl catechol, whereas, toluene grown cells of *P. putida* PaW1 respire catechol as a key diagnostic intermediate. Cells of *A. xylosoxidans* KR induced for toluene metabolism utilize p-cresol and 4-hydroxybenzyl alcohol, whereas toluene induced cells of *P. cepacia* G4 utilize o-cresol. Using these key intermediates as diagnostic features for the estimation of toluene metabolic pathways, we analyzed several of the isolates obtained from the groundwater-GAC slurries from the northern Michigan gas plant GAC treatment site. As shown in Table 2, many of the isolates have toluene catabolic profiles similar to that found in *P. putida* F1 and thus would be expected to metabolize toluene via a *cis*-toluene dihydrodiol intermediate. *Pseudomonas fluorescens* 711 and *P. fluorescens* K1-1 have toluene catabolic profiles indicative of more than one of the archetypal pathways for catabolism of toluene. Because neither isolate polymerizes indole to indigo, a reaction that is diagnostic for the toluene oxygenase of *P. putida* F1,[18-20] we excluded pathway B (see Figure 2) for these strains. Further analysis will be required to determine whether these strains utilize pathway C or D. It should be noted that none of the GAC isolates analyzed to date have shown a toluene catabolic profile similar to that found in *P. putida* PaW1.

Pseudomonas pickettii PKO1 as a Model Organism

P. pickettii PKO1 was previously isolated by us in a microcosm experiment in which benzene, toluene, and *p*-xylene were degraded by an inoculum of sandy aquifer material.[15] *Pseudomonas pickettii* PKO1 was shown to have the same BTX degradation kinetics, when added as a monospecific inoculum to microcosms, as found in the original microbial population from the sandy aquifer material.

As shown in Table 3, *P. pickettii* PKO1 can grow on toluene, benzene, and ethylbenzene as sole carbon source under aerobic or denitrifying conditions. This strain also grows on phenol and *m*-cresol; however, it cannot utilize any of the isomers of xylene nor *o*- or *p*-cresol as a growth substrate. The co-occurrence of the ability to utilize phenol or cresols together with toluene or alkyl-substituted benzenes is a pattern that we have observed repeatedly among many of the isolates from the GAC treatment columns despite the fact that there is no evidence for anthropogenic groundwater contamination by phenol or cresols at the northern Michigan gas plant site. For this reason we selected *P. pickettii* PKO1 as a model microorganism for more detailed physiological and genetic studies.

We have recently reported[26] on the molecular cloning of a 27

Table 3
Growth Substrates for *P. pickettii* PKO1 and *P. aeruginosa* PAO1(pRO1957)

		TOL	BZE	E-BZE	XYL	PHL	CRE
PKO1	Ar	+	+	+	–	+	m
	An	+	+	+	–	–	–
PAO1	Ar	+	+	–	–	+	m
(pRO1957)	An	+	–	+	–	–	–

Abbreviations: TOL, toluene; BZE, benzene; E-BZE, ethyl benzene; XYL, xylene; PHL, phenol; CRE, cresol; Ar, growth under aerobic conditions; An, growth under anaerobic (denitrifying) conditions; *m*, meta. Growth (+) was determined by the formation of discrete, isolated, opaque colonies on solid media.

kilobase *Bam*HI restriction endonuclease DNA fragment from total genomic DNA of *P. pickettii* PKO1 that contains genes required for utilization of phenol. This recombinant plasmid, designated pRO1957 (see Table 3) allows the heterogenetic cloning recipient *P. aeruginosa* PAO1 to grow on phenol, *m*-cresol, toluene, and benzene under aerobic conditions, and on toluene and ethylbenzene under denitrifying conditions. *P. aeruginosa* PAO1 will not grow on any of these substrates in the absence of plasmid pRO1957 (data not shown in Table 3).

Oxygen uptake studies of toluene- or phenol-grown cells of *P. pickettii* PKO1 and *P. aeruginosa* PAO1(pRO1957) show that prior growth on toluene allows for metabolism of benzene and all three isomers of xylene, but there was only marginal respiration of phenol or cresols (Table 4). Similarly, prior growth on phenol allowed cells to respire cresols, but there was only marginal activity against toluene and no activity against benzene and xylenes. These results suggest that although genes encoding enzymes for catabolism of phenol and toluene are present on plasmid pRO1957, these catabolic activities are clearly induced separately and thus are likely to represent separately regulated gene clusters. Molecular genetic analyses of toluene and phenol degradative genes encoded on plasmid pRO1957 are currently in progress in our laboratory.

Table 4
Oxygen Uptake for Toluene or Phenol Grown Cells of *P. pickettii* PKO1 and *P. aeruginosa* PAO1(pRO1957)

Bacterial strain	Inducer	TOL	PHL	BZE	E-BZE	XYL	CRE	CAT	3MCAT
PKO1	TOL	++	+/–	+	–	+ _o,m,p_	+/– _o,m,p_	+++	+++
	PHL	+/–	++	–	–	– _o,m,p_	++ _o,m,p_	+++	+++
PAO1 (pRO1957)	TOL	++	+/–	+	–	+ _o,m,p_	– _o,m,p_	+++	+++
	PHL	+/–	++	–	–	– _o,m,p_	++ _o,m,p_	+++	++

Symbols represent μM oxygen consumed per min per cell suspension normalized to a density (A_{425}) of 1.0; – = 0.00; +/– = 0.00-0.02; + = 0.02- 0.05; ++ = 0.05-0.10; +++ = >0.10. Abbreviations: TOL, toluene; PHL, phenol; BZE, benzene; E-BZE, ethyl benzene; XYL, xylene; CRE, cresol; CAT, catechol; 3MCAT, 3-methyl catechol; *o*, ortho; *m*, meta; *p*, para.

A salient feature of the data presented in Table 4 is that toluene-induced cells of *P. pickettii* PKO1 and *P. aeruginosa* PAO1(pRO1957) were capable of metabolizing *o*-, *m*-, and *p*-xylene even though xylenes were not growth-supporting substrates (see Table 3). Similarly, induction with phenol allowed for utilization of all three isomers of cresol even though only *m*-cresol was a growth substrate. These results indicate that *P. pickettii* PKO1 is capable of degrading a broader range of aromatic substrates than can be accommodated by the specificity of induction of individual catabolic pathways.

Conclusions and Perspectives

The ability of indigenous microorganisms to degrade petroleum hydrocarbons *in situ* following aquifer contamination is often regarded as being limited by the availability of oxygen in the subsurface environment.[27,28] Field analyses at the gas plant facility in northern

Michigan have demonstrated that BTX disappearance was directly related to the availability of dissolved oxygen in the groundwater.[12] However, the low solubility of oxygen in groundwater, together with the technical difficulties associated with attempted dispersion of oxygen into contaminant plumes, has limited the utility of oxygen-dependent *in situ* remediation. Nitrate is an alternate electron acceptor used by numerous microorganisms in respiration when oxygen is depleted, and several studies[29-31] have shown nitrate-dependent biodegradation of aromatic hydrocarbons in aquifers. Our studies on the groundwater remediation efforts at a gas production facility in northern Michigan have demonstrated the presence of considerable catabolic diversity among microorganisms present on granular activated carbon particles from a GAC filtration train. Some of these microbial isolates showed both oxygen-dependent as well as nitrate-dependent degradation of the aromatic hydrocarbons that contaminate the aquifer. The dissolved oxygen levels in the GAC filtration train have not been monitored; however, operation of the unit would result in periodic oxygen recharge (following backwashing of the carbon) followed by oxygen depletion as a result of biodegradation as well as adsorption of dissolved oxygen by the carbon. Thus, the GAC filtration train has functioned as a selective enrichment vessel for indigenous aquifer microorganisms capable of degrading BTX under oxic as well as anoxic conditions.

In addition to the problems already discussed associated with availability of appropriate electron acceptors for *in situ* biodegradation of petroleum hydrocarbons, very low substrate concentrations also pose problems for biological treatment. Substrate concentrations in the range of 100 µg/l or less may be insufficient to induce the transcription of genes encoding necessary catabolic enzymes. Such a "threshold" effect for enzyme induction has been suggested by some researchers.[32,33] Our studies on enzyme induction patterns in *P. pickettii* PKO1 have shown that xylenes can be metabolized by toluene-induced cells and that cresols can be metabolized by phenol-induced cells but that xylenes and cresols do not induce the enzymes required for their own catabolism. Therefore, the metabolic diversity of aquifer microorganisms is significantly broader than the induction specificity for the catabolic pathways used by these microorganisms for degradation of aromatic hydrocarbons. This relationship may have evolved as a result of the co-occurrence of such families of compounds.

Acknowledgments

This research was supported through a roundtable research agreement with the Michigan Oil and Gas Association (MOGA CoBioReM, Inc.). Additional partial support was provided by the National Institute of Environmental Health Sciences Superfund Research and Education Grant No. ES-04911 and the Office of Research and Development, U.S. Environmental Protection Agency under Grant No. R815750-010. The content of this publication does not necessarily represent the views of the agency. We thank Tracy Boyd for assistance in obtaining granular activated carbon samples.

References

1. R.A. Freeze and J.A. Cherry, Groundwater (Prentice-Hall, Inc., Englewood Cliffs, NJ, 1979), pp. 6-9.
2. T.C. Voice, in Standard Handbook of Hazardous Waste Treatment and Disposal, H.M. Freeman, Ed. (McGraw-Hill Book Co., New York, 1989), pp. 6.3-6.21.
3. W.G. Characklis, *Biotechnol. Bioeng.* **23**, 1923 (1981).
4. J.D. Lowry and C.E. Burkhead, *J. Water Poll. Cont. Fed.* **52**, 389 (1980).
5. K.P. Olmstead, Ph.D. Dissertation, (University Michigan, 1989).
6. E.J. Bouwer and P.J. McCarty, *Environ. Sci. Technol.* **18**, 836 (1982).
7. J. DeLaat and F. Bouanga, *Water Res.* **19**, 1565 (1985).
8. G.E. Speitel et al., *Environ. Sci. Technol.* **23**, 68 (1989).
9. W.-C. Ying, Ph.D. Dissertation, (University Michigan, 1978).
10. J.G. den Blanken, *J. Environ. Engin.* **108**, 405 (1982).
11. C.Y. Chiang et al., *Proc. Petrol. Hydrocarbon Org. Chem. Ground Water* (National Well Water Association/American Petroleum Institute, 1986).
12. C.Y. Chiang et al., *Proc. Petrol. Hydrocarbon Org. Chem. Ground Water* (National Well Water Association/American Petroleum Institute, 1987).
13. H.J. Vogel and D.M. Bonner, *J. Biol. Chem.* **218**, 97 (1956).
14. R.Y. Stanier, N. Palleroni, and M. Doudoroff, *J. Gen. Microbiol.* **43**, 159 (1966).
15. T.L. Gibson, A.S. Abdul, and R.H. Olsen, *Environ. Sci. Technol.*, in press.
16. R.C. Bayly and G.J. Wigmore, *J. Bacteriol.* **113**, 1112 (1973).

17. C.F. Feist and G.D. Hegeman, *J. Bacteriol.* **100**, 869 (1969).
18. D.T. Gibson, J.R. Koch, and R.E. Kallio, *Biochemistry* **7**, 2653 (1968).
19. D.T. Gibson *et al.*, *Biochemistry* **9**, 1631 (1970).
20. B.D. Ensley *et al.*, *Science* **222**, 167 (1983).
21. M.S. Shields *et al.*, *Appl. Environ. Microbiol.* **55**, 1624 (1989).
22. T. Nakazawa and T. Yokota, *J. Bacteriol.* **115**, 262 (1973).
23. P.A. Williams and K. Murray, *J. Bacteriol.* **120**, 416 (1974).
24. G.M. Whited, Ph. D. Dissertation, (University of Texas at Austin, 1986).
25. L.N. Ornston and D. Parke, *Curr. Top. Cell Regulation* **12**, 209 (1977).
26. J.J. Kukor and R.H. Olsen, *Abstr. Annual Mtg. Amer. Soc. Microbiol.* **89**, K-58 (1989).
27. J.F. Barker and G.C. Patrick, *Ground Water Monitor. Rev.* **7**, 64 (1987).
28. R.C. Borden and P.B. Bedient, *Water Resources Res.* **22**, 1973 (1986).
29. G. Battermann and P. Werner, *Wasser/Abwasser* **125**, 366 (1984).
30. E.P. Kuhn *et al.*, *Appl. Environ. Microbiol.* **54**, 490 (1988).
31. E.P. Kuhn *et al.*, *Environ. Sci. Technol.* **19**, 961 (1985).
32. R.S. Boethling and M. Alexander, *Appl. Environ. Microbiol.* **37**, 1211 (1979).
33. R.S. Boethling and M. Alexander, *Environ. Sci. Technol.* **13**, 989 (1979).

Discussion

Schink: I am a little surprised that one of your isolates is able to degrade xylenes in the absence of oxygen. When you talk about anaerobic conditions, what does that mean in your case?

Kukor: Anaerobic conditions to me mean a nitrogen-carbon dioxide-hydrogen atmosphere in which nitrate is present at 10mM as an electron acceptor and in which a known aerobe that cannot denitrify, like strain mt-2, is the control that we are using. The control will not grow under a comparable regimen.

Schink: So do you have an idea of the leftover oxygen in that system?

Kukor: No, we have not monitored that at the present time. You are thinking perhaps that there is residual oxygen for oxygenase to use?

Schink: Well, it could be that it is just sufficient for the oxygenase to run but not enough for the respiratoy oxidases to use.

Kukor: I would expect that you would see some degradation then from strain mt-2, which is certainly going to be a very good scavenger of oxygen under those conditions. That is the only control that I have now because we are just now setting up the anaerobic batch experiments with monitoring for oxygen present in the system. We use a methylene blue indicator to tell us that the oxygen has been scrubbed from the system, but we do not actually have any more sophisticated monitor than that right now.

Omenn: If the strain that you are working on now, that is, strain PK01, is induced by toluene, then it no longer needs toluene added and will presumably be effective to reduce the 200ppb xylene out in the field. Is that the strategy?

Kukor: Yes, unfortunately I am expecting that if toluene is actually the effector molecule and if it is required for activation of transcription, then when toluene gets down below some threshold concentration, if there is such a thing, that you would get shutdown of the operon and that xylene would not then be utilized. At the site in Michigan, toluene is now down to 10ppb, whereas the xylenes are about eight times higher than that.

Omenn: Another strategy, of course, as has been used for strain G4, is to take a strain that is induced, in that case by phenol, and then to maintain its induction with some innocuous intermediate.

Kukor: For strain G4, we have not been told what the innocuous inducer is. We know phenol will work, but we are not going to get permission to add phenol to the ground in order to clean up xylenes. My approach has been to obtain a constitutive mutant that will continue, even at some low level, to transcribe rather than to have to put another carbon source in the ground that is a potential contaminant.

Omenn: But if you can make a constitutive mutant, it would solve the problem.

Kukor: As long as there is sufficient total organic carbon to allow for some growth and to enhance expression of enzymes.

Young: Just a point of information. Your initial isolations were never direct for denitrifiers, right? It appeared as if you would isolate under aerobic conditions and then test them under denitrifying conditions.

Kukor: No, there was direct selection on toluene media with nitrate under anaerobic conditions and also enrichments under anaerobic conditions. We did aerobic as well as anaerobic isolations in parallel.

Omenn: What level of toluene do you use when you do your selection?

Kukor: Toluene is used at 0.5mM.

Ecological Considerations and Risk Assessment

22

A Comparison of International Approaches to Biotechnology Risk Assessment

Daphne Kamely

U.S. Army Chemical Research,
Development and
Engineering Center
Aberdeen Proving Ground,
MD 21010-5423

and

Department of Biochemistry
School of Hygiene and
Public Health
Johns Hopkins University
Baltimore, MD 21205

Advances in molecular biology have enabled researchers to insert genes into microorganisms and to clone the genetic material to a desired quantity. It is now possible to isolate drugs, chemicals, and other rare molecules in significant quantities. Researchers are now also gaining insights into gene regulation, gene expression, and the molecular mechanisms underlying enzymatic and hormonal action. At the same time, biotechnology may pose hazards to human health and the environment. Whereas existing regulations can be used to regulate new biotechnology applications, little is known about the risks resulting from these new products and processes. This study contrasts biotechnology risk assessment in the major regulatory agencies of the United States with those in Europe and Japan, where major advances have taken place over the last decade. In European countries, there is a spectrum of approaches to the risk assessment of biotechnology, varying anywhere from no regulation and voluntary compliance to a total ban. The release of genetically engineered organisms and the various environmental statutes governing such releases are discussed and compared in the various countries.

Introduction

Gypsy moths and killer bees were the results of well-intentional efforts that went awry. Although in both of these cases the mishaps resulted from errors in breeding rather than gene splicing, the negative effects have been perceived by the public as reason to be wary of genetic experimentation. Is it any wonder then that the public fears that the deliberate release of genetically altered organisms into the environment could result in new infestations that might bring devastating consequences?

Advances in molecular biology have enabled researchers to insert genes into microorganisms and to clone the genetic material to a desired quantity. At a fraction of the cost and time of previous processes, it is now possible to isolate drugs, chemicals, and other rare molecules in significant quantities. Using biotechnology, laboratory researchers are gaining further insights into gene regulation, gene expression, and the molecular mechanisms underlying enzymatic and hormonal action. At the same time, recombinant DNA technology may pose hazards of harmful consequences to human health and the environment. For example, nonpathogenic genetic material initially inserted into microbes could evolve through the cloning process to become pathogenic. Although it is easy to clone genetic material to desired quantities and specifications, once the organism is released into the environment, it is difficult to contain this altered organism. It is these kinds of scenarios that have raised concern and led to the proposal of regulatory policies, legislation, and regulation of biotechnology.

Initially, biotechnology was limited to basic biomedical research, which was adequately covered by the National Institutes of Health (NIH) Guidelines. The intervention of regulatory agencies became necessary as biotechnology expanded to include products and processes, some of which involved environmental releases. Whereas existing regulations can be used to regulate new biotechnology applications, little is known about the risks that these new products pose to human health and the environment.

This study focuses on approaches to biotechnology risk assessment in three major regulatory agencies, the Food and Drug Administration (FDA), the U.S. Department of Agriculture (USDA), and the U.S. Environmental Protection Agency (EPA). Regulatory procedures and risk assessment programs in these agencies are discussed in terms of their strengths and weaknesses.

Approaches to risk assessment in the United States (U.S.) are contrasted with those in Europe and Japan, where major advances in biotechnology have taken place over the last decade. In European countries, there is a spectrum of approaches to the risk assessment of biotechnology, varying anywhere from no regulation whatsoever to voluntary compliance and at the other extreme, a total ban. Japan, on the other hand, benefits from a cooperative system among government, industry, and academic institutions, which greatly facilitates that country's regulatory process and allows it to advance rapidly in biotechnology.

Background

In order to understand regulatory approaches to biotechnology and risk assessment in the United States, it is important to describe the events that led to the initial public response and the subsequent regulatory framework in the United States.

With the discovery of restriction enzymes, laboratory scientists began to cut and recombine the genetic material of microorganisms. They were able to create new deoxyribonucleic acid (DNA) molecules, some of which exhibited altered properties. Scientists also learned to isolate individual genes, insert those into microbial DNA, grow the microbes, and thus clone the spliced gene to the desired quantity. Later, it was the scientists themselves who realized that this powerful recombinant DNA technique, with its numerous possibilities and advantages, might also pose unknown risks to human health and the environment. The scientists called public attention to a meeting that took place at the Asilomar Conference Center, Pacific Grove, California, in 1976,[2] where they self-imposed a moratorium on all recombinant DNA research. The moratorium remained in effect until the NIH published guidelines to cover this research.[3] Because the initial recombinant DNA experiments were limited to basic biomedical research, all of which was funded by the NIH, the NIH guidelines ensured that no organisms escaped the laboratory. In fact, the effects of the NIH guidelines extended beyond the scope of government-funded research: other research institutions and subsequent industries performing recombinant DNA research voluntarily agreed to abide by the NIH guidelines. This voluntary control worked well without established regulations until local citizens became aware of recombinant DNA experiments that were carried out in their immediate vicinity. In cities and municipalities such as Cambridge, Massachusetts, where university research was particularly active, community organizations formed, and some campaigned against all gene-splicing research.

In the early days of recombinant DNA research when experimentation was still confined to the laboratory environment, scientists would have been better served had they attempted to educate the public about their research and paid more attention to safety and risk assessment. However, many investigators who had lost valuable time during the initial moratorium on DNA research felt that they could not wait for public acceptance. Because the NIH guidelines covered all aspects of public safety, many scientists opted to focus on their research rather than on public policy issues. As a result, the public was not assured that recombinant DNA research was safe. This and divided opinions among expert scientists only focused more attention on possible health hazards and raised concerns about the safety of the new genetic technology. Increasing public pressure prompted some local governments to impose restrictions beyond the NIH guidelines. When the federal government finally intervened and started to sponsor conferences and risk assessment research in this area, it was almost too late to halt the regulatory developments. Furthermore, because the few risk assessment experiments that were conducted[4] yielded ambiguous results, they had little effect on quelling public concerns. Congress introduced over a dozen bills to regulate recombinant DNA research, none of which ever became law. The NIH Recombinant DNA Advisory Committee (RAC) spent numerous hours reviewing research proposals and setting containment levels for laboratory experiments. Universities established Institutional Biosafety Committees charged with assuring the safety of the research in their respective institutions. Still, there were few instances where the public was informed and educated about the scientific progress and the safety of the research. The public perception that recombinant DNA research was hazardous to human health and the environment forced molecular biologists to continue their research under much stricter conditions than were necessary. The RAC proceeded well into the late 1970s, carefully reviewing all risk assessment data on a case-by-case basis before it began to relax the NIH guidelines. To date, there has not been a single accident of harm due to recombinant DNA experimentation.

Renewed concern surfaced as recombinant DNA technology moved from the public to the private sector. Recombinant DNA research was expanded to include other biotechnical advances such as hybridoma research; the large-scale production of new drugs, hormones, chemicals, enzymes, diagnostic and detection devices; and novel process technology. Scientists were no longer experimenting with small 10-liter quantities; large-scale fermentation processes were required. In agriculture and in industrial areas, research started to move from the laboratory into the open field. The NIH guidelines could no longer cover this rapid growth. The intervention of regulatory agencies became necessary as products moved from the laboratory to the marketplace.

Regulation of Biotechnology in the United States

The regulatory process surrounding biotechnology has been a long and arduous process, which has not been resolved to the satisfaction of either industry or the academic institutions. In order to understand why the regulatory process has been so cumbersome and complicated, it is important to review the role of the federal agencies in the regulation of biotechnology.

In the United States, federal agencies play different roles in the regulation of biotechnology, depending on the nature of the product.

The agencies regulating biotechnological products and processes are the FDA, USDA, the EPA, the Consumer Product Safety Commission, the Occupational Safety and Health Administration, and the Department of Commerce. Thus, whether the product is biomedical or diagnostic, agricultural or industrial, it falls under the regulatory authority of one or more federal agencies.

All agencies adhere to a common procedure when conducting a biotechnology review. As a first step, technical and scientific information provided by the manufacturer is reviewed. The proper federal agency performs and provides a risk assessment. It may choose to go back to the manufacturer to request additional information or opt to work with the data as submitted by the company. On completion of the technical review, the scientific information is evaluated in view of the economic and other safety concerns. All federal agencies are increasingly concerned with safety issues, yet at the same time do not wish to stifle technical innovation and progress. Because of the multidisciplinary nature of biotechnology products, it is not always clear which agency will handle the submission. For example, a given pesticide can be regulated either by the EPA or the USDA, depending on the agent's use. In some cases, this puts an additional burden on the company to obtain permits from more than one agency for the same product.

Ironically, the agency with the most knowledge and experience in biotechnology is the NIH, an agency that funds scientific research but has no regulatory authority. The NIH can only act in an advisory capacity and cannot authorize an environmental release. Among the federal agencies, the FDA regulates the production of human and animal drugs and cosmetics. Because most products that come under FDA jurisdiction are manufactured in the laboratory, the FDA continues to regulate biotechnology products under its existing authority, which is derived from the Federal Food and Drug Acts; the FDA uses the NIH guidelines to review each pending application on a case-by-case basis. The FDA uses two separate statutes to regulate biotechnological products and processes: the Food, Drug and Cosmetic Act and the U.S. Public Health Act. The production of all human drugs, biologics, diagnostics, and medical devices is regulated by the FDA. Furthermore, certain food and food additives also fall under the jurisdiction of the FDA. Although the USDA regulates the production of animal vaccines and biologics, the FDA is responsible for veterinary drugs.

It takes approximately seven years to approve a drug through the FDA process which allows the FDA to evaluate the incoming requests on a case-by-case basis. Despite the growing number of recombinant drugs and vaccines submitted to the FDA for approval, the FDA has sufficient time for a careful review and risk assessment. Moreover, the FDA has been in existence for more than 80 years. The agency is staffed with competent scientists who have experience in the evaluation of drugs, diagnostics, and vaccines. Because the procedure for approving a drug is so cumbersome, companies try to submit their best available data. As a result, the FDA receives better data than most federal agencies. In addition, the process of evaluating genetically engineered drugs and diagnostics is similar to the process used for the nonengineered counterparts. In fact, most testing is conducted in a contained laboratory rather than in an uncontrolled environment.

By far the most burdened agencies are the USDA and EPA. The USDA has broad jurisdiction over plants, insects, animals, animal vaccines, and animal biologicals. It uses a variety of statutes to regulate biotechnological products. These include the Federal Plant Pest Act, the Plant Quarantine Act, the Federal Noxious Weed Act, and the Virus Serum Toxin Act. The EPA regulates chemicals, pesticides, and environmental releases. The USDA has a more difficult task than the FDA. Its jurisdiction is broader, yet the data it receives is incomplete. Unlike the FDA, where most drug manufacturing is confined to the laboratory, the USDA receives mostly field applications. Over 50 applications on the environmental release of genetically engineered plants and microbes are currently being processed at the USDA. All are examined on a case-by-case basis, and all are processed within 120 days. In order to facilitate the safe testing of genetically engineered organisms and assure compliance with federal regulations, the USDA has issued an Electronic Bulletin Board, which serves as a gateway to 11 databases. The databases serve as sources of information, Institutional Biosafety Committee contacts, and biosafety knowledge bases. In addition, the USDA is sponsoring the publication of protocols for monitoring field testing as well as providing guidance to biotechnology investigators. The USDA has some in-house expertise in biotechnology. It is currently staffing its biotechnology office with more experts. Rather than streamline the biotechnology review process, the USDA hopes that with an increased number of approved releases, more risk assessment results will become available. Consequently, more and more future products may be exempt from the regulatory process.

The agency with the least defined role in the regulation of biotechnology is the EPA. Yet the nature of the statutes and responsibilities of the EPA allows it to regulate a broad range of biotechnological products and processes. The EPA has 13 environmental statutes, two of which are currently used to regulate biotechnological products. The Federal Insecticide, Fungicide and Rodenticide Act (FIFRA) is used to regulate most genetically engineered pesticides, whereas the Toxic Substances Control Act (TSCA) is used to regulate all other engineered biological and biochemical products and processes. Because biotechnology is being developed as a tool in waste management and cleanup of hazardous substances, two other statutes may be activated: the Resource Conservation and Recovery Act, and the Comprehensive Environmental Response, Compensation and Liability Act. The EPA has a short time limit on the approval of products. Under TSCA, the agency is required to act on an application within 90 days. This can be extended, but with over 100,000 registered chemicals (biological molecules are considered chemicals under the broad definition of the EPA), the agency can hardly afford to regulate them on a case-by-case basis. Moreover, the EPA does not have scientific expertise in biotechnology. Often, it needs to seek outside advice in order to approve a genetically engineered product.

Deliberate release is clearly the area of the EPA. To date, more than twenty microbial pesticides have been approved and registered with the EPA; most of them are natural products for use in agriculture, forestry, and insect control. When the EPA began to examine genetically engineered microbes, it became clear that there was no risk assessment data to support the release of these novel microbes. From a scientific point of view, the appropriate approach would have been to conduct a controlled physical scale-up of risk assessment experiments, starting with an enclosed laboratory environment, then testing in a greenhouse, next in a small field plot, and finally in the open environment.

Alternatively, the EPA could require that the company submit biologically contained microbes for approval. An example of biologically contained strains are crippled microorganisms into which a replication-defective gene has been introduced. Once the organism has gone through one or two replication cycles in which it has carried out its function, it dies off. Another example of a biologically contained strain is a microorganism that grows on a toxic substance as its sole source of food, thereby degrading it. Once the pollutant is depleted, the organism can no longer survive. Finally, the use of suicide genes can serve as another form of biological containment. This is an inducible gene incorporated into the microorganism. Once triggered, it will kill the organism and thereby halt its spread in the open environment.

Physical and/or biological containments are options that the EPA can consider. Yet the EPA could not afford to base its approval process on containment information alone. Under FIFRA, the EPA requires risk data to assure that the release is safe to human health and the environment. If the data is insufficient, the EPA can either require additional test data or disapprove of the release pending additional information. Given the regulatory constraints that the EPA faces, the agency cannot permit a release unless more risk assessment information is available. Should there be an adverse effect to human health and the environment, the EPA will have to answer for its actions to Congress, the American public, and numerous lawsuits, all of which may result in more stringent regulations. As in the case of chemicals that were initially underregulated such as asbestos, the costs of regulating products once they are out in the market are staggering. Therefore, in the case of biotechnology products and processes, the EPA has opted to be more cautious. Moreover, there is an increased public involvement with the EPA regulatory process. As a result, the EPA tends to overregulate rather than proceed with the approval process. The EPA opts to require more risk assessment data, thus placing the burden of proof on the manufacturing companies. Some industry and policy experts argue that if the United States government does not make an effort to advance this technology, the country will lag in international competitiveness. In 1984, Congress began once more to examine the issues; the Office of Technology Assessment took interest in deliberate release; and the scientific institutions, among them the National Academy of Sciences, began to conduct risk assessment studies. However, none of these actions helped speed up the process. Many genetically engineered products are still not moving fast enough through the regulatory process.

More and more small biotechnology companies are not able to keep up with the regulatory pressures; the smaller companies either have to shut down or merge with larger corporations.

What are the options that the regulatory agencies have for handling biotechnology more efficiently?

With the increased number of incoming applications, the regulatory agencies can conduct a less efficient and less stringent review process. They can request less risk assessment information and extrapolate and estimate some of the toxicity data rather than require further testing. However, with increasing concern over environmental and health safety, the public could hardly approve of this option.

The other option is to request a larger budget from Congress and to put more resources into the regulation of biotechnology. This will involve the hiring and training of experts, the sponsoring of expert committees, and the conduct of further on-site testing. In this age of federal deficit, the federal agencies cannot anticipate an increased budget. Even large environmental disasters such as the Alaskan oil spill cannot receive an increased federal budget for cleanup efforts.

A third option is to standardize and streamline the review process, an approach that the EPA has decided to take. Rather than handle each application on a case-by-case basis, the EPA is trying to approve classes of pesticides or similar products under one assessment. To further facilitate the process, all agencies have issued guidance to biotechnology investigators and manufacturers. Although the EPA hopes to cluster similar petitions under one approval process, the USDA will continue its case-by-case approach, with an attempt to exempt an increased number of applications as more risk assessment information becomes available. Because the FDA is not under the same time constraints as the other regulatory agencies, it will continue the review process on a case-by-case basis.

Yet another approach would be to establish a committee to oversee all biotechnology regulatory activities. To an extent, the Biotechnology Science Coordinating Committee (BSCC) fulfills this function. Established as an interagency coordinating committee, the BSCC ensures consistency among regulatory agencies and provides guidance for the conduct of biotechnology risk assessments and the development of regulations.

However, other than an oversight function, the BSCC lacks the regulatory authority required to move biotechnology from the laboratory to the marketplace. The final responsibility still lies with the federal agencies, whose task is not becoming easier. The staggering number of applications in the rapidly growing field of biotechnology further complicates their task. Sound risk assessment information is urgently needed to expedite the regulatory process.

Biotechnology in Europe

Although Europe is striving toward uniform regulations and economic policies, biotechnology is handled in a different manner in each one of the Western European countries. Biotechnology regulations range anywhere from no controls in Italy to a total ban in West Germany. Nevertheless, European concern with risk aspects of biotechnology is growing.

Of the western European countries, Great Britain has started to invest in biotechnology early on. It had an advantage over the United States because the public supported advances in biotechnology from the beginning. Biosafety committees were established, and petitions were approved. To date, several environmental releases have taken place in Great Britain, and more are being considered. Several multinational companies with manufacturing capabilities both in the United States and in Great Britain have opted to market their biotechnological products in Britain because the approval process seems to be shorter and less cumbersome. Industry also attempts to choose a coherent explanation and a suitable image when it addresses the public. Published last year in Great Britain by Hobsons Scientific, Biotechnology in Focus[5] is aimed at the lay public and explains the complexities of biotechnology in a simple language. Other rationally targeted follow-ups are in preparation.

Similarly, France has authorized environmental releases and approved several genetically engineered products. In France, industry works closely with the government and the academic institutions. Just as nuclear energy faced no public objection in the past, the French public does not regard biotechnology as a threat but rather as an innovative tool to advance technology and improve the quality of life. There is very little public involvement in any genetic release experiments. Nevertheless, French industry, together with the European Economic Community and several French ministries, maintains an active interest in keeping the public abreast of developments in biotechnology. As recently as April 1989, the French Association for the Development of Bioindustry organized an international conference entitled "Risk Management in Biotechnology." With the participation of leading international experts, the meeting explored technical expectations, economic and social issues, possible biotechnology risks, risk management, and international biosafety guidelines.

Some of the most innovative biotechnology companies have established operations in the Netherlands. Over the years, biotechnology regulations in the Netherlands have become more stringent due to public concern and influence from neighboring Germany. However, because the approval process within the government is uniform, it is still possible to obtain manufacturing permits for genetically engineered products. Companies in the Netherlands are primarily interested in drugs and diagnostics. There are only a few petitions for environmental releases.

The most stringent countries are Denmark and Germany. Both countries have biotechnology companies who are interested in marketing biotechnology products and processes and need to release genetically engineered microbes into the environment. Denmark has banned all releases but is still allowing the manufacturing of drugs and diagnostics under strict regulations. In Germany, the Green Party is officially opposed to any genetic research and has managed over the past few years to bring genetic research to a halt. In fact, no environmental releases are permitted in Germany. Biotechnology has become a political issue. Several companies are moving their biotechnology operations out of Germany and are looking to invest elsewhere. The German government is concerned that technical innovation has come to a complete halt in their country and that they may no longer be able to compete in the open market. For the same reasons, universities are losing important faculty positions. Because of the strict regulations governing genetic research, prominent German scientists are accepting appointments in other countries where they can conduct research more freely and keep up with their field of research.

In contrast, Italy has not enforced any regulations in biotechnology. The Italian government has proposed several approaches in international meetings, but to date, there is no legislation on environmental releases in that country. Several companies have contemplated moving their operations to Italy to avoid strict government controls. However, it is difficult to predict whether Italy will opt to impose regulation in the future, an action that may prevent these companies from operating their manufacturing plants as originally planned.

Biotechnology in Japan

By far the most successful country in conducting biotechnology research is Japan. As in other research areas, the Japanese government works closely with industry and academic institutions through its Ministry of International Trade and Industry. There is close collaboration between the various sectors of industry and government, and conflicts seldom arise. Biotechnology is projected to be at least a $100 billion international market by the year 2000, and Japan is targeting to control 75 percent of this market.

Interestingly enough, Japan does not conduct environmental releases of genetically engineered organisms. Most of their efforts are focused on the manufacturing of drugs, diagnostics, and upscale technology for industrial purposes. There is strict adherence to the Japanese Recombinant DNA Guidelines so that the enforcement of regulations is not necessary. The containment standards are extremely stringent, but most institutions and manufacturing plants are able to work efficiently under these stringent conditions. Clinical tests proceed at a faster rate than in the United States.

The Japanese also invest in foreign companies throughout the world, acquiring licensing and patent rights. Thus, if they wish to market a product in the future and subject themselves to the regulations of foreign countries, they have the tools to do so. At present, it is easy to conduct risk assessment experiments in Japan so that there is no need to go abroad.

Conclusions

Biotechnology has advanced rapidly in the last few years and has branched into many industrial sectors. Several environmental releases of genetically engineered microbes have been conducted throughout the world, yielding additional safety data and risk-assessment information. Most of the data indicates that the releases are safe. However, in view of other unknown parameters associated with the genetic engineering of novel microbes, the authorities are not convinced that the research is safe.

In many countries, public opinion is divided on biotechnology. Although some people believe that the research is safe and holds promise for great technological innovation, others fear the hazardous consequences of biotechnology and demand that the research be banned. Undoubtedly, biotechnology has tremendous potential to improve current technology and the quality of life. Using biotechnology, cure and treatment for several major diseases may be possible. In the future, hepatitis may be prevented, leukemias may be cured, and cancers of microscopic dimensions may be detected. In the agricultural area, frost damage may be retarded, crop-destroying pests may be killed without chemicals, and toxic waste may be effectively treated using biotechnology degradation products. Already, progress has been made in the drug, vaccine, and diagnostic fields. Greater promises are in store for the agricultural and upscale technologies.

Biotechnology needs to be pursued in a safe manner, with sound risk assessments backing up experimental and manufacturing data. Moreover, a scientifically based regulatory policy is required that encourages innovation without compromising sound environmental management. Initially, products of genetic engineering may require greater scrutiny than products of traditional breeding. Ultimately, the world may be sufficiently interested in this technology to weigh the risks against the benefits and favor biotechnology and its numerous applications, provided sufficient safeguards are taken. Furthermore, regulations should be updated on a regular basis as more risk-assessment information becomes available. This will not only facilitate the task of the federal agencies but also help expedite the review process and minimize unnecessary regulatory burdens.

Better risk-assessment communication, including public education programs, public presentations, and open debates, will contribute to the understanding of the numerous advantages that biotechnology can offer. Through protective measures, a careful approach, and by addressing the risks that biotechnology poses to human health and the environment, industry and academia can benefit from this tremendous technology and its applications in the biomedical, agricultural, and industrial areas. Every technology has its growing pains, and biotechnology is no exception. Yet these pains can be minimized by proceeding in a safe and controlled manner. Public perception is as important as the development of biotechnology itself. Industry knows and has emphasized repeatedly that if there is no public acceptance of their product, there may not be a product. Concerns raised by scientists, environmentalists, and public interest groups require the continued communication of risks and benefits. Both science and the public will benefit from a cautious stepwise approach.

References

1. Office of Technology Assessment, *Public Perceptions of Biotechnology*, press release, May 27, 1987.
2. Report of the Organizing Committee of the Asilomar Conference on Recombinant DNA Molecules, *Science* **185**, 303 (1974).
3. National Institutes of Health Guidelines for Research Involving Recombinant DNA Molecules, *Federal Register* June, 1976.
4. DNA Experimentation with *E. coli*-K1, *J. Infect. Dis.* **137**, (1978).
5. *Biotechnology in Focus*, (Hobsons Scientific, United Kingdom, 1988).

Discussion

Lugtenberg: With respect to crippled strains, you gave the example of Chakrabarty's pollutant as a food source. You claimed that the strain died out when the pollutant was depleted. I do not see why the strain should die.

Kamely: Even if it does not die, it becomes inactive, and in some cases you can show that the strain resumes growth once the pollutant is added back.

Lugtenberg: Why could it not use something else as a food source?

Kamely: Because it is dependent on this particular pollutant as a sole food source.

Lugtenberg: How safe is that?

Kamely: That is a matter which needs to be taken into consideration.

Lugtenberg: I do not know the background, but I hardly believe in safe strains. I think that sometimes a single mutation can break through the safety mechanism.

Kamely: I agree. Many people share this view. If you remember, I asked Dr. Bedard whether her strain that grows on biphenyl died or whether it could be reactivated. In many cases, a given strain can be activated once it is given the proper food source. This phenomenon can occur several months later. In fact, Chakrabarty's strains behave in a similar manner, especially the *Pseudomonas* strains that grow on 2,4,5-T. This is what makes the task of regulation so difficult. If the strain is dormant, it may exhibit other unsafe properties once it is reactivated. As a result, regulatory agencies take a long time to do risk assessments. The companies are anxious to get the product on the market. It is my belief that the more data we gather, the more we can clearly demonstrate the safety of engineered microorganisms.

Lugtenberg: One more comment on crippled strains, especially those pertaining to vaccines. If you want to put strains out in the environment, the major problem in planned microinteractions is to get the manipulated strains established in the environment. If at the same time you also want the strains to be crippled, then I think it will never work.

Kamely: Many people share this view with you.

Chakrabarty: Just to continue what Dr. Lugtenberg said. He said that he does not consider the strain safe. The problem is, "What is a safe strain"? Even if a particular bacterium does not die quickly, does that mean that it is unsafe? People have been using biususium in this way for a long time, and there has been no great catastrophy. So long as a microorganism is nonpathogenic, isolated from nature, and thrown back into nature, it will eventually get in phase with nature and the other microorganisms. Incidentally, I might mention that we did careful experiments with photogenetic *matters* in them so that we could follow their path carefully. In fact, the bacteria very rapidly ceased growing. When you add back the pollutant after five or six weeks, they will start to grow. So we know that there is a minimum number that are maintained in the soil. However, with regard to safety, the implication is that if your bacterium does not die off very quickly, it is unsafe. Throwing harmless bacteria into nature, even in large numbers, has not caused, as far as I know, any disaster in the environment. In fact, there are natural bacteria that are a lot more pathogenic than the genetically engineered bacteria proposed here.

Kamely: Let me comment on that. What you and your colleagues believe may sound logical to you but may not be agreeable to other members of the public. Let me give you an example of a gene therapy experiment that was recently approved at the National Institutes of Health. The researchers designed as a vector a retrovirus that is replication-defective, for example, it goes through one or two cycles of division and then dies off. Yet a retrovirus can also be a potent cancer causing virus. Moreover, one kind of retrovirus, human immunovirus, can cause acquired immunodeficiency syndrome. Because of the risks involved, it took several years to approve this simple experiment. Now, imagine you are going to send a similar virus into the uncontrolled, open environment. There is no way to contain its spread, should it prove harmful. This is why Jeremy Rifkin and prominent scientists such as Jonathan King and Keith Yamamoto are opposed to environmental release. The arguments they make are valid. I believe the only way to counter that is to obtain good risk-assessment data and demonstrate that the benefits outweigh the dangers to the environment. There is no risk-free environment, but the risks can be minimized.

23

Risk Assessment for Biodegradation in Pollution Control and Cleanup

Gilbert S. Omenn
Al W. Bourquin
*University of Washington
School of Public Health and
Community Medicine
Seattle, WA 98195, and
Ecova Corporation
Redmond, WA 98052*

Risk assessment for biodegradation must investigate the survival, proliferation, function, transport, and effects of introduced organisms and the expression and transfer of their genomes. This paper reviews methods for achieving those objectives, addressing both genetically engineered organisms and organisms isolated or selected by traditional means. Strategies for minimizing any risks of untoward effects include selection of organisms from habitats to which they will be applied and containment of organisms in bioreactors or larger enclosures. Several examples of practical bioremediation work in the field in controlled environments are described.

Introduction

Evaluation of potential risks from deliberate release into the environment of genetically engineered organisms or other microorganisms requires systematic, stepwise gathering of relevant empirical data. Risks are of two complementary categories: (1) that the organisms will fail to achieve their intended effects; and (2) that unintended adverse effects on the environment may occur. Others authors in this book have addressed the first type of risk. In fact, many of the methods required will serve both types of risk assessment.

Speculating about and modeling potential risks will not suffice; a growing data base is essential for informed speculation about potential risks that need to be investigated and for modeling the survival, proliferation, function, and transport of introduced organisms and the expression and transfer of their genomes. The experience of the National Institutes of Health during the past 15 years with orderly development of risk assessment experiments provides a sound analogy for the broader questions that have been raised as this work moves beyond the controlled laboratory setting and industrial fermentation to field applications in agriculture, forestry, and pollution control and cleanup.[1-6]

The special attraction of recombinant DNA technology, and probably its inherent safety feature, is its specificity. Gene splicing can involve just one or very few specific genes for a specific purpose, contrasted with crossing the entire genome of two plants or fused protoplasts or treating organisms with chemical mutagens. Success depends on knowing the genes responsible for biologically significant functions; being able to isolate, clone, and introduce the gene into the desired recipient; having means to grow recipient cells into full plants or effective microbes; and being certain that the function of the introduced gene can be regulated as desired without negative effects on the recipient or the ecosystem in which it is expected to function. Genetic engineering strategies already employed include plasmid-mediated transfer of genes between bacteria or from Agrobacteria to plants, transposon-mediated transfer of chromosomal genes, and deletion of specific genes for undesired functions.

Microorganisms must be found or modified to meet demanding requirements of unusual environments, and they must survive and proliferate in competition with the existing flora, predators, and sometimes extreme or widely fluctuating chemical and physical conditions. Biochemical capacities in nature most likely to be useful are dehalogenation, deamination, denitration, and ring cleavage. Even partial detoxification of compounds identified as hazardous under toxic waste and clean water regulations would be a useful step in overall disposal strategies. Thus, lists of regulated chemicals may be considered directories of opportunity for genetic engineering (see the appendix in reference 3). Enhanced, ecologically adapted *in situ* biodegradation may be useful in sediments, soils, and sumps.

Recommendations that surely can reduce the likelihood of any risk to the environment from use of genetically enhanced organisms in pollution cleanup include the following:

1. Gain maximal information about the recipient and donor organisms utilized.
2. Assure high specificity and precision in the genetic change introduced.
3. Use recipient organisms well adapted to the habitat in which they are to be employed to express their newly endowed specific attributes.
4. Identify and enumerate introduced organisms in the ecosystem.
5. Monitor the fate of introduced organisms, including persistence, proliferation, and dispersion.

Methods must be developed for the following objectives:

1. Detection and enumeration of the introduced organism.
2. Detailed description of the patterns of release and spread of the organism.
3. Detection of gene transfer to and from other organisms.
4. Orderly recognition of toxicity, both acute and chronic, for nontarget species of many kinds.
5. Detection of disruption of biogeochemical environmental processes.

In every case, specific organisms, sites, and applications will be involved. Thus, it is no surprise that the U.S. Environmental Protection Agency and the National Institutes of Health have called for case-by-case assessments.[7-9] Nevertheless, certain methodologies are at the base of this field.

The first purpose of this chapter is to evaluate the suitability of empirical methods for assessing potential outcomes of environmental release of genetically modified organisms and to identify strengths, limitations, and research needs in these subfields that must be brought together, both for risk assessment and for improving the capabilities of bioremediation technologies. The second part of the chapter will illustrate the state of the art in field applications and propose a risk-minimization strategy.

Methods for the Detection, Identification, and Enumeration of Introduced Organisms

Sampling. Strategies for sampling depend on the purpose. To ascertain whether an introduced organism has persisted and carried out its desired functions, one must know the density and activity of the organism in the target field; thus, sampling must be intensive, local, and quantitative. To cast a wide net over potential problems from transport beyond the site of application, a larger geographic area must be sampled with methods that qualitatively identify the organism or its special genome and provide clues to the partitioning of the organism in various potential habitats or microhabitats. Sampling should include tissues and excreta from potential animal hosts. We will generally prefer a combination of these approaches.

Sediments and soils present problems for sampling because of the adsorption of microorganisms to various surfaces, from which desorption is unpredictable. Cells can be dissociated from solid phases by physical or chemical means and then be subjected to selective plate counting. Alternatively, the sediment or soil itself can be placed into broth enrichment medium, using replicated enrichments and replicated isolations from each flask. In either approach, molecular analyses can be grafted onto the culture method. The enrichment approach is likely to detect genetically engineered microorganisms at lower densities than is possible with direct plate counting, and it is compatible with quantitation using most-probable-number (MPN) methods.[10] Designing an economical but sufficient sampling strategy is a general problem in ecology; a performance curve of density against sampling effort can be a useful guide.

Microbiological culture methods with marker genes. Specific, convenient, reliable, and sensitive tracer methodologies are a prerequisite for the entire process of risk assessment in environmental biotechnology. Microbiologists have relied on the principles of selective enrichment or enhancement culture and differential media for nearly 100 years to recover and type organisms from various ecosystems. Media are available for detection and differentiation of organisms according to their natural characteristics, especially metabolic requirements. The use of strains that are tagged with a particular metabolic activity or resistance attribute greatly facilitates the identification and enumeration of organisms of interest. For example, lactose fermentation might be a useful marker gene for bacteria other than *Escherichia coli* (which is unusual in being able to metabolize lactose).[11] To make marker genes more specific, convenient inducible promoter-operator sequences can be used, including also the tryptophan promoter-operator region (tryptophan) and the phage lambda right operator (high temperature or ultraviolet irradiation) for induction of the marker trait.

Markers may be introduced conveniently on plasmids. Obviously, if the plasmid is unstable and the DNA sequence of interest is not also carried on the plasmid, the marker will be unreliable. Sometimes, the biodegradative activity itself may be usefully detected with special color reactions, as noted by other authors. There are limitations in the genetic markers available. The most convenient markers often are expressed as resistance to inhibition of growth, including the following list of candidates for resistance markers: novobiocin, aristocitin, hygromycin B, kasugamycin, bacitracin, fusidic acid, pimaricin, virginiamycin, nalidixic acid, bambermycins, tylomycin, and oleandomycin, plus such heavy metal ions as mercuric and cadmium.[12] It is essential to choose antibiotics that are not in use in humans or animals, because plasmid-mediated multiple resistances to clinically useful antibiotics are a major public health problem. In order to avoid extensive interspecies transfer, it is important to use resistance genes that are located in the chromosome, not carried on easily transmissible extrachromosomal plasmids, and preferably not located in close proximity to repeated sequences that may function with transposable elements. Some strains resistant to an antibiotic or a heavy metal ion do not grow well in the absence of that selective agent. Also, certain pesticides may interfere with heavy metal markers by inducing resistance among indigenous organisms. Finally, it is desirable to have two markers, so that a spontaneous mutation will not lead to disappearance of the singly tagged organism from the detection system.

Immunological Methods. Immunofluorescence techniques have been applied in microbial ecology for strains of *Rhizobium* species, *Azotobacter, Beijerinckea, Azospirillum*, nitrifiers, sulfur oxidizers, fungi, and other organisms.[13,14] However, there are several limitations to this approach. First, minimal countable densities in soils are 10^6 to 10^7 organisms per gram of soil,[14] depending on desorption. This is too insensitive for our purposes. Second, other particles in the environment may fluoresce; certain materials autofluoresce; inorganic particles may bind nonspecifically to the fluorescent antibody; and there may be truly cross-reacting surface proteins on other organisms, or cross-reactions with contaminants present in the material in which the antiserum was produced. Third, the genetically engineered microorganism may not fluoresce due to organic slimes, as in the case of a fixed-bed wastewater treatment reactor,[15] or because its antigen is not stable. Finally, immunofluorescence may not distinguish between living and dead cells and will not track the recombinant DNA gene itself, unless the antigen is specified by that DNA sequence.

Use of monoclonal antibodies offers substantial improvements in specificity, although not necessarily in sensitivity. Autofluorescence, interference by bacterial slimes, and inability to distinguish living and dead cells remain problems.

Genetic analyses: restriction enzyme mapping and sequencing. Restriction enzymes, which specifically cleave DNA into easily separated and recognizable fragments, can be quite helpful in identifying and monitoring recombinant organisms. These naturally occurring enzymes have been the backbone of recombinant DNA advances in recent years; they cleave double-stranded DNA at specific sites determined by nucleotide sequences of four or six base pairs. Depending on the presence and location of the specific sequences, each restriction enzyme will yield a number of distinct fragments that can be separated according to their size on agarose gel electrophoresis. This approach is simplest with plasmids (limited amount of DNA). Restriction fragment patterns must be determined both for the nonrecombinant and recombinant plasmids (or chromosomal DNA). Inserted and deleted DNA are identified through the changes in size of particular DNA fragments. Restriction enzymes are numerous and relatively expensive. Manufacturers should be expected or required to perform the initial analyses of the sequences, ascertaining which enzyme (or enzymes) would be best for subsequent monitoring needs.

Restriction enzymes also are critical tools for sequencing genomes or plasmids. Chemical sequencing of DNA has been combined with hybridization (Southern blotting) to yield a rapid, direct method for sequencing regions of chromosomes from whole genomic DNA.[16] Its applications in the near term will be limited to very special characterizations of fine structure. Another target for nucleotide sequencing, however, may be useful sooner, namely, the 5S ribosomal RNA. Several studies of *Vibrio cholerae* strains from marine environments have utilized sequencing methods to compare organisms from different sites or time periods or from the same environment with a notable difference in function.[17] Prokaryotic 5S rRNA sequences vary between species by five to 15 percent, and within species a range of variation of about two percent has been found. rRNA analysis, in conjunction with probe analysis for the recombinant gene, may become an efficient molecular means for showing that the gene has been transferred to a strain or species other than the one deliberately introduced.

Genetic analyses: DNA probes. When the specific DNA sequence is prepared for insertion into a recipient organism, a probe sequence complementary to the introduced sequence can be constructed for use in future monitoring efforts. The length and sequence of the probe depend on the host-vector system that is utilized. If the recombinant DNA is an altered gene that normally is present in that host, the differences in sequence may be as small as a single nucleotide, so that very carefully defined hybridization conditions will be necessary to demonstrate the difference. The methodology is much simpler when a wholly new gene is introduced. The probe can be labeled for radioactive or fluorescent readout and can be hybridized to colonies growing on the surface of a nitrocellulose filter in contact with appropriate media. This technique is relatively expensive, and it depends on adequate colony growth. Probe techniques do not enhance selective growth, nor do they provide a selective differential medium. Thus, the specificity of probe hybridization must be coupled with traditional culture techniques.

The colony hybridization method currently has a sensitivity capable of detecting one colony in 10^6 of a nonhomologous DNA background.[18] Amplification methods for labeled probes tied to fluorescent, luminescent, or colorimetric products of enzyme cascades can increase the sensitivity by two orders of magnitude or more. Probe analysis can be combined with the restriction enzyme mapping just described to test whether the organism isolated from the environment, compared with the restriction fragment pattern for the original recombinant organism, still has the recombinant sequence in the original position and to determine whether it has undergone any detectable alterations or deletions. Additional tests, using monoclonal antibodies for detecting metabolic or resistance properties, are necessary to ascertain that the recombinant gene actually is producing its gene product.

Methods for Assessing Fate and the Effects of Genetically Engineered Organisms

In striking contrast with the situation of organisms that may be released accidentally into the environment from laboratory or industrial applications, organisms released deliberately to function in the environment must be able to survive, proliferate, and express their desired functions. Many microbial ecologists have emphasized what an enormous challenge it will be to introduce truly novel organisms into well-adapted habitats.[2,3,19] Nevertheless, some troubling examples are known of invading organisms that became pests or strikingly changed a particular habitat. The mongoose, *Herpestes auropunctates*; the gypsy moth, *Lymantria dispar*; chestnut blight due to a parasitic Asian fungus, *Endothia parasitica*; the Japanese beetle; and kudzu are classic examples,[20,21] having occurred in 1872, the late 1800s, 1900, 1911, and the 1930s, respectively.[22] There should be lessons that can be applied from these unusual negative experiences. Perhaps the two most important are that broad host range is undesirable and that introduced organisms need not be genetically engineered to become dominant invaders.

Empirical assessment of the fate, transport, gene transfer, and ecosystem effects of introduced organisms should begin with totally contained systems that simulate terrestrial or aquatic environments of interest. These environments range from flasks, mason jars, and growth chambers on the laboratory bench to fully contained greenhouses and systematically sampled natural areas sometimes termed mesocosms. As will be discussed shortly, fully controlled environments for bioremediation may be preferred over releasing organisms into open environments.

Of two types of microcosms,[23-25] the first is naturally derived, representing an excised natural community. Samples of soil, lake water, or marine sediment may be brought into the laboratory for analysis. The second type of microcosm is synthesized or standardized with chemically defined media. Indicator organisms must be chosen and introduced to make a biologically meaningful and ecologically instructive multitrophic system.

Naturally Derived Microcosms. The U.S. Environmental Protection Agency (EPA) has developed microcosm programs for both terrestrial and aquatic research. As several other authors have illustrated, this approach has readily been adapted to study samples from chemically contaminated sites. The work builds on several decades of studies on the persistence of certain microorganisms in natural ecosystems, especially organisms associated with animals and plants as pathogens or pollution-indicator bacteria. More contemporary information needs to be gained about persistence, cell densities, and fate of species such as *Pseudomonas, Alcaligenes, Vibrio, Nitrosomonas, Actinetobacter, Aeromonas, Klebsiella, Enterobacter,* and others found in fresh and marine water systems and soils.

Terrestrial models are being developed for the following five ecosystems: (1) *Rhizobium*-legume-soil; (2) root rhizosphere of easily manipulated and cultivated plants (radishes and potatoes); (3) soil-plant systems for investigating fate and effects of engineered organisms capable of biodegrading certain pesticides; (4) vegetables undergoing microbial decay; and (5) plant leaf surfaces. Natural terrestrial habitats have been selected that support high natural cell density. For example, an average legume nodule contains 10^7 to 10^9 viable cells, and plant root rhizospheres contain 10^6 or more bacteria per centimeter length of root surface. The spray application of herbicide-degrading bacteria onto soil and plants will probably not achieve high cell densities unless there is a significant regrowth of the organism. However, many of the indigenous soil bacteria may have been killed by the herbicide, making both nutrients and niches available for the resistant engineered or selected plasmid-containing microbe. The natural decay of vegetation in the pesticide model and in the postharvest vegetable leaf-decay model will lead to marked changes in terrestrial microflora, especially plant-pathogenic soft-rot bacteria of the genera *Erwinia*, *Pectobacterium*, and *Pseudomonas*. Because these organisms undergo promiscuous plasmid transfer, they are ideal for following the fate of well-marked novel genomes.

Studies with naturally derived aquatic systems may utilize ecocores taken from the sediment of lakes, streams, and estuaries. Bourquin and Pritchard of the EPA used such ecocores to determine degradation rates of xenobiotics by the organisms present in the sediments.[2,23] Ecosystems with high microbial densities are most likely to foster gene flow between species; these include certain aquatic sediments, salt marsh sediments, and various liquid-to-surface interfaces. Cell-to-cell movement of genes is thought to depend more on ecological intimacy than on evolutionary relatedness. Such a conclusion can be investigated in aquatic microcosms, admittedly with many simplifying assumptions.

Grimes, Singleton, and Colwell[26] reported an instructive use of microcosms to investigate a hypothesis based on observations in the natural marine environment. The Puerto Rico Trench surface water of the Atlantic Ocean was the dump site for some 3.6×10^8 liters of composite pharmaceutical waste (CPW) per year from 1972 through 1981. Contrary to expectations, the culturable bacterial community in the dump site was dominated by *Vibrio* species rather than by *Pseudomonas*. It was hypothesized that the pharmaceutical wastes had led to a restructuring of the culturable heterotrophic bacterial community. To test this hypothesis of allogenic succession, laboratory experiments were conducted. Culturable bacterial flora of Chesapeake Bay water samples, when treated with CPW, showed no apparent toxic effects and an increase in the number of bacteria. Next, microcosms containing two-species communities (*Vibrio* PR-110 and *Pseudomonas* AO-17 or AO-66) were studied; *Vibrio* was dominant and increased its dominance in relation to dose of wastes added. Of course, it is a long way from recognizing these shifts in marine bacterial communities to understanding the direct and indirect consequences on the overall ecosystem.

Synthesized or standardized microcosms. Synthetic microcosms are composed of distilled water; silica sand; reagent-grade chemicals; and a variety of algae, grazers, and detritivores that are easily reared in the laboratory.[27,28] These systems provide a nonsite-specific, ecosystem-level bioassay with interspecies competition within primary, secondary, and recycling trophic levels. Replicate microcosms (in 3-liter bottles) can be set up to allow for manipulation of physical and chemical variables of interest, dose-response studies, and reproducibility of observations. The microcosms display nutrient depletion, algal competition and succession, and algal depletion through grazing and nutrient depletion. External agents, such as malathion, copper sulfate, and streptomycin, have been assayed in different phases of maturation of these synthesized ecosystems.[27] Thus, these microcosms represent a significant step toward revealing complexity in ecosystem responses and effects.

A variety of measurements and observations can be made over the course of an extensive protocol in the microcosm, and recovery from temporary toxicities can be demonstrated because of the periodic (usually weekly) reinoculation of small numbers of organisms. Considerable sophistication in data management[27] and modeling[28] has been achieved, but more extensive biochemical measurements need to be developed. The operational costs are low, with all the supplies and highly standardized cultures readily available. To introduce microorganisms instead of chemicals in these systems, the sampling techniques would have to be altered extensively to prevent escape of the test organisms and to assure aseptic technique. Large organisms would have to be sampled without removal, and resultant counts would be approximate. Microscopic counts would have to be handled quite differently. Scraping of wall surfaces presumably could be managed externally with magnetic control of internal scrapers.

Mesocosms. Well-controlled environments outside the laboratory are a critical step before open field trials. The greenhouse and the controlled field site are well-established tools of biologists for planting species of interest,and observing them and their responses to microbial and chemical sprays, irrigation schemes, and other manipulations. For aquatic environments, flowthrough systems with bags or tanks are often utilized; however, these are not closed environments. With regard to microbial agents, the extensive, much-debated record on ice-nucleation mutants of *Pseudomonas syringae* and *Erwinia herbicola* to prevent frost injury is the leading example. Survival, lateral dissemination, and population dynamics of nucleation-negative mutants and nucleation-positive populations, and the specificity of their interactions on leaf surfaces, could be studied much better in controlled field sites than in greenhouses. Antibiotic and DNA sequence markers have been utilized.[29]

For pollution control applications, there should be an analogous scaling up from the laboratory to pilot simulations of waste treatment facilities, agricultural and forestry decomposition sites, contaminated soil sites, mineral ore leaching site, or oil sump cleanup sites. The ecocore microcosm approach can be combined with *in situ* fully contained tests in which the desired microorganisms can be introduced and monitored for their fate and effects. As in the example of ice-nucleation negative mutants, markers for following the organism and its genome and multiple measures of effects in the target environment must be built into case-specific protocols.

Before toxic waste sites are sealed, incinerated, or removed, there are appropriate and varied opportunities for testing either organisms with specific degradative capabilities, or mixed cultures of organisms with a variety of capabilities, in an effort to detoxify, at least partially, the more intractable and toxic agents in the site.[2,3] It should be possible to use a well-demarcated portion of the site and to monitor the fate and effects of the introduced organisms, always with the capacity to seal the operation as previously planned. Less-controlled field sites represent an enormous array of site-specific needs, opportunities, and potential risks. There must be assurance that the organisms have shown no cause for concern in microcosm studies, have highly specific properties, preferably are drawn from a site to which they may be returned or a similar ecological habitat, and that decontamination of the entire operation is feasible. It is possible that organisms could be modified to "disarm" them ecologically, so they will not be likely to spread beyond the range where they are intended to be effective, or so that they can be "recalled" through sensitivity to certain antibiotics or bacterial phage[30] or "suicide" metabolites. We must take care, however, that the protection does not introduce greater hazards than the organism itself. Many worries about possible ecological effects are mitigated at hazardous waste sites, which are already ecological disasters.

Methods for Assessing the Genetic Stability of Genetically Engineered Organisms

Genetic stability studies must address some of the more speculative concerns about genetically engineering microorganisms. It is conceivable that even a seemingly precise recombinant DNA experiment might carry along transcription signals or coding sequences that would have unpredicted effects in additional host organisms. Repeated sequences or transposons might lead to multiple and unintended insertions, with disruption or conceivably activation of certain host genes. Some of these speculations are difficult to operationalize, but it is possible to investigate the likelihood of transfer of DNA sequences between species. This is particularly true in cases when the inserted DNA sequences are carried on extrachromosomal plasmids, which are known to be readily transferred across species. An empirical approach is needed to address issues of host range, because theory is weak, both for gene transfer and for toxicity.

Organisms initially can be grown to high cell densities in laboratory media and combined with bacteria likely to be encountered in nature. Using routine selective media and specific assays for the markers or marker DNA sequences, such mixed cultures can be examined for recombinant organisms receiving the marker genes. Comparable studies can be carried out with naked DNA sequences in plasmids and chromosomal sites, with checking for transfer frequencies due to transformation, transduction, or conjugation mechanisms. Because plasmid DNA is certain to be released from lysed bacterial cells, it is useful to inquire about the fate and effects resulting from release of plasmid DNA into specific niches such as pollutant degradation sites in water or soil systems or legume root nodules and root rhizospheres.

Helper plasmids in terrestrial microcosm flora, contributions of transposons, and triparental matings may be essential to analyze. Combining special microcosms with effective markers may permit studies of considerably higher complexity and specificity than two-species or even mixed-culture chemostat experiments. The combination is central to the stepwise, systematic, empirical investigation of these organisms.

Genera of bacteria likely to be exchanging broad host range plasmids in the respective ecosystems are listed in the following classifications:[25]

1. Soil: *Pseudomonas, Alcaligenes, Klebsiella, Enterobacter, Rhizobium*
2. Aquatic: *Pseudomonas, Escherichia, Klebsiella*
3. Marine: *Vibrio*

We have powerful tools for developing this field. However, very few applications can be cited thus far with organisms of interest for environmental applications. As noted, care must be exercised in the choice of marker genes and phenotypes to avoid introducing unnecessary risks from the monitoring process. In many situations, the growth of introduced organisms will be so limited and the dilution by natural flora will be so great that DNA probe or monoclonal antibody reagents will be useful only after successful selection and enrichment for the desired organism. Obviously, it will be even more difficult to use the same diagnostic tools to trace the genome into minor species in the environment. On the other hand, should gene transfer occur into an organism that becomes a dominant species, these diagnostic tools might be highly effective.

Minimizing Potential Risks by Working in Controlled Environments

Many of the approaches described previously to characterize the survival, function, proliferation, transport, and gene transfer of introduced organisms for assessment of potential risks to the environment are useful also to characterize the functional performance of the organism in biodegradation. Thus far, there has been minimal interest in exploiting R-DNA–engineered microorganisms for the twin reasons that (1) existing or classically selected organisms may suffice in well-managed sites and (2) use of R-DNA–engineered organisms may elicit unpredictable regulatory review.

The main bioremediation technology in the field today involves engineering applications of basic principles of aerobic metabolism: optimizing the concentrations of oxygen and nutrients and assuring adequate moisture within a given environment to enhance the indigenous microbial population. Generally, there is little or no knowledge of the organisms present at the site. Better understanding of microbial ecology and genetic enhancement of biodegradation as described by the authors in this book should accelerate advances in bioremediation.

The most common form of bioremediation of contaminated soil has been known as "landfarming." In many cases, landfarming has been little more than dumping contaminated waste onto land and letting nature work its way. Modern management of such sites might better be termed "solid-phase bioremediation." The main advances come from addition of nutrients and active aeration, plus a slight increase in the release of chemicals adsorbed to soil particles. The Ecova Corporation, (Redmond, Washington) for example, has used this technique very effectively to clean up fuel oils, diesel fuels, pesticide contamination, and other types of easily degraded n substrates in several states in the United States High molecular weight petroleum-based contaminants often remain. In several sites, Ecova has compared this basal approach to an alternative that includes inoculation of pertinent strains (for example, 2,4-D–degrading strains of *Pseudomonas*, generously provided by Chapman); generally, no further increase in rate of degradation has been obtained.

For example, an experiment was carried out on a petroleum-contaminated site in California. A gridwork map was prepared, and test squares were compared. An organism with constitutive biodegradative activity against polynuclear aromatic compounds (PNAs) was inoculated; dibenzofuran served as the marker compound. The concept was that if constitutive organisms that did not require induction by lower molecular weight (MW) compounds could be isolated, then those organisms might degrade more of the heavier MW PNAs, thereby reducing residuals of the 4-6 ring compounds. Such an organism, *Pseudomonas* strain DBM101, isolated from a creosote-contaminated site, was constitutive for dibenzofuran and gave yellow ring-cleavage products for this compound as well as other PNAs, including benzo(a)pyrene. The organism was quite active and survived well in the laboratory with soil cores from the site. In the field, it did grow for a short period of time, but then rapidly died off, as demonstrated by enumeration techniques. Even without enhancement, concentrations of high MW compounds were reduced to mandated cleanup levels over time.

Bioreactors provide a practical means of assuring a controlled environment for biodegradation. For groundwater sites contaminated with chlorinated or mixed solvents, the approach involves empirical development in the laboratory of a site-specific bioreactor with a consortium of indigenous organisms plus laboratory stock cultures.

Then we move to the field in combination with an air stripper so that nonbiodegradable solvents are air-stripped while the biodegradable solvents are treated in a continuous stir bioreactor. For example, after only eight days, all the influent contaminants at a particular California site were reduced below the effluent discharge limits and have remained so over a two-year period, with very few breakthroughs. Furthermore, the underground plume has been contained.

Similarly, to contain leachate as well as volatile compounds in solid-phase bioremediation, a liner with leachate control system is laid down, covered with clean sand, and then the contaminated soil is brought into a completely enclosed facility where all the air exiting the system is handled either through bioreactors or through carbon filtration systems. Unfortunately, this approach may be complicated by pending regulations in the United States. Under the Resource Conservation and Recovery Act (RCRA) "Land-Ban" provisions, as of August 1989, management of many types of contaminated soils, especially refinery wastes, will have to be carried out so as to eliminate both emissions to the air and movement of contaminated soils. Even on-site manipulations to bring huge batches of soil into these controlled bioremediation environments might be disallowed. Objections to such inappropriate regulations are pending.

Large bioreactors can be used to remediate contaminated surface waters or contaminated soils in soil water slurries. At a North Dakota site, Ecova utilized 50,000-gallon tanks that can handle up to 40 percent soil slurries. This system also permits adding a specially designed organism under full containment.

Multistep systems may include pumping contaminated water through pretreatment systems on the surface (either air-stripping or biodegradation) and then final treatments after readjusting the effluent for optimal oxygen and nutrients and reinjecting into the subsurface. For example, a site in Montana was contaminated with chlorinated phenolic waste; initial assessment showed particularly high concentrations of chlorinated methylchlorphenol. A site map after drilling and analysis of prepared samples demonstrated movement of the contaminated subsurface to the north. Ecova installed a series of pumping wells along the property line and reinjection wells at the head end of the plume. No surface bioreactor was needed in this case, because the subsurface was very porous and merely needed an optimized subsurface environment in order to stimulate aerobic biodegradation of the contaminants by the indigenous microflora. In fact, the environment was not even limited by nutrients; oxygen alone maximized the degradation.

Roles for genetically engineered organisms. Given such results, one might ask in which circumstances addition of organisms might be needed to stimulate biodegradation. Nelson and colleagues[31] at the EPA and Ecova have developed strain G-4 to degrade trichloroethylene (TCE) and other chlorinated solvents; this strain's addition greatly outperforms uninoculated controls in laboratory natural microcosms. However, the addition of such an organism directly into the subsurface at adequate cell densities is very difficult. Therefore, we envision pumping the contaminated groundwater to the surface, then treating in a bioreactor that activates the organism. In this particular case, the G-4 organisms grow on phenol, which induces a phenol monooxygenase that is also active in the degradation of TCE. The activated organisms can then be reinjected into the subsurface with another compound the company has developed that maintains the stimulation of these specific enzymes for TCE degradation while avoiding the need for any further phenol. An alternative genetically engineered solution, which avoids the need for phenol altogether, is the development of a constitutive toluene monooxygenase-producing *Escherichia coli* strain. Winter, Yen, and Ensley[32] at Amgen, Inc. used recombinant DNA techniques to introduce the toluene-oxidizing pathway genes from *Pseudomonas mendocina* KR-1.

Conclusions

Molecular, microbiological, and ecological tools are already available for empirical studies that should steadily advance our knowledge and narrow our uncertainties about the effects of genetically engineered indigenous organisms. It will be more difficult to anticipate the behavior and effects of nonindigenous organisms, whether genetically engineered or not.

Despite the paucity of published papers in our literature search, the microcosm-mesocosm approach must be considered a promising strategy. We should encourage investigations of the actions of naturally occurring and introduced microorganisms in ecocores from contaminated environments and in synthesized microcosms.

Nevertheless, the complexity of ecosystems is such that site-specific naturally derived communities and convenient multitrophic synthesized microcosms represent only snapshots in a dynamic panorama. The site chosen, the species introduced, and the physical and chemical conditions tested all greatly influence the results. The challenge is to find sensitive and meaningful correlation in microcosms with the effects seen or not seen in controlled field sites and eventually perhaps in open field applications. It would be helpful if we knew more about the complex ecological responses to chemical pesticides and to the dozen EPA-approved nongenetically engineered microbial pesticides (of which the most used is *Bacillus thuringiensis* for control of the gypsy moth). It is clear that expansion of research and training in many aspects of ecology will be necessary in order to address these questions. It is not likely, however, that genetically engineered organisms, especially when drawn from habitats into which they will be reintroduced, carry any greater risk than the agents with which we consider ourselves familiar.

A report from the National Academy of Sciences[4] reached the following conclusions:

> **1.** There is no evidence of unique hazards from the use of rDNA techniques or in the movement of genes between unrelated organisms.
>
> **2.** Risks associated with introduction of rDNA-engineered organisms are the same in kind as those associated with introduction of unmodified organisms or organisms modified by other means.

3. Assessment of potential risks should be based on the nature of the organism and the environment, not on the method by which the organism was produced.

Another National Academy of Sciences report on environmental problem-solving recommended involvement of ecological scientists from the beginning of projects, treatment of projects as experiments, collection of natural history information on the sites and neighboring or comparable sites, search for interactions and indirect and cumulative effects, recognition of heterogeneity in space and time, and need to think probabilistically about uncertainties.[33] I think this generic advice is highly applicable in environmental biotechnology.

In the meantime, models and speculations about risks from deliberate release of genetically engineered organisms are informed minimally by actual observations. As always, confidence is lower and estimates of risk are higher when data are poor. This field can surely be advanced, and the models can be made much better if the lead regulatory agencies of the government, namely the EPA and the Department of Agriculture, and the major facilities-operating agencies, the Department of Defense and the Department of Energy, would carry out and stimulate orderly biotechnology research and development on pollution control and cleanup. Such developmental work can be combined with the stepwise investigation of potential ecological effects, demonstrating for others how to advance the field responsibly.

We are impressed with the effectiveness of combined technologies that accelerate biodegradation under field conditions without resort to genetically engineered organisms. Thus, we recommend that controlled treatment environments be encouraged and that potential regulatory obstacles, such as the pending RCRA "Land-Ban," be removed or modified to encourage use of biological systems. Controlled treatment environments of the kind described here, both for natural organisms and for organisms with genetically introduced special capabilities in cases of resistant substrates or resistant partial degradation products, should be encouraged and exploited for their efficacy and safety.

References

1. B.R. Levin, *Recombinant DNA Tech. Bull.* **7**, 107 (1984).
2. G.S. Omenn and A. Hollaender, Eds., *Genetic Control of Environmental Pollutants.* (Plenum Press, New York, 1984), pp. 408.
3. G.S. Omenn, Ed., *Environmental Biotechnology: Reducing Risks from Environmental Chemicals Through Biotechnology* (Plenum Press, New York, 1988), pp. 505.
4. National Academy of Sciences Council, *Introduction of Recombinant DNA-Engineered Organisms into the Environment: Key Issues* (National Academy Press, 1987), pp. 24.
5. J.M. Tiedje *et al., Ecology* **70**, 298 (1989).
6. W. Klingmuller, Ed., *Risk Assessment for Deliberate Releases: The Possible Impact of Genetically Engineered Microorganisms on the Environment* (Springer-Verlag, Berlin, 1988), pp. 193.
7. U.S. Environmental Protection Agency. *Federal Register* **49**, 50880 (1984).
8. E. Milewski and S.A. Tolin, *Recombinant DNA Tech. Bull.* **7**, 114 (1984).
9. E.A. Milewski, *Recombinant DNA Tech. Bull.* **8**, 102 (1985).
10. E. Russek and R.R. Colwell, *Appl. Environ. Microbiol.* **45**, 1646 (1983).
11. F. O'Gara, B. Boesten, and S. Fanning, in *Risk Assessment for Deliberate Releases: The Possible Impact of Genetically Engineered Microorganisms on the Environment* (Springer-Verlag, Berlin, 1988), p. 50.
12. S.E. Lindow and N.J. Panopoulos. Request for permission to test *P. syringae* pv. syringae and *Erwinia Herbicola* Carrying Specific Deletions in Ice Nucleation Genes Under Field Conditions as Biocontrol Agents of Frost Injury to Plants, Revised Protocol for Recombinant DNA Committee (National Institutes of Health, Washington, D.C., 1983).
13. D. Glaser *et al.,* in *Biotechnology and the Environment*, G.S. Omenn, and A.H. Teich, Eds., (Noyes Data Corporation, New Jersey, 1986) p. 114.
14. B.B. Bohlool and E.F. Schmidt, *Adv. Microb. Ecol.* **4**, 203 (1980).
15. H. Szwerinski, S. Gaiser, and D. Bardtke, *Appl. Microb. Biotechnol.* **21**, 125 (1985).
16. G.M. Church and W. Gilbert, *Proc. Natl. Acad. Sci. USA* **81**, 1991 (1984).
17. M.T. MacDonnell and R.R. Colwell, *Appl. Environ. Microbiol.* **48**, 119 (1984).
18. G.S. Sayler *et al., Appl. Environ. Microbiol.* **49**, 1295 (1985).
19. M. Alexander, *Ann. Rev. Microbiol.* **35**, 113 (1981).
20. F.E. Sharples, *Recombinant DNA Tech. Bull.* **6**, 43 (1983).
21. W.J. Brill, *Science* **227**, 381 (1985).
22. C.A. Franklin, E.R. Nestmann, and L. Ritter, *Risk Assessment and Regulation of Genetically Engineered Products*, Biotechnology in Agricultural Chemistry (ACS Symposium Series, Vol. 334, 1987, p. 336.
23. H.P. Pritchard and A.W. Bourquin. *Adv. Microb. Ecol.* **7**, 133 (1984).
24. D. Dean-Ross, *Recombinant DNA Tech. Bull.* **9**, 16 (1986).
25. G.S. Omenn, in *Biotechnology Risk Assessment*, J. Fiksel and V.T. Covello, Eds. (Pergamon Press, New York, 1986), p. 144.
26. D.J. Grimes, F.L. Singleton, and R.R. Colwell, *J. Appl. Bacteriol.* **57**, 247 (1984).
27. F.L. Taub *et al.,* in *Aquatic Toxicology and Hazard Assessment: Sixth Symposium*, W.E. Bishop, R.D. Cardwell, and B.B. Heidolph, Eds. (American Society of Testing and Materials, Philadelphia, 1983), p. 5.

28. G.L. Swartzman and K.A. Rose, *Ecol. Modeling* **22**, 123 (1983).
29. J.B. Wyngaarden, *Lindow and Panopoulos Proposal Concerning Ice Nucleation Bacteria: Environmental Assessment and Finding of No Significant Impact* (National Institutes of Health, January 21, 1985).
30. J.H. Brown *et al., Bull. Ecol. Soc. Amer.* **65**, 436 (1984).
31. M.J.K. Nelson, P.H. Pritchard, and Al W. Bourquin, in *Environmental Biotechnology: Reducing the Risks from Environmental Chemicals Through Biotechnology*, G.S. Omenn, Ed. (Plenum Press, New York, 1988) p. 203.
32. R.B. Winter, K.-M Yen, and B.D. Ensley, *Biotech.* **7**, 282 (1989).
33. National Research Council, *Ecological Knowledge and Environmental Problem-Solving: Concepts and Case Studies* (National Academy Press, Washington, D.C., 1986).

Discussion

Salkinoja-Salonen: When you looked at the survival of the organisms in soil did you use an MPN (most-probable-number) method, or did you use a plate assay?

Omenn: These were plate assays.

Salkinoja-Salonen: It surprises me that you could detect as low as 100 organisms per gram of soil unless you have a very strong counter selection. Usually, the bacteria in a plate assay suffocate in excess of the heterogeneous flora.

Omenn: That is a good point. In these soil environments, most of the organisms were hydrocarbon degraders; there were very few other heterotrophic degraders, due to low organic carbon. Mahaffey and Bourquin used selective media to detect and quantitate the *Pseudomonas* strain DBM101. The organisms were grown on succinate media and detected by formation of yellow ring-cleavage products from dibenzofuran.

Salkinoja-Salonen: My experience is that with an MPN assay, you can go to $10,^2$ but with a plate assay, you never go below $10,^4$ and often you remain at 10^6 organisms per gram. I think that this is relevant to our discussion of survival in soil. Also, I want to comment on Dr. Kamely's statement about Dr. Chakrabarty's strain, that it would die off in soil because it uses 2,4,5-T as a carbon source. It does not die of hunger; it is just not competitive against the indigenous flora unless there is a toxic substance around. I think this is true for many of the organisms that do not die but are just less competitive, so their numbers decrease. Therefore, the survival in soil is very much dependent on the method of assay and the conditions that prevail in the soil. If it is natural soil with no toxic compounds against survival, relevant abundance would be very much lower than where there are toxicants around.

Also, I have another question. Did you induce with phenol to obtain trichloroethylene oxidation in groundwater?

Omenn: Not in ground water. The scheme is to use the specially developed organism in a bioreactor. Phenol is well contained and induces a phenol monooxygenase that also functions in TCE (trichloroethylene) oxidation. Then the organism is introduced into the flow of the groundwater through the bioreactor; that phase does not see the phenol.

Salkinoja-Salonen: What is the purpose of using the phenol?

Omenn: In this strain, phenol is essential to induce the TCE-degrading enzymes, as published by Nelson, Pritchard, and Bourquin (see reference 31).

Salkinoja-Salonen: What is the biochemistry behind it?

Chakrabarty: It has been shown that dioxygenases or monooxygenases such as phenol oxygenase can allow complete oxidation of TCE. A gene has been cloned by Bert Ensley (see reference 32), put in *Escherichia coli* under a constitutive promotor, and then *E. coli* completely degraded TCE. So, you do not really need phenol.

Kukor: In the case of G4, because it is a prototroph, the reason you have to supply phenol or some other intermediate in the pathway is because it is a fully regulated pathway and needs an appropriate effector molecule to induce the operon. That is why phenol was used for induction. Actually, the Ecova system then uses an intermediate in the pathway that is not phenol. You do not want to keep using phenol, a toxic material, for the biodegradation in the bioreactor.

Omenn: The Ecova system uses an inducible monooxygenase; the Amgen system uses a constitutive mutant, which we believe to be the same enzyme or a similar monooxygenase. However, the regulatory hurdles of the genetically altered organisms do not allow the use of the Amgen organism at this time. The Ecova system is being implemented in the field.

24

Concept of a Safe Marker to Track Gram-Negative Bacteria in the Environment and Allow Later Reisolation

correspondence

Ben Lugtenberg
Ruud de Maagd
Bas Zaat

Leiden University
Department of Plant
Molecular Biology
Nonnensteeg 3, 2311
VJ Leiden, The Netherlands

Markers used to follow the fate of bacteria released in the environment should fulfill a large number of requirements. We present here the concept for the construction of a novel marker that is safe, specific for the released bacterium, easy to detect, and generally applicable to a variety of gram-negative bacteria. Moreover, because the marker is located at the cell surface, the released bacteria can specifically be collected from the environment using immunofishing and can subsequently be analyzed without further culturing.

Introduction

Release of genetically engineered microorganisms in the environment for the purpose of cleaning up chemical waste is a subject of increasing importance. Our knowledge about the fate of such organisms after release is limited, partly because reliable and safe marker genes are lacking. The presently considered or used marker genes have the following disadvantages:

1. Transposons, stable and easily detectable markers, often encode antibiotic-degrading enzymes. (Although massive

amounts of bacteria encoding the same genes have been released deliberately for decades as feces by men and animals treated with antibiotics, the release of limited numbers of such organisms in field experiments is presently considered by many colleagues as a threat to the environment.)

2. Transposons are jumping elements that can pick up genes, which subsequently can be transferred to other microorganisms.

3. Detection after sampling usually requires growth of the microorganisms in laboratory media for many generations (for example, antibiotic resistance, utilization of lactose). Consequently, the bacteria are not isolated with their native makeup, which eliminates the possibility to collect information about their growth conditions *in situ*.

4. The use of cell surface–exposed markers like lipopolysaccharides (LPSs) and some other polysaccharides does allow the reisolation of bacteria in their native makeup by immunofishing. Although LPSs are often very specific for a particular strain,[1,2] the biosynthesis of LPS is so complex that it requires approximately 30 genes (scattered over the chromosome). Therefore, the use of LPS as a generally applicable marker is not feasible.

5. The immunological detection of the only other general class of cell surface molecules, the outer membrane proteins, is sterically prevented by the long O-antigen chain of LPS.[5] Soil bacteria often produce O-antigen.[1,2]

6. Detection of most other markers (for example DNA, nonexposed epitomes) is only possible after disruption of the cell.

7. Detection is often not very sensitive (for example, *lux* genes).

8. The safety mechanism of most safe markers can easily be blown up by point mutations or deletions that spontaneously occur in nature.

We propose the construction of a novel marker that lacks the mentioned disadvantages. It is based on the use of two proteins that are naturally produced by soil bacteria. By genetic manipulation, a chimeric protein will be constructed that is expressed at the cell surface of living cells, which therefore can be specifically isolated by immunofishing.

Strategy for the Construction of an Improved Marker

The improved marker that we propose has the following features:

1. It must be generally applicable for gram-negative bacteria. Therefore, it should be genetically simple. The molecule of choice is a protein (in contrast to LPS).
2. It should allow the isolation of a bacterium from the environment in its native makeup by immunofishing. This would allow the specific reisolation of the released bacteria and, by analysis of its protein profile, identification of the factor that limits bacterial growth in the studied environmental condition.[4,5]

Binding of immunoglobulins to outer membrane proteins is sterically hindered by the O-antigen part of the LPS molecule.[3] Many soil-borne gram-negative bacteria carry such an O-antigen. Therefore, an outer membrane protein can only be used as a suitable marker when it contains one or more epitopes that extend far enough from the outer membrane to avoid shielding by the O-antigen. This goal can be fulfilled by the construction of a chimeric protein of PhoE protein and NodO protein. The former protein is a transmembrane protein of which the topology is known in great detail. The latter protein can only be produced by specific strains of *Rhizobium*, which, on induction by plant flavonoids, secrete the protein into the medium. By genetic manipulation, we want to link (part of) the normally secreted NodO protein as a long, extended tag to the PhoE outer membrane protein. Antibodies directed against the exposed part of the chimeric protein can then be used to specifically detect the released bacteria in the environment. We consider this system environmentally safe because both the PhoE protein and the

NodO protein naturally occur in the environment. All sensitive methods [immunological ones, polymerase chain reaction (PCR)] can be used to detect it. The system has the additional advantage that analysis of these bacteria collected by immunofishing can then be used to reveal information about the conditions under which the cells grew in the environment.[5]

3. To allow the general use of this chimeric marker in various gram-negative bacteria, the chimeric gene will be inserted into a transposon-derivative that lacks the antibiotic resistance marker as well as the transposase. Transposase activity can be complemented by a certain unstable plasmid that carries the transposase gene. Prior to release, the bacterium must be cured from the latter plasmid, which can easily be done by omitting selection pressure. The chimeric gene can be placed under control of a chosen promoter that is active in a wide range of gram-negative soil bacteria.

4. Specific detection of the cells expressing the chimeric protein can be taken care of by using the suitable antiserum. The antiserum should not be cross-reactive with the PhoE protein and should be directed to either the NodO protein (which, in its wild type form is *secreted* by the producing *Rhizobium* cells and therefore will not be collected by immunofishing) or to a novel epitope specific for the exposed part of the chimeric protein.

Choice of the Chimeric Protein

PhoE protein is an outer membrane protein of *Escherichia coli* and other *Enterobacteriaceae*, for example, the soil bacterium *Enterobacter*, which is induced as part of the *pho*-regulon by phosphate limitation.[6,7] The *phoE* gene has been cloned. The topology of the protein is known in detail. Sixteen ß-sheets span the membrane. The membrane-spanning segments are separated from each other by usually short hydrophilic loops at the periplasmic and outside faces.[8] Using genetic engineering, information encoding foreign epitopes has been inserted in surface-exposed loops without interfering with the biogenesis of the protein.[9] *E.coli* PhoE protein has already been expressed in the unrelated *Pseudomonas* bacteria (J. Tommassen *et al.*, unpublished). It is thus clear that PhoE protein can be considered as an anchor in the outer membrane in which stretches of foreign proteins (up to at least 20 amino acids) can be inserted without disturbing the protein's biogenesis.

NodO protein is produced on induction of *nod*(ulation) genes by flavonoids (plant products) by only Rhizobium *leguminosarum* strains of the biovar *viciae*. The protein, apparent molecular weight 50kD, is secreted by the producing cells.[10] The *nodO* gene has been cloned and sequenced (R.A. de Maagd *et al.*, in preparation). The protein has been purified, and anti-NodO protein antibodies are available.[10]

Conclusions

The described marker can be considered safe because it is a hybrid of two proteins that naturally occur in the environment. The NodO part of the hybrid is unique for the released bacteria because NodO protein is only produced by certain rhizobia that do not carry it on their cell surface but secrete it. By inserting the chimeric gene in a disarmed transposon derivative, it can be incorporated in a variety of gram-negative bacteria. Expression conditions can be chosen to be high or low, inducible or constitutive. The marker is the first described marker that is both generally applicable and allows recovery of producing cells.

References

1. L.A. de Weger *et al.*, *J. Bacteriol.* **169**, 1441 (1987).
2. R.A. de Maagd, C. van Rossum, and B.J.J. Lugtenberg, *J. Bacteriol.* **170**, 3782 (1988).
3. P.A. van der Ley *et al.*, *Microbiol. Pathogenesis* **1**, 43 (1986).
4. B. Lugtenberg and L. van Alphen, *Biochim. Biophys. Acta* **737**, 51 (1983).
5. B.J.J. Lugtenberg, in *Enterobacterial Surface Antigens: Methods for Molecular Characterization*, T. Korhonen *et al.*, Eds. (Elsevier, Amsterdam, 1985) pp. 3-16.
6. N. Overbeeke, G. van Scharrenburg, and B. Lugtenberg, FEBS Lett. **112**, 1229 (1980).
7. J. Tommassen and B. Lugtenberg, *J. Bacteriol.* **143**, 151 (1980).

8. P. van der Ley, PhD Thesis, (University of Utrecht, The Netherlands, 1988).
9. M. Agterberg, H. Adriaanse, and J. Tommassen, *Gene* **59**, 145 (1987).
10. R.A. de Maagd *et al., J. Bacteriol.* **171**, 1151 (1989).
11. B. Lugtenberg, L.A. de Weger, and C. Wijffelman, in *Safety Assurance for Environmental Introductions of Genetically Engineered Organisms, Vol. G18,* J. Fiksel and V.T. Covello, Eds. (Springer Verlag, Berlin, NATO ASI Series G., 1988), pp. 129-162.

Discussion

Chakrabarty: Have you carried out the whole project?

Lugtenberg: We have done part of it: we have cloned and sequenced the two genes, and we know what strategy we are going to use; we have the disarmed transposon, but we have not carried out the rest of the project yet.

Chakrabarty: Do you know if the inserted peptide of the hybrid protein will be exposed enough so that the antibody would actually bind it. After all, it is a protein that is secreted, and there are a number of *Rhizobium* strains that produce the protein. I am trying to find out whether you can demonstrate that monoclonal antibodies would specifically pick up the introduced cells or whether cells that might specifically absorb some of the secreted protein will also be detected in your test.

Lugtenberg: We still have to do this experiment and see if we can really insert part of the NodO protein in there. Perhaps that will give rise to new antigenic determinants that will be very specific. There is also a possibility, if one introduces a larger part of the NodO protein, that native antigenic determinants of NodO protein are present. I think that, using immunofishing, you may end up with a contamination of secreted NodO protein but never with contaminating cells because by changing the localization of NodO protein from a soluble protein to a cell surface–bound protein, the only cells carrying (part of) NodO protein are of the introduced bateria. The major problem is perhaps whether we could successfully introduce such a large part of NodO protein that it is indeed recognized by antibodies in whole cells.

Chakrabarty: It depends on on the conformation of the hybrid protein. It is possible that your antigenic determinant might still be hidden?

Lugtenberg: We have not tried it yet. But so far a stretch of 20 amino acids has successfully been inserted in PhoE protein by others, and my guess is that an insertion of between 20 and 50 amino acid residues is sufficient for the experiment to work.

Janssen: This question is related to the previous one. Has immunofishing been developed as a technique for fishing specific material out of complex mixtures?

Lugtenberg: Several laboratories are working on it, and I have been aware of this approach for many years now, although I have hardly seen any publications on the subject. If you use soil, I think there will be complications. In principle, I believe that the technique can be used successfully in aqueous systems because it is relatively simple and similar to approaches that are normally used in the laboratory. In soil and in the rhizosphere, it may be less successful.

Salkinoja-Salonen: I agree that in soil you will have complications. For instance, I know that the technique has been used in water systems. In soil we have seen in the electron microscope that bacteria penetrate in very, very narrow pores in soil structures. Because the pores are narrow, we cannot extract bacteria alive from there. We had to sonicate the soil in order to get them out. I do not see how to recover bacteria with antibody probes either. The accessibility is just as big a problem for the antibody as it is for the microbes that try to biodegrade a chemical in the environment. Do you think so?

Lugtenberg: You might well be right. In our case we will first try to apply it to the rhizosphere; that will not be easy, but it will be less difficult than in soil.

Eveleigh: Could I just make a comment. One, I think the methodology has been well worked out, and it is very good. However, in selecting your system, what about dead cells and live cells that can be a critical factor here; presumably everything will show up positively.

Lugtenberg: In the case of successful immunofishing, we will fish out everything that looks like an epitope, whether dead or alive.

Chakrabarty: But is that what you want? Do you actually want to fish out both the dead and the living cells?

Lugtenberg: What we want to do is actually two things. One is to develop a safe marker for risk assessment purposes. The second aim is that we want to have more information about conditions in the rhizosphere. In our laboratory we do experiments on the attachment of **Rhizobium** bacteria to root hair tips as one of the first stages in nodulation. We have indications that under laboratory conditions limitation from manganese ions is an important signal for successful nodulation. It would be extremely interesting to see whether there is also manganese limitation in the rhizosphere. To test this, and it is just a theory so far, we could isolate in the laboratory promoters that are turned on specifically by manganese limitation. We could then use the promoter in combination with immunofishing to see whether in bacteria reisolated from the tips of root hairs this promoter is indeed turned on.

25

A Perspective on the Development of Regulations for Release of Genetically Engineered Microbes

Douglas E. Eveleigh
Department of Biochemistry and Microbiology,
Cook College,
Rutgers University,
New Brunswick, NJ
08903-0231

The bases for gaining appropriate data that assess the safety of the release of genetically engineered microbes (GEMS) into the environment are gradually being clarified. No untoward changes have been recorded following the release of GEMS in model systems. However, there can be no absolute predictive methodology to assess the release of novel organisms into a new environment, and this brings into focus the importance of assessing such subtle effects as climatic changes. Such needs for monitoring the release of GEMS have spawned several exciting new ecological methodologies. One restrictive aspect is that current high costs associated with field testing of GEMS restrict their development to a few companies that have major financial backing. Despite the fact that the scientists involved with the development of genetically engineered microbes have communicated poorly with the lay public, a national survey has indicated that the overall public perception of the application of genetically engineered organisms is quite positive.

Introduction

Microbes are usefully employed in the food and beverage industry and in the production of pharmaceuticals; their omnivorous appetites have been corralled for man's benefit in sewage treatment plants and degradation of noxious chemicals. Development of genetically engineered microbes (GEMS) can further enhance their uses in such diverse spheres as crop development, pest control agents, fertilizers[1], improved waste treatment[2] and removal of pollutants.[3] These applications of GEMS also raise a variety of practical, administrative, and even moral concerns[4-13]

Regulatory Development

The development of the regulations regarding gaining approval for release of GEMS organisms into the environment has an intriguing history. The relaxation of the National Institutes of Health (NIH) Recombinant DNA (rDNA) Guidelines in 1979 permitted consideration of the dramatic change of position from "containment of GEMS" to their "Planned Introduction into the Environment." The need immediately became apparent for regulatory guidelines from which the basis for environmental release of GEMS could be rationally assessed. In the United States, the regulatory agencies were overwhelmed by the novel nature of the genetic and ecological sophistication thrust upon them and were understaffed in coping with this new situation. However, the agencies fully recognized the importance of GEMS (scientifically and politically) and battled to decide which agency should have the appropriate regulatory authority. For instance, were GEMS used in pest control of food crops to be the domain of the Food and Drug Agency or the Environmental Protection Agency? The U.S. Executive Branch set up a "Coordinated Framework for the Regulation of Biotechnology" (June 1986), and after public discussion the relative roles of each agency were clarified.[14] In retrospect, the time frame in which the agencies deciphered their relative roles was slow.

Although the NIH rDNA Guidelines sanctioned the release of GEMS, the was critical need for identifying the type of data necessary for such objective decision making resulted in considerable public discussion regarding the pros and cons of environmental release.[15-27] Opinion was manifestly divergent regarding the potential dangers of the release of GEMS, especially concerning the lack of data on the indirect ecological effects that molecular biologists tended to gloss over (see list that follows). Most recently the Ecological Society of America (ESA) published a well-received position paper on the release of genetically modified organisms.[12] Input was from more than 100 scientists plus that from an open as ESA discussion meeting. The ESA document recommended that all genetically engineered organisms should receive regulatory approval but not necessarily in a burdensome manner, that is, case by case but with due consideration of past experience with equivalent GEMS. This document went further than prior reports in defining a list of areas and factors to be considered in risk assessments and also in weighing the importance of those areas and factors.[28] A basic list entitled "Attributes of Organisms and Environments for Possible Consideration in Risk Evaluation" is sub-divided into:

1. Attributes of genetic alteration
2. Attributes of parent (wild type) organism
3. Phenotypic attributes of engineered organisms compared to the parent organism
4. Attributes of the environment

Each section lists attributes classified according to a proposed level of scientific consideration. Thus, if there is selection pressure for an engineered trait (for example, antibiotic resistance), greater consideration of the ecological effects of such traits is given in comparison to nonselected traits. The table has over 30 broad ranging yet specific attributes which are considered in relation to their immediate and *in toto* effects, for example, the pleiotropic effects of the introduced genes on the host, unintended lateral transfer genes to other species, and the scale and frequency of application. The final ESA assessment is not radically different from prior deliberations such as the U.S. National Academy of Sciences report (1987), yet it differs in that it is definitive in its recommendations. In this regard it has been given high marks by Congress plus the warmest welcome so far by Environmental Groups. However, Kingsbury[29] perspicaciously comments that this welcome could be an indirect response arising through a "distrust of the executive branch of Government by the environmental groups, and secondly agency disagreements within the government." In a similar context there is a perceived mistrust of industrial positions due to the conceived focus on commercial interest. In contrast, over the years the ESA has developed a position of trust from its "proenvironmental stands." In April 1987, the first United States legally sanctioned environmental release was approved: the use of the ice-minus *Pseudomonas syringae* by Advanced Genetic Sciences, Oakland, CA. (Frostban®), and also by Dr. Lindow, University of California, for strawberries and potatoes.[30] In summary, the formulation of practical federal guidelines for the release of GEMS traveled a rocky road but has finally advanced dramatically through cooperation between government agencies and integrated public debate.

International development of guidelines similarly emerged only after considerable debate and a range of interpretations from strict to liberal. In the United Kingdom, the first release was for an engineered baculovirus used to control the moth *Panolis flammea,* a pest of lodgepole pines. The genetically engineered modification was done simply to gain a marker to distinguish the virus from its parent.[31] No major objection was raised following the initial debates. In contrast, in the European Parliament the concept of planned release of GEMS is still receiving strong opposition.[32,33] Kamely[34] reviews the current status in Europe in Chapter 23 of this Book. These are well-intentioned discussions, but perhaps the strongest need is for international accord. Microbes know of no international boundaries.

What has been learned from an exciting decade of debate?

1. Programs have advanced steadily and cautiously based on general risk probabilities, that is, assessment of risks of the release of GEMS both sequentially and additively, and their survival, multipli-

cation, dissemination, transfer, and potential to cause harm.[35] Evaluations have been on a case-by-case basis and this status is recommended to continue. However, as data and assessments accumulate, complete new and duplicative data will not be required for the release of each proposed application of a GEM.

2. The complexities of predictive ecology have been brought to the fore. Currently one cannot completely predict the impact of even the controlled introduction of GEMS into the environment. There is no data base for new organisms. However, a corollary "objective" is that a predictive methodology will be developed. Because bacteria can grow rapidly and are extremely adaptable and hardy, they assume initial importance in these early predictive assessments of controlled released of genetically modified organisms. One important corollary is the rekindling of the debate of whether or not macroecological principles apply to prokaryotes.

3. For the protagonists of the release of GEMS, it is encouraging to observe that no untoward changes due to GEMS tested in model systems have been recorded after a decade of testing.

4. For the antagonists, they note that even with an abundance of negative evidence, it is difficult to render advice to regulatory agencies, or for them to define guidelines. The practical position can be summarized by May's[36] comment on the predictive applications of ecological theory noted:"The choice is not between perfect and imperfect advice to managers, but between crudely imperfect advice and no advice at all."

Although there is an abundance of negative data, that is, no untoward effects, it must be remembered that obviously GEMS do have an impact on the local sites because this is the rationale for employing them. Perhaps most perplexing is the possibility that changes may have already occurred that are too subtle to detect. For example, would the release of frost-negative bacteria change weather patterns and how could such changes in climate be evaluated or predicted? In such negative longer term scenarios will modification of rain patterns occur due to the release of ice-minus bacteria, and could the domain of plants that require overwintering freezing cycles in order to gain seed germination move closer to the North or South

Poles? In a different context, the effects of cloning the gene for the *Bacillus thuringiensis* insect toxin into plants has been questioned. Advocates note that *B. thuringiensis* has been employed as a "spore dust" for many years without untoward effect. However, in this instance the spores are washed from the food products. With major expression of the *B. thuringiensis* toxin gene in the plant, the food product and perhaps all plant organs can have a high concentration of the toxin, which could have an effect on animals fed such plants in the long term. There is also the increased possibility that as the toxin remains undegraded for long periods, that this situation would favor selection of resistance insects.

5. The need for monitoring GEMS in the environment has spawned several novel approaches. Some are relatively simple extensions of prior systems. Antibiotic resistance genes have been inserted in the chromosome of fluorescent soil pseudomonads in order to gain stability of the gene and when combined with the use of lactose (*lac*ZY gene) yield an effective color-selective analytical method.[37,38] Monitoring approaches independent of cultivation include analysis via gene-cassette product, immunofluorescence, nucleic acid sequence analysis, and nucleic acid hybridization. Atlas and Steffan[34] using DNA amplification to detect GEMS, were able to identify as low as 1 cell/gram soil even with a background of 10^9 nontarget bacteria. A spin off of this technology can be the routine monitoring of *E. coli* and *Salmonella* sp. by use of specific DNA probes.

A further positive aspect associated with monitoring is the development of the use of "suicide" (conditionally lethal) genes to gain post-release control of GEMS. For instance, the *hok* gene produces a small protein that results in collapse of transmembrane potential and death of the cell.[40] In certain *E. coli* strains, the parB locus on plasmid R1 gives stable maintenance through regulation of *hok* by *sok* (suppression of killing) coding for antisense RNA binding to the *hok* message. If loss of the plasmid occurs at cell division, it results in cell death as the *sok* product is less stable than the lethal *hok* product. Early on, it was proposed to develop this system for containment in industrial fermentations by putting the *hok* gene under control of a nutritional promoter, for example, tryptophan. When the tryptophan is fully utilized, the *hok* gene is turned on, and the bacterium dies. This is especially industrially attractive because the *hok* membrane protein is lethal to both gram-positive and gram-negative bacteria.[40] The suicide principle is also being developed for the control of released GEMS, for example, through regulatory control using a promoter sensitive to an environmental toxicant/regulator. Several scenarios are possible. For instance, Stephen Cuskey [Environmental Protection Agency (EPA), Gulf Breeze, FL][41] is developing the lethal RK2 *kil*A(lethal)/*kor*A (kill override) based system. Here the suicide *kil* gene is constitutively switched on, but its lethal activities are inactivated by the *kor* gene product whose production is under the control of a promoter that is recognized by a toxicant. Thus in the presence of the toxicant, *kor* is switched on, and the cell survives. Following complete degradation of the toxicant, the *kor* activities are terminated, and the GEM then dies. These *hok* and *kil* based systems are extensions of the original biological control concept.[42] Cuskey notes that a system based on a single suicide gene may not be foolproof; for instance, a single mutation could disrupt such regulatory systems. However, he notes that there are perhaps even thousands of analogous genes, and through their combinational use, stability of a suicide-based system is a reflection of the researcher's ingenuity.

Suicide genes are an attractive model for studying specific microbial populations, in combination analysis of genetic perturbations that will doubtless occur;[26,43,44] but suicide genes have the additional attribute of a lethal control at hand. Minimally, this is an excellent risk assessment model. Conceptually this approach is attractive to regulatory agencies (the target GEM is killed). The approach also offers considerable economic advantage to industry *sensu* continued sales of their product.

6. Initial costs of this research for full field trials evaluating GEMS are staggering, in the realm of hundreds of thousands of dollars. These costs will drop dramatically in the second and third trials. Even so, universities can participate in such exciting experiments only with predominantly industrial backing. The costs are prohibitively expensive for government funding such as in the U.S. Department of Agriculture Competitive Grants Program of $50-$100,000/year.

In summary, the bases for gaining appropriate data for assessing the safety for the release of GEMS into the environment is gradually being clarified. It is encouraging to note that no untoward changes have been recorded following the release of GEMS in model systems. However, it is clear that there can be no absolute predictive methodology to assess the release of novel organisms in a new environment, and this brings to focus the importance of assessing perhaps such subtle effects as changes in the climate. These needs for monitoring release have spawned several exciting new ecological methodologies. Currently, the high costs associated with field testing of GEMS restrict their development to a few companies that have major financial backing.

The Public Awareness of Genetic Engineering

One outcome of the tempestuous scientific debates that occurred regarding the benefits and risks of genetic engineering was that the United States Congress requested a nationwide survey to answer the question "What does the public think of Genetic Engineering?" (U.S. Congress, Office of Technology Assessment (OTA).[45] The results regarding the awareness of the American public and their assessments of the risks and benefits are briefly reviewed.

Thirty five percent of the respondents in the survey responded that they had heard a fair amount regarding genetic engineering, which contrasted with the 39 percent who had heard relatively little, and a further 24 percent recorded that they knew almost nothing about the topic. Among college graduates, only 61 percent had heard or read a fair amount about genetic engineering. This result should be tempered because it was clear that even amongst the nonscientifically inclined, a substantial group (17 percent) stated that they were aware of genetic engineering. Indeed, the final assessment was that about half of the American public has a good general sense of what genetic engineering means. The assessments of benefits from genetic engineering were viewed positively. A clear majority of Americans approved diverse proposed applications, including treatment of cancer and development of vaccines and cures for human genetic dis-

Table 1
Concern Level of Some Environmental Issues[1,2]

	Very to somewhat	Not too concerned	Never heard of
Radioactive discharge from Nuclear power plants	70	15	15
Acid rain	72	13	24
Greenhouse effect	33	10	55
Antibiotic resistant bacteria	32	6	61
GEMS for agricultural use	20	8	70

[1]Modified from the OTA report.[45]
[2]Data represent percent of the respondents.

eases, frost and disease resistant crops, more productive farm animals, and larger game fish. This degree of approval was clearly related to the immediacy of personal benefit (cancer treatments (75 percent) or new vaccines (57 percent) than to a utilitarian philosophy for the general good (more productive farm animals 37 percent).

Public perception of the risks associated with genetic engineering was less than those associated with nuclear power plants, antibiotic resistant bacteria, and the greenhouse effect (Table 1).

It must be cautioned that only 19 percent of the population had heard of the potential dangers of genetic engineering. Within this group a diversity of potential problems were recognized: uncontrolled spread of modified organisms (16 percent), health hazards (12 percent), creation of mutations/monsters and environmental contamination (seven percent). Chemical warfare ranked as one potential outcome although only at the one percent level of responses, whereas interestingly germ warfare was not cited. In contrast to this well-informed group, in the total survey of all participants, including the 81 percent claiming no knowledge of the potential dangers, over half responded to say that genetic engineering was a somewhat serious danger to both people and the environment. This somewhat negative response was interpreted to perhaps reflect a general public concern for science and technology, the well-known Frankenstein monster syndrome. Although the seven topic areas cited above were clearly given approval, the perception of risk was evident by the majority of the public. Four of the seven topics were considered "somewhat likely to be dangerous" (for example, antibiotic resistance, 61 percent; endangerment of food supply, 52 percent). A greater proportion of respondents (63 percent) believed that genetically altered bacteria pose a greater threat than genetically altered plants or animals (47 percent).

Public perception of acceptance of risk regarding genetic engineering. The OTA survey indicated that a majority of Americans (55 percent) approved genetically engineered plants, animals, or microbes for increased farm production if the risk level of danger of extinction of a plant or fish were put at 1:1000. This approval rating rose to 66 percent with a risk level of 1:10,000. In contrast, roughly one-fifth of the respondents stated that they would never approve of genetically engineered products. Overall, if there were no human risks, the American public accepted the other risk factors and approved the use of genetically engineered organisms (Table 2).

This OTA study reflected opinions (October to November 1986). At that time, roughly half the population described themselves as very interested, concerned, or knowledgeable about science and technology. A similar proportion believed that genetic engineering could present serious dangers to the populace or to the environment but with the corollary that an even greater number (two thirds) opine that it will make a better life for all people.

The OTA report raises a further issue, namely the ability of scientist to communicate with the lay person. Any such survey taken can be jaundiced by preconceived notions, and this situation was emphasized in the report through citing the following disparate quotations:

"A substantial majority of Americans do not have sufficient vocabulary or comprehension of concepts to utilize a wide array of scientific communication..." (Jon D. Miller, *The Washington Post*, June 2, 1986)

"The public...can assimilate an astonishing amount of technical information if they feel that it's necessary to protect themselves in a

Table 2
**Approval Rating* of Environmental Applications of
Genetically Engineered Organisms Under Remote Risk Conditions[45]**

	Approve	Disapprove	Not Sure
Disease -desistant crops	73	23	4
Bacteria to clean oil spills	73	23	4
Frost-resistant crops	70	27	3
More effective pesticides	56	40	4
Larger game fish	53	43	4

[1]U.S. Congress, Office of Technology Assessment, from reference 45.
[2]Percent response.
[3]No direct risk to humans: remote risk to the environment.

dispute." (Robert C. Forney, *Christian Science Monitor*, Sept. 26, 1986).

With such disparate viewpoints, it is appropriate to discuss the ability of scientists to present their views to the lay public. Unfortunately, once again scientists have shown themselves inept in dealing with the news media. When Advanced Genetic Sciences first publicized their legal spraying of Frostban®, the news release in national newspapers showed the spray operator wearing a "moonsuit," plus a caption "claiming" that this new GEM was completely safe to man. The caption and the photo were incongruous. A recent article on genetic engineering from *The Boston Globe* pictured a transgenically altered Chinese pig whose features were so distant from American strains that an antivivisectionist group could have used the picture for their political gain. Scientists also have communication problems simply through use of jargon. For example, the U.S. Congress OTA report notes that the public gave approval in the range of 53-73 percent (Table 2) for the environmental application of GEMS if the risks were one to a thousand. However, when the risks were "unknown but very remote" (which was assumed scientifically as a much lower risk than $1:10^3$), less of the public (45 percent) gave their approval. Thus, a term such as "very remote" was not understood let alone the use of laboratory jargon. Analogously, the term "Deliberately Released GEMS" has poor connotations. Why not "Planned Introduction" as emphasized by Kingsbury[14] which although perhaps a euphemism, implies confidence?

Furthermore, scientists are "honest and pure" and generally present complete details of a study when often interim judgments and broad perspective are more appropriate. In a similar manner, the slow response by federal agencies for general guidelines on the necessary criteria for assessment of the release of GEMS resulted in several states going ahead and developing their own laws. Eight states have initiated development of their own guidelines, and those of Hawaii, Maine, and Maryland have been enacted.[46] In New Jersey, State Senator Dorsey introduced a Bill S.1123 to "regulate the release of genetically engineered microorganisms" and although the bill was never enacted, Dorsey's efforts have resulted in seven communities passing new town laws banning genetic engineering within their bounds. Such complexity of interacting town, state, and federal statutes does not engender efficiency in facilitating the planned introduction of GEMS.

Conclusions

In overview, the release of genetically engineered microbes into the environment is controversial and has stirred considerable debate. Governnmental agencies have had to develop a dialogue with both scientists and the public. They have used the diverse opinions in gradually formulating a sound set of guidelines for the release of genetically engineered microbes. During this period, and despite scientists poor communication with the lay public,[47] a congressionally mandated national survey has indicated that the public perception of the application of genetically engineered organisms is quite positive.

Acknowledgments

This study was supported by the U.S. Department of Energy, Washington, DC, the Solar Energy Research Institute, Golden, CO, and the New Jersey Agricultural Experiment Station, Publication No. D-01111-05-89.

References

1. P.R. Day, in *Engineered Organisms in the Environment—Scientific Issues*, H.O. Halvorson, D. Pramer, and M. Rogul, Eds. (American Society of Microbiology, Washington, D.C., 1985), pp. 4-10.
2. J. Todd, *Whole Earth Review* **62**, 36 (1989).
3. R.K. Jain and G.S. Sayler. *Microbiol. Sci.* **4**, 59 (1986).
4. S. Crawley, *TREE* **3**, S2 (1988).
5. J.R. Fowle III, Ed., *Issues Amer. Assoc. Adv. Sci. Selected Symp.* (Washington, D.C., 1987), pp. 242.
6. Y. Grossman, *Bio Science* **39**, 229 (1989).
7. H.O. Halvorson, D. Pramer, and M. Rogul, Eds., *Engineered Organisms in the Environment*. Scientific Issues (American Society of Microbiology, Washington, D.C., 1985), pp. 442.
8. Organization for Economic Cooperation and Development, *Recombinant DNA Safety Considerations: Safety Considerations for Industrial, Agricultural and Environmental Applications of Organisms Derived by Recombinant DNA Techniques*. (Paris, 1986).
9. S. Stearns, J. Meyer, and J. Shykoff, *Tree* **3**, S2 (1988).
10. M. Sussman *et. al.*, Eds.,*The Release of Genetically-Engineered Micro-organisms. Proceedings of the First International Conference of the Release of Genetically-Engineered Micro-organisms*, (Academic Press, London, 1988), pp. 306.
11. A.H. Teich, M.A. Levin, and J.H. Pace, Eds., Biotechnology and the Environment. Risk and Regulation.(American Association for the Advancement of Science, Washington, DC, 1985).
12. J.M. Tiedje *et al.*, *Ecology* **70**, 298 (1989).
13. U.S. National Academy of Sciences, *Introduction of Recombinant DNA-Engineered Organisms into the Environment: Key Issues*, (National Academy Press, Washington, DC, 1987).
14. D.T. Kingsbury, *Tib Tech.* **6**, S39 (1988).
15. S. Baumberg, *Tib Tech.* **6**, 107 (1988).
16. W.J. Brill, *Science* **227**, 381 (1985a).
17. W.J. Brill, *Science* **229**, 115 (1985b).
18. W.J. Brill, *Issues in Science and Technol.* **5**, 44 (1988).
19. P.N. Campbell, *Biotech. Appl.Biochem.* **10**, 483 (1988).
20. J.J. Cohrssen, *Biotechnol. Lab.* **6**, 22 (1988).
21. R.K. Colwell, *Science* **229**, 111 (1985a).
22. R.K. Colwell, in *Engineered Organisms in the Environment, H.O. Halvorson, D. Pramer, and M. Rogul, Eds.* (American Society of Microbiology, Washington, DC, 1985b), pp. 230-232.
23. B.D. Davis, *Genetic Eng. News* **8**, 21 (1988).
24. B.R. Glick and Y.C. Skof, *Biotech. Adv.* **4**, 261 (1986).
25. M. Rogul, in *Biotechnology and the Environment. Risk and Regulation*, A.H. Teich,

M.A. Levin, and H. Pace, Eds. (American Association for the Advancement of Science, Washington, DC, 1985), pp.1-13.

26. J.H. Slater, in *Engineered Organisms in the Environment. Scientific Issues,* H.O. Halvorson, D. Pramer, and M. Rogul, Eds. (American Society of Microbiology, Washington, DC, 1985), pp. 89-98.

27. J.T. Trevors, T. Barkay, and A.W. Bourquin, *Can. J. Microbiol.* **33**, 191 (1987).

28. A.M. Campbell, *Tib Tech.* **7**, 109 (1989).

29. D.T. Kingsbury, *Tib Tech.* **7**, 110 (1989).

30. J. Van Brunt, *Bio/Technology* **5**, 558 (1987).

31. D.H.L. Bishop, *Nature* **323**, 496 (1986).

32. J. Hodgson, *Tib Tech.* **7**, 107 (1989).

33. F.E. Young and H.I. Miller, *Gene* **75**, 1 (1989).

34. D. Kamely, in *Biotechnology and Biodegradation,* D. Kamely, A. Chakrabardy, and Gilbert S. Omenn, Eds. (Portfolio Publishing Company, The Woodlands, TX, 1989).

35. M. Alexander, in *Biotechnology and the Environment Risk and Regulation,* A.H. Teich, M.A. Levin, and J.H. Pace, Eds. (American Association for the Advancement of Science, Washington, D.C.,1985), pp. 115-136.

36. R. May, in *Ecological Communities: Conceptual Issues and the Evidence,* D.R. Strong *et. al.,* Eds. (Princeton University Press, Princeton, N.J., 1984), pp. 3-16.

37. G.F. Barry, *Bio/Technol.* **4**, 446 (1984).

38. D.J. Drahos, B.C. Hemming, and S. McPherson, *Bio/Technology* **4**, 439 (1986).

39. R.M. Atlas and R.J. Steffan, in *The Release of Genetically-Engineered Micro-organisms. Proceedings of the First International Conference of the Release of Genetically-Engineered Micro-organisms,* M. Sussman *et al.,* Eds. (Academic Press, London, 1988), p. 224.

40. S. Molin, *et al., Bio/Technology* **5**, 1315 (1987).

41. J.L. Fox, *ASM News* **55**, 259 (1989).

42. R. Curtis III, in *The Release of Genetically-Engineered Micro-organisms. Proceedings of the First International Conference of the Release of Genetically-Engineered Micro-organisms,* M. Sussman *et al.,* Eds. (Academic Press, London, 1988), pp. 7-20.

43. R. Lewin, *Science* **219**, 478 (1983).

44. J. Lederberg, *Social Res.* **55**, 343 (1988).

45. U.S. Congress, Office of Technology Assessment, *New Developments in Biotechnology—Background paper: Public Perceptions of Biotechnology* (OTA-BP-BA-45, Washington, DC, U.S. Government Printing Office, May 1987).

46. G.J. Mossinghoff, *Tib Tech.* **7**, 79 (1989).

47. B. Iglewski, *Amer. Soc. Microbiol. News.* **55**, 306 (1989).

Discussion

Dr. Kamely: You said initially that you differ with me on the fact that the agencies got along very well. I do not differ with you. I agree with you completely. Initially, there were tremendous battles among the regulatory agencies. Especially on pesticides, the EPA and USD fought long and hard. The work load is so heavy that regulatory agencies are more than happy to share the regulatory responsibilities. (As a matter of fact, when I outlined the procedure for risk assessment in the Toxic Substance Control Act), the internal committees that evaluate the risks are composed of several scientists from the USDA and the FDA who sit regularly on these committees even though the final decision belongs to the EPA's. Another point that was made by you and Dr. Omenn is that on the one hand, the regulatory agencies are asked to come up with sound risk assessments, and on the other hand the research is poorly funded. I do not know a single regulatory agency that has biotechnology research funding. Instead, when risk assessments are performed, the funds are always diverted from other programs and are usually not sufficient. The only agency that has sufficient funds is the NIH and the NIH is not a regulatory agency. The NIH does not call its research biotechnology. The NIH calls it biomedical research, and as we all know, biomedical research involves genetic engineering. In contrast, what I see at DoD is a powerful lobby. Scientists on the other hand are poor lobbyists. The DoD on the other hand teams up with supporting industries and makes a convincing case. Every time there are budget cuts, research suffers first. If biotechnology can be established as a funding element, then risk assessment should be included as an integral part of the biotechnology program.

Dr. Eveleigh: I think it was just the way we expressed it, I do not think that there is any disagreement. Again, I do feel though at a meeting like this that we have got to get together a statement, a statement to the agencies that there is a need for a budget for risk assessment internationally, not just the United States. There really is a need for this sort of input.

Summation

Gilbert S. Omenn

I applaud the organizers and the host committee of this International Research Workshop on Biotechnology and Biodegradation for a fine program with 28 very good presentations and active discussions.

Gunsalus set our challenge when he asked: "How can we help Nature's cycles keep up with the waste streams of the growing population on Spaceship Earth?" *Newsweek* (June 19, 1989, pp. 52-53) provided a dramatic answer in its lead science story: MICROBES TO THE RESCUE! In fact, the response must be a complex combination of science and technology, government action, individual responsibility, and community actions.

I believe the guiding principles must be (1) to detoxify, preferably to detoxify *in situ*, and (2) to minimize the production and toxicity of new wastes. We cannot continue to rely on removal of hazardous wastes to that wonderful place called "Elsewhere."

Smith got us launched on the basic sciences aspects and biotechnology techniques. His focus on heme proteins that are oxidases and peroxidases provided an introduction to the many oxidative heme-containing enzymes that play a central role in biodegradation pathways. These enzymes, therefore, are of special interest for detailed structure-function analyses and for potential genetic modification of their properties.

Young was the first of several speakers to address anaerobic environments. Many of the most important environmental compartments that have become contaminated are largely anaerobic. The dechlorination and ring fission approaches were highlighted. On a laboratory scale, at least, they are quite useful. After many years of bias from microbiology colleagues that only pure culture studies should be pursued, she presented with considerable pleasure the growing interest in mixed culture approaches for biodegradation. All through the Workshop there was a recognition that there must be greater interrelationship between basic research and applied work. The practical world requirements for mixtures of active organisms to deal with the mixtures of chemicals in contaminated sites need to be combined with the basic research capacity to isolate pure cultures so that the metabolic pathways themselves might be identified and dissected. Only then can the powerful tools of modern genetics be utilized to enhance the capabilities of organisms that would then be applied, probably in mixtures, to specific field sites.

I have highlighted in Table 1 the two-way interaction between basic science and field applications.

It is a serious fallacy to think of research progress only going from basic science to applied research to field demonstrations. Very often thoughtful and experimental assessment of the bottlenecks and intractable problems in the practical world can refocus our basic science efforts in ways that enable us to ask new and more interesting basic science questions, as well as to obtain research findings that become useful for applications. It is clear that microbiology and microbial ecology have been greatly stimulated by the biotechnological interest in biodegradation. As Dr. Young commented, there has been an explosion of new genera and species in the most recent edition of *Bergey's Manual of Determinative Bacteriology*.

Whether to aerate and use aerobic organisms, including organisms in bioreactors, or whether to work in the anaerobic environment will be a continuing challenge in the years ahead. A variety of approaches will be required. In many cases, it will be desirable to find ways to combine anaerobic and aerobic biodegradative actions.

Many speakers addressed particular classes of target chemicals of high priority for pollution cleanup. Davison described pathways of degradation for vanillate and sodium dodecyl sulfate, including genetic engineering methods that might be applied. Vanillate and especially catechols later were mentioned frequently as key intermediates in oxidative pathways. Janssen took us through multiple pathways for dechlorination and metabolism of the chloroaliphatics. These compounds include some of the best known and most widely prevalent toxic contaminants. He emphasized that multiple enzymes

Table 1
Summary Themes

- Diverse capabilities in nature but pathways more complex than anticipated
- Basic science and field applications: two-way interactions
- More interconnections needed
- Combine aerobic and anaerobic growth and biodegradation (qualitative and quantitative)
- Target key classes of chemicals
- Gain experience with different types of environmental compartments, settings, sites
- Build experience stepwise to earn public confidence for *in situ* bioremediation and microbial detoxification of wastestreams

---

and multiple pathways can be involved. Their relative roles and their feasibility of manipulation are still to be explored. DeFrank addressed the organophosphorus compounds, which are of special importance in agriculture and military uses. There is a clear need from these and other presentations to focus on the energetics of recalcitrant compounds. We need to understand better the cometabolism of growth substrates and target substrates and how to combine aerobic and anaerobic capabilities.

Ward, speaking on behalf of several attending colleagues, gave us a useful introduction into the many interests of Department of Defense agencies in biotechnology applications. These range from generic areas of bioreclamation to more specific areas of decontamination, decommissioning, and explosives modifications. Many, but not all of these needs, are likely to have promising applications for biotechnology.

Anderson stimulated much discussion about screening methods for the bioreactivity of various sites, including emphasis on quantitative aspects, rates of biodegradation, and influence of environmental conditions *in vitro* and *in situ*. Ribbons turned the approach around and focused on catechols and other dihydrodiols as starting materials for synthesis of novel bioactive compounds with chiral features that may generate useful pharmaceutical applications. This opportunistic approach may help pharmacologists proceed beyond routine screening of compounds for biological and clinical activity to more rational design of drugs and, with microbial ecologists, rational design of biodegrader organisms.

We should recognize the classic contributions of Chakrabarty to this field as well as the continuing plasmid and transposon studies he presented here. His development of patentable oil-degrading organisms was highlighted in the *Newsweek* article already mentioned. His chemostat scheme that produced *Pseudomonas cepacia* strain AC1100, active against 2,4,5-trichlorophenoxyacetic acid should be utilized by others for additional recalcitrant molecules. His concept of directed evolution and recruitment of genes and their functions is central to much of the genetic engineering approach that we hope will be pursued by chemostat selection or, more likely, by recombinant DNA techniques.

Timmis explained and illustrated the complementary approach of rational pathway construction, sharing some very impressive developments to date. His emphasis is on selection or design of broad-spectrum proteins. Consider the problems identified by many of you arising from bottlenecks in pathways. We must realize that these pathways are turning out to be much more complex than anticipated; more steps, more genes, more complicated regulatory mechanisms. Thus, the focus on regulatory elements, on permeases, and on enzymes for common steps in multiple pathways seems highly appropriate and productive. Timmis's plan to develop "modules" of genes for key coordinated steps is a quite promising approach for mobilizing genetic techniques for these problems.

It is a tall order. The more we learn about these biological systems, the more complicated the pathways become and the more daunting becomes the challenge of designing rational schemes for constructing active pathways without feedback inhibition and other important limitations. Nevertheless, critical common pathways for particular high-priority chemicals such as chloroaliphatics and chloroaromatics may be amenable to these modern biotechnological techniques.

Schink described methoxy compounds. Ether linkages turn out to be quite important in several classes of chemicals, especially lignins, which I will mention shortly. As a human biologist, I was fascinated to learn of the role of vitamin B_{12}. He particularly emphasized the quantitative relationships that should be estimated and measured closely as we try to assess functional performance and the cometabolism that may bring together growth and biodegradation, or anaerobic and aerobic combinations. The concept that any particular organism may be incapable of generating the energy required for growth, but that combinations of organisms may together do so, is a nice example of "social biology."

We turned next to the toluene-xylene systems. Zeyer emphasized overcoming bottlenecks in key metabolic pathways. I thought the switching from nitrate to nitrous oxide, thereby avoiding the inhibitory effect of the accumulating nitrite, was particularly felicitous. Kukor carried on with results from the benzene-toluene-ethylbenzene-xylene (BTEX) cleanup in a Michigan field site. The consortium of microbiologists, ecologists, engineers, and others recently assembled at the University of Michigan and Michigan State University with substantial support from federal, state, and industrial sources can become a leading example of the combination of basic science and practical applications. His example stressed the difficult challenge of cleaning up xylene in a site where biodegradation of the benzene, ethylbenzene, and toluene was easy.

Neilson discussed anew the important class of halogenated phenols, in this case emphasizing those compounds arising from the bleaching of pulp and contaminating mostly anaerobic aquatic sediments. The key intermediate compounds are chlorocatechols and chloroguaiacols. The point was well made that different dichlorocatechols vary markedly in their susceptibility to biodegradation by particular organisms or enzymes. This further example of the complexity of our challenge shows that although there is capability for dechlorination, many of the compounds present may be difficult to degrade because of the position of substitutions on the benzene rings and because of the concentrations in the environment in relation to K_ms of the enzymes for those substrates. Finally, many of you mentioned that other steps, in this case methylation, may cause disappearance of the target compound yet mask the failure to dechlorinate. If the toxicity is primarily related to the halogens, such limited biotransformation is not sufficient for detoxification. Salkinoja-Salonen focused on chlorophenols from sawmills and wood treatment plants that contaminate soils. It was impressive how many routes of inoculation are available for introducing the active microorganisms into the contaminated environment: liquid phase, wood chips, immobilized solid supports.

We covered multiple environmental compartments and key target classes of potentially toxic chemicals (see Table 1). Buswell, Glaser, and Gunsalus discussed some of the many interesting features of lignins and their biodegradation. In the discussion, Smith and others urged that a concerted effort at mutant analysis be mobilized to elucidate some of the many poorly understood steps in lignin metabolism. It is interesting that the first steps of lignin metabolism take place extracellularly and must produce sufficiently small fragments that they readily penetrate to intracellular sites for further metabolism. The utilization of a mutant of *Phanerochaete chrysosporium* that grows well on glycerol was a notable development as was the recognition of glyoxal oxidase as an endogenous source of production of the hydrogen peroxide that is necessary for the lignin peroxidases. As I noted previously, many speakers returned to the theme of the central role of heme proteins that are peroxidases and oxidases. The postulated role of veratryl alcohol also seems to be a promising area for further investigation.

Municipal solid wastes are an enormous problem, especially in volume. In Italy there is an elaborate scheme of six categories of decreasingly hazardous wastes. To the extent that large volumes of solid wastes (as well as contaminated soils and other sites) are classified as "hazardous" and require disposal, usually in well-managed hazardous waste landfills, we are unwisely wasting valuable resources. In the United States, there is a limited number of such landfills and great resistance in most communities to establishing new landfills or building hazardous waste or solid waste incinerators. Therefore, it is very important for our environmental objectives in the intermediate and longer term that these waste disposal resources be used as parsimoniously as is consistent with the significant hazards of particular wastes. Detoxification, permitting lower categorization of hazard, and minimization of waste production deserve high priority. In any case, the joint Venice/Barcelona project of Cecchi and Mata-Alaveraz demonstrated that there is considerable capability to detoxify the organic fraction of municipal solid waste, especially if the wastes are well sorted, preferably at the sources. The step diffusional model seemed to me to provide a pretty good correlation with the categories of chemicals, not chemically defined, but defined by ease of degradation under the conditions of activated sludge treatment.

Bedard described the extensive information obtained at the General Electric Company research laboratories on the many congeners of PCBs. Some of the strains seem quite promising for dechlorination, yet the progress from field demonstrations has been rather disappointing. The system is still dependent on induction by biphenyl. One might hope that other inducers could be found or high-constitutive producers might be isolated, as has been feasible in other systems.

Multiple applications for bioreactors were described by Visscher for waste gases, contaminated soils, and wastewater treatment. In my own talk, I emphasized that *in situ* use of bioreactors as closed and controlled systems should be highly acceptable and, from evidence to date, is really quite effective. These bioreactors also have the attractive feature for the combination of interests expressed at this conference of allowing well-controlled introduction of specific organisms, including genetically engineered organisms.

Finally, under the banner of risk assessment and risk communication, we must recognize the increasingly open societies of all western countries and even the Communist countries, or at least some of them. The public has a legitimate and active interest in these environmental topics. We need to justify the optimism expressed in the *Newsweek* article about environmental microbiology and the potential of genetic engineering for cleaning up environmental contaminations and wastestreams. There is an opportunity for those of us in the emerging field of environmental biotechnology to lead the way with regard to public acceptance for the rest of genetic engineering of organisms that might be released into the environment. We must proceed in reassuring ways, by making clear our objectives and by undertaking appropriate measurements and publishing the results. We must respond to the clear and compelling public interest in reducing risks from existing and future environmental chemical contaminations. Here is an obvious benefit-risk trade-off, with large potential benefits. The public opinion poll results Eveleigh presented were a bit less comforting to me than to him. From my experience in government and as an involved citizen, I think a 23 percent negative opinion might represent a disproportionate opposition, if well organized, perhaps overriding the impressive 73 percent positive responses. However, the results certainly do show positive public interest.

Lugtenberg's presentation of genetic and immunologic methods and my emphasis on stepwise progression from benchtop to pilot scale to closed systems to environmental applications of microorganisms should help convince governments and the public that scientists are proceeding in a responsible fashion. We are adapting to a society in which it is not sufficient to have good intentions; we must have good and demonstrably safe results as well. We recognize that it is necessary to work with the regulators and the environmentalists to achieve early field tests and effective utilization of these really remarkable scientific advances.

I hope that these themes that I have emphasized (see Table 1) capture much of what have been your interests and your conclusions from the workshop. In nature there are diverse capabilities of which we have still identified relatively few. As we explore these pathways, we find that they are not so easily transferred into manipulated systems as might be hoped. Many of the organisms with the most interesting capabilities have totally unknown genetics, and there is very little known about their metabolism.

I have emphasized the interrelationships between basic science and field applications. There is no doubt we need more interconnections. We must ask those basic scientists who are interested to provide organisms for earlier field application tests and, in turn, provide information to them about the problems and debottlenecking that might be addressed. The reductionist approach of pure cultures must be complemented with studies of combinations for growth and biodegradation, for aerobic and anaerobic pathways, and of qualitative and quantitative investigations. In the future, I am confident that the identification of pathways and intermediates will be complemented by more information on rates, including rates in relation to environmentally significant conditions and time scales.

Experience from various settings and with different kinds of chemicals will grow. I hope that the pace of progress continues to accelerate. I applaud your efforts and thank you for this opportunity to summarize and comment on an instructive week of environmental science.

Participants

J.P.E. Anderson
Bayer, AG, PF-F/CE
Institut fur Okobiologie
Zentrum Landwirtschaft, D5090
5000 Leverkusen
Federal Republic of Germany

Donna Bedard
G.E. Research and Development Center
Building K-1, Room 3B23,
P.O. Box 8
Schenectady, New York 12301

Bruce W. Brodman
Advance Concepts Team
U.S. Army Armament Development and
Engineering Center
SMCAR-AEE-BR, B455T
Picatinny Arsenal,
New Jersey 27806-5000

John A. Buswell
Complex Carbohydrate Research Center
University of Georgia
220 Riverbend Road
Athens, Georgia 30602

Robert Campbell
Chemical and Biological Sciences Branch
European Research Office
223-231 Old Marylebone Road
London NWI5TH England

Franco Cecchi
Department of Environmental Science
University of Venice
Calle Larga S. Marta 2137
30123 Venezia, Italy

Ananda M. Chakrabarty
Department of Microbiology
University of Illinois College of Medicine
835 South Wolcott Avenue
Chicago, Illinois 60612
Jimmy Cornette
HQ, AFEFC/RDV
Tindall Air Force Base,
Florida 32403-6000

Ronald Crawford
Department of Bacteriology
Institute for Molecular and Agricultural
Genetic Engineering
University of Idaho
Moscow, Idaho 83843

John Davison
Molecular Biology
International Institute of Cellular and
Molecular Pathology
75 Avenue Hippocrate
1200 Brussels
Belgium

Joseph J. DeFrank
Decontamination Technology Branch
U.S. Army Chemical Research,
Development and Engineering Center/
SMCCR-PPD
Aberdeen Proving Ground,
Maryland 21010-5423

Douglas Eveleigh
Biochemistry and Microbiology
Cook College
Rutgers University
New Brunswick, New Jersey 08903

John Glaser
Environmental Protection Agency
26 Martin Luther King Drive
Cincinnati, Ohio 45268

I.C. Gunsalus
International Center for Genetic
Engineering and Biotechnology
Padriciano 99
34012 Trieste, Italy

Dick Janssen
Department of Biochemistry
Gronigen University
Nijenborgh 16
9747 AG Groningen, The Netherlands

Daphne Kamely
U.S. Army Chemical Research,
Development and Engineering Center
SMCCR-TDB
Aberdeen Proving Ground,
Maryland 21010-5423

David L. Kaplan
U.S. Army Research and Development
Engineering Center
Biotechnology Branch
Kansas Street
Natick, Massachusetts 01760-5020

Jerome Kukor
Department of Microbiology
University of Michigan Medical School
M5605/0620 Medical Science 2
Ann Arbor, Michigan 48109

Ben Lugtenberg
Department of Plant Molecular Biology
Leiden University
Nonnensteeg 3, 2311 VJ Leiden
The Netherlands

Joan Mata-Alvarez
Department of Enginyeria Quimica
Facultat Quimica
University of Barcelona
08028 Barcelona
Spain

Manuel Mota
Oporto University
Oporto,
Portugal

Alasdair Neilson
Swedish Environmental
Research Institute
Institute for Vatten-Och
Luftvardsforskning
IVL:STH, Box 21060
S100 31 Stockholm, Sweden

Robert Newburgh
Biological Sciences Division
Office of Naval Research
Arlington, Virginia 22217

Julio M. Novais
Biotechnology Section
Instituto Superior Technico
1096 Lisbon Cordex
Portugal

John Obringer
DFB U.S. Air Force Academy
Colorado Springs,
Colorado 80840-5701

Gilbert Omenn
Medical and Environmental Health
School of Public Health and
Community Medicine
University of Washington
Seattle, Washington 98105

Douglas Ribbons
Department of Biochemistry
Imperial College of Science, Technology,
and Medicine
Enzymatix Ltd. & Halogenerate Ltd.
Cambridge, U.K. SW7 2AZ
England

Isabel Sa Correia
Department of Chemical Engineering
Instituto Superior Tecnico
1096 Lisbon Codex
Portugal

Mirja Salkinoja-Salonen
Department of General Microbiology
University of Helsinki
Mannerheimintie 172
Helsinki,
Finland 00280

Bernard Schink
Lehrstuhl Mikrobiologie 1
University of Tubingen
Auf der Morgenstelle 28,
D7400 Tubingen
Germany

Michael Smith
Biochemistry Department
Biotechnology Laboratory
Room 237 Wesbrook Building
6174 University Boulevard
Vancouver, BC Canada V6t 1W5

James Spain
Biotechnology Research
HQ, AFEFC/RDVW
Tindall Air Force Base,
Florida 32403-6000

Kenneth Timmis
Division of Microbiology
National Research Center for
Biotechnology
Mascheroder Weg 1
D-3300 Braunschweig,
West Germany

Klaus Visscher
RIVM
Antonie van Leeuwenhoeklaan 9
P.O. Box 1, 3720 BA Bilthoven
The Netherlands

F. Prescott Ward
U.S. Army Chemical Research Develop-
ment and Engineering Center
SMCCR-TD
Aberdeen Proving Ground,
Maryland 21010-5423

Lily Y. Young
Department of Microbiology and
Department of
Environmental Medicine
New York University Medical Center
550 First Avenue
New York, New York 10016

Josef Zeyer
WAWAG
Federal Institute of Technology
CH-6047 Kastanienbaum
Switzerland

Index